Inside Russian Medicine

Inside Russian Medicine

An American Doctor's First-Hand Report

William A. Knaus, M.D.

with research assistance by
Nicholas A. Petroff

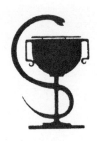

New York   EVEREST HOUSE   *Publishers*

Library of Congress Cataloging in Publication Data:
Knaus, William A
    Inside Russian medicine.
    Bibliography: p. 379
    Includes index.
    1. Medicine—Russia. 2. Medicine, State—Russia.
3. Russia—Description and travel—1970—
    Biography. I. Petroff, Nicholas A. II. Title.
    [DNLM: 1. Medicine   USSR. WB 50 GR9 K67i]
    R532. K55 1981 362.1′0947 80-29372
    ISBN 0-89696-115-X

To Jan, with special remembrance of
Dr. William Horsely Gantt, 1893–1980,
physician, scientist, author, and friend
who went to Russia first.

ACKNOWLEDGMENTS

Three writers—Michael Halberstam, Karen Hunt, and Bill Riviere—provided personal inspiration, guidance, and direction to this book and to my writing career.

My research associate, Nicholas Petroff, worked with me for over a year providing full-time expertise, enthusiasm, and inspiration. This would have been less of a book without him.

A substantial part of the information on women and children in Chapter 5 comes from a detailed analysis of Soviet infant mortality rates carried out by Murray Feshbach of the U.S. Bureau of the Census and from Christopher Davis, an economist from the University of Birmingham. I am grateful for their expert guidance, generosity, and enthusiasm.

This book was five years in research and over a year in actual writing. Over this time, many individuals offered their assistance and expertise. With the unfortunate but necessary exclusion of the many ordinary Soviet citizens and physicians who contributed the most, the following is an alphabetical listing of some of the individuals to whom I am grateful:

Dr. Yury V. Astrozhnikov, All-Union Research Institute of Clinical and Experimental Surgery, Moscow, USSR; Albert Berkowitz, National Library of Medicine, Washington, D.C.; Dr. Mikhail Borisov, Medical Counselor, Soviet Embassy to the United States, Washington, D.C.; Dr. Martin Cherniack, Stanford University School of Medicine, Palo Alto, California; Dr. Christopher Danis, University of Birmingham, Cambridge, Massachusetts; Dr. Michael DeBakey, Baylor University School of Medicine, Houston, Texas; Dr. Murray Feshbach, U.S. Department of Commerce, Washington, D.C.; Dr. Robert Fisher, Office of International Health, Department of Health and Human Services, Washington, D.C.; Dr. Richard Friedman, Harvard Medical School, Boston, Massachusetts; Dr. W. Horsley Gantt, Johns Hopkins University, Baltimore, Maryland; Dr. Ariel Hollinshead, George Washington University School of Medicine, Washington, D.C.; Dr. Andrey K. Kiselev, USSR Ministry of Health, Moscow, USSR; Dr. Aleksander Leaf, Harvard Medical School, Boston, Massachusetts; Dr. Sam Linn, Office of International Health, Department of Health and Human Services, Washington, D.C.; Dr. Urii P. Lisitsin, All-Union Scientific Research Institute, Moscow, USSR; Dr. John G. Mair, The Fairfax Hospital, Falls Church, Virginia; Dr. James Muller, Harvard Medical School, Boston, Massachusetts; Dr. Nikolai Gavrilov, Semashko Research Institute, Moscow, USSR; Dr. Carl C. Nydell, Jr., U.S. Department of State, Moscow, USSR; Dr. Georgii A. Popov, Moscow State University, Moscow, USSR; Dr. Joseph Quinn, Fogarty International Center, Department of Health and Human Sciences, Washington, D.C.; Dr. Mark M. Ravitch, University of Pittsburgh School of Medicine, Pittsburgh, Pennsylvania; Aleksandr Solzhenitsyn, New Cavendish, Vermont; Dr. Patrick Storey, University of Pennsylvania School of Medicine, Philadelphia, Pennsylvania; Dr. Vadim B. Tsybolsky, Semashko Research Institute, Moscow, USSR; Dr. Edward N. Vantsian, All-Union Research Institute of Clinical and Experimental Surgery, Moscow, USSR; and Dr. Marty Wolfe, U.S. Department of State, Washington, D.C.

Drs. Jack Zimmerman and Mohammed Shavari, my associates at the George Washington University Hospital, unselfishly worked while I wrote. Ms. Karen Hunt edited the final draft. Many of the good sentences are hers. Ms. Gerri Arnold, Ms. Francis Liu and Ms. Ann Conway typed the manuscript.

Special thanks to Jerry Gross, my editor, and Mike Cantalupo of Everest House, and to John Schaffner, Victor Chapin, and Barney Karpfinger, my agents. Despite all this help, I alone am responsible for all material in this book.

Contents

We must not lose sight of the fact that according to an important biological law living organisms can not only degenerate but also regenerate and return to their original states . . . and that some diseases will cure themselves.

—Gavriil Sergeevich Pondoev
in *Notes of a Soviet Doctor*

PREFACE

I went to the Soviet Union for the first time in June 1973 and stayed for twelve months. During that year, I worked as a physician for two groups of American guides on a traveling exhibit called "Outdoor Recreation in the U.S.A." One of a series of exhibits sponsored by the former United States Information Agency, it was designed to bring Soviet citizens in one-to-one contact with Russian-speaking Americans.[1]

The snowmobiles, water skis, camping equipment, and photographs of outdoor scenes served as a backdrop for the actual questions Soviets came to the exhibit to ask: "How much does an automobile cost? Is it true you don't need a passport to travel from one American city to another? Why do all the newspapers hate President Nixon? Can you really buy your own house?"

Many of the most frequent questions and statements were about medicine, Soviet and American: "Is it true that American medicine discriminates against the poor? Why does it cost so much to be sick in America? In the Soviet Union all medicine is *besplatno* [free of charge]. Soviet medicine is the best in the world, isn't it?"

"Outdoor Recreation in the U.S.A." moved to a different Soviet city every two months. It opened in Moscow, went some six hundred miles east to Ufa in the central plain of the USSR, then more than four thousand miles farther east to Irkutsk in Siberia, then back west to the more European parts of the country, with showings in Yerevan, the capital of Soviet Armenia, and Kishinev, capital of the Moldavian Republic. The exhibit closed in Odessa, an old Ukrainian city on the Black Sea.

Because we lived in each city for two months, there was time to meet many of the more than one million Soviet citizens who visited the exhibit and to learn firsthand about their everyday lives. On most evenings I had invitations to the homes of Soviet friends, where

[1] Throughout this book, with the exception of the title, I use the word *Soviet* to refer to citizens, concepts, or characteristics of the Union of Soviet Socialist Republics (USSR) and its government. The word *Russian* is used only in reference to persons or properties of that nationality. Currently, Russian citizens account for only half (approximately 51 percent) of the population of the USSR.

11

food and conversation seemed unlimited. As a doctor, I became friends with many of my medical counterparts, young and old. With the younger Soviet doctors I compared experiences of medical school and internship. Through these friendships I was able, unofficially, to spend time observing the day-to-day routine in Soviet hospitals and clinics.

During my first year in the Soviet Union there were, fortunately, only a few times when an American guide needed admission to a Soviet hospital. When this did happen, however, I was able to work directly with my Soviet colleagues. On those occasions I met older Soviet physicians, professors and doctors of medical science who, while equally cooperative, treated me formally, maintaining a safe distance.

Regardless of age and situation, by the end of the year I was close friends with dozens of ordinary Soviet citizens, physicians, workers, and students, most of whom had never spoken with an American before. None were dissidents, at least not in the Western definition, and few had thought of emigrating.

We exchanged gifts, compared notes, and promised to stay in touch. Throughout the year, and on return visits when I contacted many of them, I was remarkably free to go where I wanted, talk to whom I wanted, to watch and to learn.

Between visits I added to my knowledge by reading Soviet medical journals, textbooks, and newspapers and by following announced changes in official policies. The growing number of Soviet physicians visiting the United States, and Washington, D.C., in particular, through the U.S.–USSR Health Exchange agreement also helped. They kept me posted on scientific and political developments and on the most current statistics.

But before I actually began writing I knew that statistics would form only a minor part of this book. Preparing a truly scholarly work on medical care in the Soviet Union is like completing a crossword puzzle in a foreign language. There are clues to the words and numbers that fit in the spaces, but between the differences in definitions and the difficulties of translation much of the task is essentially guesswork. Furthermore, since it will be some time until Soviet scientists improve their statistical and information-gathering ability, many of the spaces have to remain blank.

Yet even as a personal portrait of Soviet medicine, my report is necessarily indistinct in certain areas, completed with broad brush strokes, not fine detail. For this I make no apologies except to admit freely that after six years of study there are aspects of Soviet medicine I do not fully understand. Anyone who has traveled to the USSR, even for a short tour, recognizes this feeling of confusion, contradiction, and bewilderment. Nothing is exactly as it seems and just when you think you understand the Soviet system, it surprises you.

One of the earliest and most lasting impressions is the loss of individual freedom. Intourist, the official government tourist agency, tells the visitor what hotel he will stay in, just as the official Soviet housing bureau assigns apartments to its citizens. To travel to another city a visitor, like a Soviet citizen, needs a visa. The government wants to know where everyone is all the time.

The government also assigns jobs. It establishes production quotas. It rations consumer goods. It organizes recreation. The government is everywhere in a Soviet citizen's life, trying to ensure that everything he does and everything that happens to him is in the best interest of the country. The same attitude extends to medical care.

In the United States and most Western countries, responsibility for and decisions about personal health, like those of job, life-style, and travel, rest with the individual. He or she is held to account for personal habits relating to his or her health and for seeking medical care when and if it is needed.

In the Soviet Union, to use the words of Professor Urii Lisitsin, Director of Medical Information for the USSR, "The health of each citizen is regarded not only as his personal affair but as part of the national wealth."

Since health is a national resource, the Soviet government wants to protect its investment. The government places physicians throughout the worker's environment, in the factory, riding the ambulances, and, when necessary, in the home. There are more doctors in the USSR than in any other country. The average Soviet citizen sees a doctor more than twice as often as his American counterpart.

The government has also built more hospital beds (3.2 million) and clinics (35,000) than any other nation. It sponsors frequent visits to Soviet sanatoriums where rest and relaxation are mixed with medical treatment. All of these services, from the clinic visit and hospital stay to the sanatorium, are free of direct charge. There are no formal medical bills in the USSR. No Soviet citizen fears the cost of a long-term illness.

At the same time, a Soviet patient cannot choose the physician or the hospital where he will be treated. He will be given little information regarding his illness, and while in the hospital he will depend on family and friends for food and other basic necessities. Despite claims of free and equal medical care, there are unofficial charges for some services. A few persons get special treatment.

Despite these obvious differences, however, this book is not meant as a comparison between the Soviet and the American, or any other nation's, medical system. Because the Soviet system is so different, it is impossible to reduce its complexity to simple one-on-one contrasts.

There is no single right answer to the challenge of providing medical care. The Soviet Union has chosen a totally government-controlled system, an approach fundamentally unlike our own mixture of private and public services. It is the day-to-day routine of the Soviet system that I have tried to make the framework of this book.

In those cases in which revealing the identity of a Soviet source could potentially damage someone's career, I have changed names and places. With this one exception, everything is accurate as I know it.

Whenever possible, I have supported my observations and those of other persons with documentation from Soviet literature. When I was confused, I asked both official and unofficial Soviet sources for help. Despite my attention to accuracy, however, I know some of my Soviet medical colleagues, especially those in official circles, will complain that my writing concentrates on the shortcomings of Soviet medical care rather than on its achievements.

This is a book about Soviet medicine written by an American physician. Just as the two countries have different systems of practicing medicine, so there is a difference in our approach to analysis and description. Negative description, when it does occur, is not directed at Soviet doctors. Like ordinary Soviet citizens, they are individually attractive and most often the instruments rather than the initiators of difficulties. I can think of no greater challenge than being a Soviet doctor. The good ones, and there are many, have my greatest respect.

Moscow, USSR and Washington, D.C.
November 1980

Inside Russian Medicine

1

Evacuation from Siberia

It is only October but a strong night wind off the Angara River has brought temperatures close to freezing. Shivering before my open window, I reach over to close the latch and recall the warning from the many Soviet visitors to our exhibit—winter comes early in Siberia. "Snow by morning" had been the finger-wagging prediction volunteered that evening by the *babushka* (older woman) who ran the hotel's café.

Pondering the prospects of my first winter in Russia, I stare out at the village, alternating sips of strong Russian tea with the remaining crumbs of chocolate chip cookies carried five thousand miles from the American Embassy commissary in Moscow.

Unlike Moscow and Ufa, the first two Soviet cities to host the United States Information Agency Exhibit to which I am assigned as physician, Irkutsk is a warm, comfortable town. Its streets are not overwhelmed by the harsh Stalinist architecture of Moscow and its character has not yet been destroyed by the high-rise efficiency of Ufa. Many of the homes here are traditional Russian log cabins built by the first exiles to eastern Siberia—noblemen sent by Peter the Great. They chose this site on the Angara River, next to Lake Baikal, the world's deepest single body of fresh water, for its beauty and tranquillity.

I am feeling secure in this remote village. But little do I realize as I close my diary that the next few hours will begin a week-long odyssey dramatizing not the beauty but the isolation of this, our temporary Siberian home. In the next seven days the small city of Irkutsk will become the center of historic negotiations between world leaders in Moscow and Washington. For seventy-two crucial hours, while the threat of war and the death of thousands grows in the Middle East, the Soviet government will, in response to my request, make unprecedented concessions to save the life of one man—an American.

Wednesday, October 17

Two A.M. Pounding on my door. I open it and Jim Torrence stumbles weakly into the room. Jim is a forty-year-old branch chief with the United States Forest Service. He is working with the exhibit in Irkutsk because of his background and the exhibit's theme—outdoor recreation. A strong, athletic person, Jim was in excellent physical shape when he arrived a month ago. Tonight he looks exhausted.

"Bill, my stomach, something's happened to it. I think I'm about to be sick."

I start to examine him but, unable to control his stomach, he runs to the bathroom. After several minutes of severe vomiting, Jim's gastrointestinal fireworks quit and although he is weak, I am able to finish my examination. I conclude that Jim's problem is a combination of food poisoning and overeating. I tell him to try to get some rest, not eat or drink anything, and call me if he has any more trouble.

Almost half the Americans with the exhibit have suffered similar, although less violent, episodes and I do not think there's any need for concern. Besides, before leaving, Jim tells me that he has just returned that night from a two-day climbing trip to a mountain close to Lake Baikal. Deep snow prevented the climbers from reaching the summit of a small mountain, but the rest of the hike was a success. Along the way they met friendly Siberians who had offered them generous portions of a heavy Russian stew. Not to slight their hospitality, Jim ate large portions along with dark-brown bread and cheese, which left him feeling full for the last two days. On the train ride back to Irkutsk he started feeling nauseated. At the hotel he immediately went to bed but was unable to sleep because of the violent stomach cramps.

In the morning I go directly to Jim's room. He is in bed, weak, but looks comfortable. He says he passed out momentarily when he walked to the bathroom in the night. This concerns me. I examine him again, looking for signs of something more serious, but I find none. I caution him not to get up again without assistance. He is to take nothing but clear fluids today and I will check him in the afternoon.

At the exhibit I talk briefly with Don Gayton, the exhibit's director, and explain that Jim will probably be unable to work for a few days but that there is no cause for concern. About 1 P.M. I receive an urgent call from Jim asking that I return immediately. I enter his room and see blood in the bathtub. Jim says he got up about noon feeling nauseated and went into the bathroom to vomit.

"I feel better now, but really weak."

I reexamine him and find his pulse rate high, an early sign of blood loss, but I am reassured to find his blood pressure does not change when I move him from a lying to a sitting position. It means that the blood loss so far has been minimal.

Nevertheless, I now have a patient who is bleeding from somewhere in his gastrointestinal system. More critical, we are in the middle of Siberia, cut off from all possible assistance. It is a long, rough, seven-hour flight from Moscow, and even phone connections with the American Embassy are extremely poor. There is only one course of action available—I will have to put Jim in the hospital.

I immediately call Don to tell him the seriousness of Jim's condition and ask him to contact our Soviet Chamber of Commerce liaison officer, whose name is Kuzmenko. Representatives of this organization travel with us throughout the Soviet Union, helping us meet local officials. I want Kuzmenko to arrange for Jim's hospitalization in the University Faculty Clinic of Irkutsk.

I have already had tours of the local medical facilities in Irkutsk and, in my opinion, this hospital (the main teaching hospital for the Irkutsk Medical School) contains the best facilities for a problem such as Jim's. In a few minutes Don returns my call. An ambulance is on the way.

Waiting for it to arrive, I tell Jim that the most likely reason for his bleeding is Mallory–Weiss Syndrome, in which vigorous vomiting creates a bleeding tear in the esophagus. There are other possibilities, I explain, such as an ulcer or gastritis, an inflammation of the stomach lining. But, considering the events of last night, I think a tear in Jim's esophagus is most likely. I also try to reassure him about his admission to a Russian hospital. This is more difficult. Although I have toured many of their hospitals and even spent a night on call with an intern, I have never taken care of my own patient in a Soviet hospital.

As far as I know, no American physician has ever been granted that privilege. Unlike the United States, a doctor educated outside Russia cannot obtain a license to practice in the USSR by simply passing a certifying examination—he must complete the entire six years of Soviet medical school.

Of course there is the American doctor at the embassy in Moscow. Occasionally, when Americans are admitted to Moscow hospitals, he visits them, but he is not consulted directly in any decisions involving their care. I have experienced good relations with the Russian physicians in Irkutsk and I resolve, somehow, not to be an observer where Jim is concerned.

In fifteen minutes the ambulance arrives, bringing a matronly Soviet *vrach* (the lowest ranking physician in the USSR) along with a *feldsher* (physician's assistant). The *vrach* glances into the bathroom, briefly examines Jim, and concurs with the need for immediate hospitalization. We load Jim onto a stretcher, cover him with blankets, and carry him down the three floors to the street.

We place Jim into the tiny Soviet ambulance and I recall the reports I had read describing the Soviet *Skoraia meditsinskaia pomoshch* (Ambulance System) as one of the best organized in the world.

In most large Soviet cities there is a central dispatcher station that receives and handles all calls. The ambulances are specialized, individually equipped to handle everything from heart attack victims to psychiatric emergencies. The ambulance today, however, is not one of their better models. It is old, has difficulty starting, and, with the exception of the *feldsher*'s medical bag, contains no medical equipment. All of this bothers Jim, and I try to joke. "It's a lot nicer than some of the cabs we've used in Russia," I tell him. Fortunately, it is a short ride to the hospital and Jim tolerates it well. But there are more problems ahead. Upon arriving at the Irkutsk University Faculty Clinic, we run headlong into Soviet medical bureaucracy. We arrived at 4 P.M., an hour after the official closing time for admissions to most hospitals in Irkutsk. After 3 P.M., I am told, all emergency admissions are referred to a single designated city hospital, and the Irkutsk Faculty Clinic is not scheduled to accept patients that evening.

While we wheel Jim into the admitting room, I am loudly informed of this fact by Vladimir Alekseyev, the doctor in charge of the intensive care unit where Jim should be admitted. But Jim is not a routine patient, I explain. There must be something we can do to change the rule. In response there is a series of shouted telephone calls over what to do with the sick *Amerikanets*. This greatly disturbs

Jim, and I am little help in calming him. Our first contact with Soviet medicine is not very reassuring.

When Vladimir stops shouting on the telephone, he explains to me that if Jim were admitted, a full staff would have to be put on duty that night. This would be quite difficult at the last minute, he explains. He suggests we take Jim to a larger city hospital. In view of the confusion we are causing, I quickly agree. After all, Jim could be bleeding while we talk. Suddenly our luck changes. Just as we are preparing to leave, a mysterious telephone conversation takes place; all the red tape is cut and Jim is immediately admitted.

Before I can follow him upstairs, I must put cloth coverlets over my shoes and drape a loose-fitting cape over my shoulders. According to the Soviets, these measures minimize the dirt that one brings in from the outside. I think they stir up more dust than they stop.

Jim is put in the hospital's intensive care unit, a dingy nine-by-twelve-foot room with faded pink walls, equipped only with three small iron-frame beds, a wall outlet for oxygen, and a small corner sink. The other two beds are empty. By now I am accustomed to the lack of medical technology in Soviet hospitals; but seeing Jim in this stark, high-ceilinged, desolate room underscores how far we are from home.

A *vrach* I do not recognize comes in and examines Jim, asking him about the events of the last few days and whether Jim has any past history of stomach problems. Thirteen years ago, Jim tells him, he had an operation to correct an abnormality he was born with. Called an annular pancreas, it is a ring of pancreatic tissue that moves from its proper location behind the stomach to form a circle around it. As a result of this encirclement, children with annular pancreas feel uncomfortably full even after small meals. Jim's operation had gone well, however, and until today, he explains, he had only occasional discomfort.

While Jim's history is being taken, I pace the room waiting for the blood tests to be ordered. I want to know Jim's hematocrit value, or the percentage of red blood cells in his blood. It would help tell us how rapidly he is bleeding. I ask Vladimir and he assures me the test will be done shortly.

A husky, handsome man with a ruddy face surrounded by a full red beard, strides into the room. No one could be more Russian than this man, Professor Aleksei Krokholev, doctor of medical sciences and chairman of the surgery department at the Faculty Clinic. He examines Jim and, in a deep resounding voice, assures him that all will be well. He speaks with such confidence that even I want to believe him. As he leaves, he motions for me to follow him to his *kabinet* (office).

The office is typical of a Soviet doctor who achieves the highest academic rank, professor. It is a large, mostly empty room with a desk at one end and chairs lining the walls. No papers clutter his desk and there are only a handful of volumes in his large bookcase.

Krokholev introduces himself as the former head of surgery at a Moscow medical school; he does not explain why he has been transferred to Siberia. We discuss Jim's case and the possible causes of his bleeding. The professor is not impressed with my theory of an esophageal tear. Jim's past surgery and what role it might play in his current problem concern him more. We decide to begin our search for the answer with a trip to the X-ray department. By this time, blood samples have been taken and, to give him fluids, an intravenous infusion started in Jim's arm.

In the X-ray department, they stand Jim in front of an X-ray screen and have him swallow thick, white, chalky barium that will outline his stomach for the gastrointestinal series. But standing is more than Jim can handle. He looks frantically around the room for a second and then collapses to the floor. We quickly lift him on the stretcher. He regains consciousness slowly and, while still groggy, vomits—barium and more blood. Regardless of the exact results of the blood test, I know now that Jim's blood level must be dangerously low.

When we get Jim back to his room, the professor comes in and assures me that, despite the brief time before the X-ray machine, he got a good look at Jim's stomach. We go back to his office to discuss the results. Krokholev tells me there was no ulcer or other obvious cause for Jim's bleeding on the X ray. "Nothing serious," he assures me. "We will not have to operate." Only at that moment does the possibility of surgery enter my mind. I feel a strange combination of fear and excitement.

I want to share his confidence that everything will be all right. After all, I think, he is a professor of surgery. Not only am I not a surgeon, but I have been a doctor for only a year, having just finished my internship when I accepted this assignment in the Soviet

Union. Feeling a mixture of foolishness and loneliness, I decide to go along with the professor—for now. But as we walk out the door, I emphasize that I have to be consulted on all decisions regarding Jim.

"Of course, *molodoi chelovek* (young man)." The professor grins and grabs me around the neck, his beard rubbing my face. "We will do everything together." The familiar and unprofessional form of greeting makes me feel even younger.

By now Jim is exhausted. I examine him and find his pulse rate rapid. I ask him to sit up, but even lifting his head slightly from the pillow makes him dizzy. I want to find the results of his blood test, but my unfamiliarity with the hospital and its personnel makes it impossible.

As night comes I arrange myself on one of the beds in Jim's room. I watch everything and try to observe any change in his condition. I explain the treatment to him and why it is necessary. Through his intravenous he is given a half-pint of blood and a pint of sugar water to increase his low blood volume. This is routine, I tell him, except we would have used more blood and fluids. Why the Soviet use such small volumes is obvious.

Soviet hospitals do not enjoy the luxury of disposable equipment so common in American medicine. The equipment for giving blood and fluid is outdated by our standards. It consists of thick, red rubber tubing and large needles, both of which have to be resterilized after each use. This makes the needle points rough. Finding a vein is like trying to cut a tomato with a dull knife. Even with initial success, the coarse needles will rapidly tear through the vein wall and stop the infusion. The tubing is sticky after repeated heatings and the blood frequently clots. That night both problems occur and Jim's intravenous stops twice. Otherwise, he is doing fine, his vital signs (pulse rate, blood pressure, and respirations) are stable, and he is able to rest.

Still I cannot relax. I am concerned whether Jim is still bleeding and, if so, how quickly. Having nothing else to do, I review the nonsurgical methods to locate bleeding within the gastrointestinal system. One is to place a needle into an artery in the patient's groin and, through it, inject dye into the vascular system. The point at which the blood is leaking will show up as a shadow or blush on the X-ray film. This is a complicated technique, known as angiography.

I remember seeing examples of this procedure in Irkutsk, but I know they do not perform angiography on emergency cases.

The other technique is gastroscopy. Jim's situation, I think, is an ideal one in which to use gastroscopy. A slender tube containing a tiny lens and light source is passed through the patient's mouth into his stomach. The doctor can look through the gastroscope and see the stomach's interior. In most cases he can tell if and where a patient is bleeding. Unfortunately, according to Vladimir, the money to purchase a gastroscope has not yet been obtained and it is not available in Irkutsk.

All evening, then, in this unfamiliar hospital, I watch Jim more closely than I have ever watched a patient before. I am without the benefit of the native language and working within a medical system few Western physicians know anything about. I lack the reassuring tests that are so much a part of American medicine.

If Jim had been my patient when I was an intern in Washington, D.C., things would have been different. I would not be sitting here, staring at him, wondering from where and how fast he is bleeding. By this time, he would have been gastroscoped and probably also had angiography. The decision to operate or not would have been made on facts, not intuition.

As the hours go by, I count Jim's pulse, measure his blood pressure, touch his forehead, feel his abdomen, and simply watch him breathe. I begin to appreciate another side to all those tests. Had I been at home, I would have spent most of my time with Jim's X rays, his test results, and making sure his chart was in order. In Irkutsk, I am spending that time with Jim.

By midnight the hospital is quiet. The transfusion is complete and Jim falls asleep. I leave shortly afterward. It has been an emotionally exciting day and I do not feel tired. But I know I should rest because of the uncertainty of tomorrow. I go downstairs, take off my boots and cape, and walk into the courtyard. As predicted, fresh snow is falling, the first of the season. The town looks like a fairyland. Moonlight illuminates each wooden house, now topped with a roof of clinging white snow. From the windows pours warm, yellow light. Despite the late hour, I walk slowly though the streets until I find myself on the bank of the Angara River.

It is at this spot that Ksenia and I often meet. Ksenia teaches Spanish at the local university. She was born in Irkutsk and still lives with her parents in a small apartment on the outskirts of town. I met Ksenia during my first week in Irkutsk at the local Soviet *Dom Kultury* (House of Culture) during a performance of *Swan Lake* that had been danced to the accompaniment of a scratchy phonograph recording. Despite the differences in our background, we were immediately attracted. By now the time we spend together is the high point of my day and I imagine her with me.

The dark eyes, thick black hair, sensual mouth, and strong emotions came from her Russian mother. From her father, a Buryat,[1] she inherited her oval face, slender body, and sharp wit. These traits make Ksenia a very special woman. She laughs often and well.

She wants to travel and hopes to get a job in Cuba teaching Russian to Cuban school children. A few weeks ago we began holding hands and kissing as we walked along the river. Last week Ksenia talked about going to a friend's apartment so we could be alone. But everyone is afraid that being caught would mean trouble. Still, we have spent most of our evenings together walking, embracing through our heavy coats. I promised to call her tonight. Now I want very much to see her. Despite my concern for Jim, she has helped me feel very much at home in this remote snow-covered city. I will call her tomorrow.

At the hotel I tell Don Gayton about Jim's condition: "He's very ill but appears to be stable and we're watching him closely." I can see Don is troubled.

I was hired to accompany the exhibit because a young male guide had died following an emergency appendectomy during the last such tour of the Soviet Union. The night of his death, the American Embassy doctor, along with a Russian specialist, was on a flight from Moscow to check on his condition. They arrived too late. Because of this unfortunate episode, our lack of understanding of Soviet medicine, and the vast distances within the USSR, it was decided to send a physician with all subsequent exhibits. I am the first to have that position.

[1] A person from the Buryat Autonymous Republic, north of Mongolia.

Thursday, October 18

I arrive at the hospital early. Superficially, Jim looks the same. As I closely examine him, however, I find his pulse is fast. Vladimir comes in and reports last night's hematocrit reading, 24; a normal value for Jim's age—46. When Jim was admitted to the hospital he had already lost half his blood volume! Now I am scared. Vladimir agrees to repeat the test immediately. I decide Jim's excellent physical condition is the reason he is doing so well. The rapid loss of so much blood would have put many persons into shock.

But the repeat hematocrit is 19, an alarming drop, especially in view of last night's transfusion. By 11 A.M. my worst fears have come true.

Jim's body is now covered with cold sweat and his pulse is getting weaker. Shock is imminent. I call the exhibit to tell Don. He attempts to relay the report to the American Embassy in Moscow. Professor Krokholev asks me into his office. When I arrive, the room is already filled with a dozen doctors. Some I recognize as attending physicians on Jim's floor. Also present is the woman radiologist who, last night, had single-handedly picked Jim up from the floor. There are representatives from the local Ministry of Health whom I had met on a recent visit to a regional hospital. Altogether it is an imposing group.

The meeting begins by a presentation of Jim's case. Vladimir describes the measures already taken at the hospital but quickly comes to the critical decision: What course of action should we now follow? Professor Krokholev stands slowly and, with one hand stroking his beard, announces in a powerful voice, "An operation is immediately necessary." The other doctors nod in silent agreement. He turns to me and, introducing me as a colleague from America, asks my opinion. I presume he is also requesting my permission to operate on Jim.

I realize this is a crucial moment in relations with my Soviet colleagues. It is by this group, and by how I handle this situation, that I will be judged. I can either gain their respect or become simply an observer.

By now I know the Russians have a great respect for dramatic presentations, even in medicine. I decide I should be confident in my delivery. I stand up and demand laboratory values that Vladimir did not include in his presentation. I review the alternatives that might be undertaken in place of surgery, although I know they are unavailable. I conclude that there is strong clinical evidence that our patient is bleeding. "In our present circumstances," I conclude, "surgery is inevitable."

I sit down exhausted. One of the female surgeons speaks, "It is a big responsibility to put on one person," she says. "Here in Russia, we make such decisions in consultation panels. We all agreed on the operation but you had to make the final decision alone. It is not fair."

Right then I thoroughly agree with her, but I am relieved that she emphasized one important point. The final decision was mine. Jim is still my patient.

The operation is to take place immediately and I suddenly remember I have not told Jim. He is already confused and frightened and I am not sure how he will react. I explain to him that all the evidence points to severe bleeding. I emphasize that there are no other approaches available in Irkutsk. "We have to operate, Jim."

"Will you be in the operating room with me?" he asks. I assure him that I will and, as I hold his hand, they come and take him away.

I hurry to call Don and tell him of the operation. Then I change into surgical scrub clothes and join the professor. We walk into the operating room together.

Krokholev is the chief surgeon, assisted by Candidate of Science Constantine Luzhnov and two assistant female surgeons, Valentina Tolstaya and Lubov Ribacka. The assistants are already gowned and gloved and stand in the back of the room waiting for Jim to be anesthetized. The induction of anesthesia is a critical point in the operation. Jim's blood volume is down, his blood pressure is dangerously low at 90/70, and his pulse is 135 and weak. When you put someone to sleep there is the definite risk of lowering blood pressure. In a patient already in shock, the risk is intensified. I wish the Russians had given Jim more blood and fluid before surgery. But the anesthesiologist nods to me that she is ready, and it is too late to turn back. Standing at the end of the table, I explain to Jim that he will soon begin to feel sleepy.

The anesthetic is given skillfully, his induction is slow and gradual, and while his blood pressure remains low, it does not fall. They drape him in sterile sheets.

The operating room is large, white-tiled, with frosted windows on two sides. The thin operating table stands alone under a large circular lamp. The equipment is quite similar to that found in America. The only difference is the amount of traffic flowing through the open door. Most of the hospital personnel are aware of Jim's admission, and more than a dozen of them crowd in the doorway. Other doctors, some of whom I know from prior meetings, also look in. I recall that one of the more common medical problems mentioned in Soviet professional journals is the high incidence of postoperative infections. In some reports, fully a third of surgical patients developed this complication. With such a relaxed attitude toward operating room visitors, I think, it is no wonder their patients develop infections.

The three assistant surgeons make a long vertical incision in Jim's abdomen. After they cut through his skin and muscle, Krokholev joins them at the head of the table. His red beard protrudes beyond the sides of his surgical mask; his blue eyes are serious. Soon he exposes Jim's stomach and begins probing for a bleeding site. I realize that frequently, even though the patient has lost a great deal of blood, the point of bleeding is never found. It can be hidden by tissue or may consist of small, oozing capillaries. In such an instance there is no way to stop the blood flow. I hope this will not be the case with Jim. A long fifteen minutes pass; nothing is found.

Krokholev extends the incision higher, into the upper abdomen. Here they can see the point where the stomach and esophagus join. If I am correct in my diagnosis, here they will find Jim's problem. Suddenly Professor Krokholev motions me to come to his side. There at the juncture of the stomach and esophagus, a torn artery is spurting blood! Now the operation becomes routine. They sew over the artery and close Jim's abdomen. The sutures are not as delicate as those used in the United States, but I am more than pleased. For the first time since morning, I feel we have good reason to anticipate a full recovery.

Professor Krokholev and I return to his office. He is also exhilarated. He knows both the Soviet and American governments are peering over his shoulder. Operating on an American citizen is bad enough; doing so while an American doctor looks on is even worse. Now we both can relax.

He orders tea, and for an hour we discuss how well the operation went. We talk of medicine and of the need for all doctors to work together. I tell him this is the main reason I came to his country. I want to meet and talk with as many of my Russian counterparts as possible. Until tonight, however, I never dreamed I would be working with them.

The professor puts his arm about my shoulder. He tells me of his early life in Russia and his lifelong desire to be a doctor. Then he sings. In a deep, low voice he sings old Russian songs of love and country, his voice filling the room. The great differences in our ages and backgrounds disappear. He takes me completely into his trust. I feel self-conscious and embarrassed, sharing emotions so openly with a man. But soon I realize the tremendous strain he has felt, and I share in the intensity of his relief. We embrace and resolve always to remember this moment.

By now, Jim is back in his room and beginning to awaken. A special nurse is there to watch him. Until tonight most nurses I had met in the USSR were easily forgotten. They usually receive two short years of training which concentrate on practical learning. They are given very little scientific background, and, with the exception of those who use nursing as a stepping stone to medical school, I had concluded that nursing attracted women with little ambition. But Vera is different. Tall with dark hair, bright, inquisitive eyes, and a warm but professional smile, she is interested and knowledgeable about Jim's surgery.

As she works, I ask about her plans. She says she wants to enter the Irkutsk Medical Institute next spring and is curious about how Jim's case would have been handled in America. I explain about the various tests we would do and she nods. "Soon, we'll have all those things here, too."

Tonight, however, Vera is forced to care for Jim without the aid of even a stethoscope with which to check his blood pressure. I lend her mine. She holds it carefully in her palm, examining it and feeling its weight. "With a stethoscope like this," she says wistfully, "I could become the best doctor in Siberia."

Vera works constantly, administering to Jim's every need. The large overhead light bothers his eyes, so we use a small corner lamp shielded by a towel. In this semidarkness, I watch her move about his bed, casting long shadows in her stiff white coat. She works with the clumsy equipment, so strange to me. I watch her graceful hands struggling with tubing and dull needles.

Hard as she tries, it seems we cannot keep an intravenous needle in Jim for longer than four hours. The blood will either clot in the tube or the needle will perforate the vein. Soon, I think, all the veins in his arms will be unusable. I hope he does not need many more transfusions.

By midnight I feel Jim's condition is stable enough for me to leave. Again I remember I have forgotten to call Ksenia. I vow to do it first thing in the morning.

Friday, October 19

My telephone rings at 8 A.M. Jim's wife is calling from Virginia. Unfortunately, the connection is so poor I can hardly understand a word she is saying. I shout the details of the operation and assure her that Jim is doing well. She tries to ask questions, but static drowns out her voice. Further information, I decide, will have to be sent by cable, which I will dictate to the State Department Medical Division. I project that I might accompany Jim home at the end of the month. The exhibit is to close in two weeks and I do not want to leave him behind.

Everyone at the hospital today is optimistic about the results of surgery. Jim's blood count is still very low at 20, but I expect it to rise by tomorrow. His blood and pulse are steady and, although weak, he is not in a great deal of pain. There is no further vomiting nor has he passed any stool—especially encouraging to me. If Jim were still bleeding, I reason, there would be visible evidence of this sort. Nevertheless we give him another pint of blood.

After the transfusion a nurse applies hot mustard plasters to Jim's chest. The small squares of tissue-thin paper give off a nauseating smell. Just as I wonder what will be next, they decide to "cup" Jim. Small glass cups, heated at the rim with an alcohol flame, are applied to his back. Heating the glass, I learn, causes a partial vacuum and, when applied, the cups pull the flesh with a suction effect, producing large blue-black welts. I am told the mustard plasters and the cups are used to increase circulation. Jim says both treatments feel good, although the cups are painful when first applied.

Vera tells me both these treatments have long traditions in Russia. Cupping for fever dates back many centuries and was used extensively by the Russian Sisters of Mercy during the Crimean War. In the Soviet Union, she says, cupping is still commonly used in the hospitals and in homes. I have to admit that, although the medical validity of cupping and mustard plasters is doubtful, their use does, as Jim says, make a person feel better. One thing I am learning: although seldom treated by a physician, Jim is frequently made to feel that something is being done for him; he is not ignored.

Saturday, October 20

I get to the hospital early again. I am anxious for the blood test results. To my amazement, the hematocrit is still 20—dangerously low. Now I realize all is not well. Since there is no evidence Jim is bleeding, I consider alternatives.

For one thing, with each transfusion Jim develops a fever. This is not the characteristic fever and chills that occur when a patient rejects the blood. I remember articles I have read about earlier attempts at blood transfusions and how rubber tubing can release a substance into the blood that causes fever but does not affect the transfusion. Perhaps Jim's fever is related to the tubing. But that does not answer the question of where all the blood is going. He has received about two quarts of blood during the last three days. Yet his blood level is failing to rise. If he bleeds again, it could well be fatal. With this very low level of red cells, especially in a patient unaccustomed to it, the heart, brain, and other vital organs do not receive enough oxygen. Permanent damage can result. We have to increase his blood level.

My calculations show that Jim is receiving only about a fourth of his daily blood and fluid requirement. Normally, in a postoperative patient, all these needs are supplied by intravenous feedings. But with the problems the Soviets are having with their equipment, giving more intravenous fluids is impossible. I decide to give Jim weak tea and water by mouth. This is not without danger since liquids could provoke further vomiting and, with fresh sutures, this has to be avoided.

The Russians and I discuss giving Jim more blood. I am concerned about the number of transfusions he is receiving, but with his low hematocrit our hand is forced, and he receives his fifth transfusion, again a long procedure. The blood repeatedly clots in the tubing and it takes all day to complete. This exhausts Jim. Having undergone a similar operation thirteen years ago, he is able to contrast what is being done to him now with that experience. He knows things are going badly.

By this time, Vladimir, the young doctor who confronted us on our admission to the hospital, and I are friends. He is on duty every third night and works each day, a schedule similar to that of my internship. In the evenings we sit together in the conference room, talking not only about Jim but about the differences in medicine in our two countries. He knows that the Soviet lack of modern equipment and their reliance on old-fashioned treatments surprise me. He explains both with a rationale I have heard many times when one contrasts medical systems in the United States and the Soviet Union.

"You must realize," he begins, "that the Soviet Union is a very young country. Before the Revolution in 1917, medical care was very poor. We have made tremendous advances. We organized a true system of free care for all people. This was difficult in a country as large as ours. There were millions of peasants scattered throughout Russia who were afraid or ignorant of medicine. It was an enormous job to reach them all, build hospitals, and train doctors. Just as we made improvements, World War II came. The United States doesn't realize how Russia suffered during the war. We lost not only money and food but most of our young men. All progress in medicine stopped during the war. We had to begin building again. We will never forget what the Nazis did to us and it will never happen again." His voice cracks.

"You in America have never suffered such a war on your land. This is why we do not yet have what you do, but we are making progress. Things are better than they were ten years ago, and they will continue to get better," he concluded.

Before leaving that evening, Vladimir and I look in on Jim together. The blood has finally been given and he is resting. I ask Vladimir what he thinks about Jim's blood level remaining so low.

"He must still be bleeding," he replies simply, shrugging his shoulders.

"But there's no indication of that," I argue.

"What else could it be?"

It is late and I am tired, so I drop the conversation. I am confident that, when the time comes, I will be able to convince the Russians I am right.

While undressing back at the hotel, I find two tickets for tonight's performance of the ballet in my pocket. Ksenia and I were to have gone and I have forgotten to call her again.

Sunday, October 21

I dial Ksenia's number the first thing. Her mother answers, "*Ksenia vyshla* [Ksenia is out]." But it is 8 A.M. Sunday, an unlikely time for her to be out. I am sure her parents know of our relationship. It is difficult to keep secrets living in a two-room apartment. I am not sure whether her mother has kept her from speaking to me or, worse yet, whether she has been officially warned not to see me. Leaving the hotel, I walk to the hospital along the river, hoping I may see her. But it is a cold morning and I meet no one along the way.

The hospital is also quiet this Sunday. Fewer people are working and there are fewer visits by the doctors, nurses, orderlies, cleaning women, and assorted Communist Party dignitaries who are always dropping by to wish Jim well. These frequent intrusions allow him little time to rest and are becoming irritating—all of them, that is, but Sasha.

Sasha is a stooped, white-haired man endlessly interested in Jim's welfare. He comes in frequently, asking Jim how he feels, and then carefully raises Jim's head to fluff his pillow. At first I assumed Sasha was an orderly, but it is now evident that his duties are more restricted. Whenever Jim needs the bedpan or a cup of tea, Sasha nods, but sends another person to handle these tasks. Walking through the hospital, I frequently notice Sasha fluffing other patient's pillows; it is all he does. This great subdivision in jobs is an important part of Soviet society. The Russians are proud that they have no unemployment. Now I realize how they do it.

The Sunday morning lull also permits me to consider a more important matter: where we stand with Jim. There are no new values available on his blood level this morning. Typical of Soviet economy, the laboratory is closed. However, Jim is scheduled for another transfusion, his sixth. If his blood level is not up tomorrow, we are in trouble. I want to talk to someone about Jim's case. Perhaps the embassy doctor in Moscow? No, the telephone connections are so poor a complicated discussion is impossible. I feel lonely and a little uncertain. Jim senses my concern and he is unusually quiet.

To make conversation I tell him of a Voice of America broadcast I heard this morning, saying Henry Kissinger was in Moscow for two days of talks with Leonid Brezhnev. He had come in on an Air Force jet.

"It sure would be great if we could get that plane," Jim says. This is the first spoken indication that Jim wants to leave.

It would be great. But I remember a conversation with Dave Millett, the embassy doctor, about evacuating patients from Russia. He made it clear that an Air Force plane could not fly into the USSR for a medical evacuation. "It's never been done in the Soviet Union," Dave explained, "I rely on Lufthansa to fly my patients to Germany."

That was fine for Dave, but there are no international flights to Germany or even Japan from Irkutsk. Besides, with Jim's condition I cannot use a commercial aircraft. On the other hand, Kissinger has just completed a series of brilliant successes in international negotiations. His Vietnam settlement, his trip to China, and his talks with the Russians have impressed the world. If the request comes from him, it just might be possible.

I tell Jim I have to send a cable and hurriedly leave. When I tell Don about asking for Kissinger's help, he is at first overwhelmed but then agrees we should explore the possibility.

"After all," he says, "the government sent all of us here and it has the responsibility to support us." Two questions, however, concern him. How would the Russians react to the request, and how critical is Jim's condition? I cannot answer the first, but insist that if Jim bleeds again and has to undergo a second operation, there is a good chance he will die.

Suddenly I am frightened. Before this I had not considered a second operation. True, we have no other options except surgery in Irkutsk. Now I am convinced we have to get Jim out of Siberia. Don calls a meeting of the staff and explains the situation. Everyone agrees to ask the embassy's help in securing either Kissinger's plane or an Air Force medical evacuation team. We call Moscow and I talk to the embassy officer. I explain the situation is stable at this time but emphasize we have no margin of safety.

"Any further complication will mean Jim's life."

"But right now, he's all right?" the embassy officer responds.

"Yes," I admit, slightly irritated. I want to tell him much more, but because of incessant static it is hopeless. He agrees to contact the embassy's Air Force attaché.

While waiting for the return call, we notify the Russians of a possible evacuation for Jim. Unlike the noncommittal answer we just got from our embassy, Mr. Kuzmenko, our Chamber of Commerce liaison, assures us that such an evacuation is possible, and that he will do everything to help. He promises to call Moscow and notify his superiors. I thank him for his support but he violently shakes his head. "We are talking about *gospodin* [Mister] Torrence's life," he says, "and for that no thanks are needed." Mr. Kuzmenko's positive attitude increases my hopes. I indulge in comfortable speculation that all will be accomplished. But my hopes soon fade. Kissinger's plane is unavailable since it is being used as a communications center with Washington. Furthermore, the Air Force spokesman at the embassy is especially discouraging: "It's unlikely that an Air Force plane would be permitted to land in the Soviet Union. It's never been done before and I suggest you take a commercial flight either to Moscow or Japan."

Anyone familiar with Aeroflot, the official Soviet airline, I answer, can appreciate the absurdity of this suggestion. Aeroflot may be the world's largest airline—linking Moscow with the entire country and the rest of the world—but Aeroflot pays little attention to passenger comfort. Every plane flies at capacity and many are only partly pressurized. I recall a terrible earache during the entire seven-hour flight from Moscow to Irkutsk.

"I'm not going to put a critically ill patient on an Aeroflot plane," I shout. "I need a military evacuation plane." We settle down to wait.

I go back to the hospital Sunday night, undecided about what I should tell Jim. The embassy has been pessimistic and I am afraid to raise his hopes. I decide to be completely honest; after all, it is his life we are discussing. I tell him Kissinger's plane cannot be moved and we have no decision regarding another Air Force plane.

"You may have to stay in Russia until you've fully recovered," I tell him reluctantly.

"But I'm not recovering, am I?"

"Let's wait for tomorrow's blood tests."

Back at the hotel I cannot sleep, so I bring my diary up to date. I write for a few hours and then walk out into the deserted, snow-covered streets. Despite the early morning hours, it is a comfortable cold, and I walk for a long time through the quiet town.

The overwhelming immensity of my request now extends well beyond the world of medicine and I begin to think of its implications. I know that, by morning, Moscow and Washington will closely scrutinize my judgment. Is Jim really sick enough to justify this action? After all, he has already made it through the toughest part—the surgery. If the morning laboratory results show improvement and I have to qualify my request, I will be accused of unnecessarily dramatizing the situation. A typical American doctor, I can hear them say, panicking the minute he doesn't have a modern hospital and fancy equipment to support him. My professional competence will be questioned, all right. Damn it though, I mutter, I know I'm doing the right thing.

Going over the situation again and again in my mind, I begin to realize that I am more concerned about my own pride than with Jim's life. It is an unfair comparison and I decide that, from now on, what happens to Jim will be my only consideration.

I begin walking back to the hotel, leaving footprints in the newly fallen snow. Maybe Ksenia will be waiting for me. But I know that is impossible. She is very careful not to be seen near the hotel. Somehow, though, I have to see her.

Monday, October 22

Walking through the courtyard to the hospital entrance this morning I have a comfortable feeling of familiarity. It is like arriving at work as an intern in Washington. By this time I know the aides, orderlies, and nurses by name and they greet me warmly. Arriving early, I join the professor on his morning rounds. I almost feel at home.

My complacency, however, is quickly dispelled. Jim's hematocrit is still 20 and, when I tell him, I cannot hide my disappointment. He becomes angry. "When are we going to get out of here?" he demands.

Since the Soviets consider bleeding a strong possibility, they want Jim's next transfusion to be fresh, rather than stored, blood. Fresh blood contains more of the factors essential for clotting than blood kept in a blood bank. If Jim is bleeding, it would be important for all his clotting or coagulation factors to be present in sufficient amounts, since normal clotting activity would reduce the amount of blood loss. In the United States we deal with this problem by quick-freezing plasma from donated blood. Freezing preserves the potency of the coagulation factors, and when the plasma is needed, it is rapidly thawed and transfused. The Soviets do not have the capability to freeze plasma in Irkutsk, so they give Jim a direct donor transfusion.

The donor in Jim's case is a Russian nurse, and she is brought directly into his room. A large glass syringe is used to draw blood from her arm and inject it into Jim's. He receives two pints of blood this way, bringing the total amount of his transfusions over the last few days to four quarts. This last procedure, because of difficulty with the syringe and needles, exhausts him. But the day's ordeal has just begun. The nurse announces it is now time for his twice-daily enema.

Enemas, colonic irrigations, *klizmy*, have a long and inglorious tradition in Russian medicine. Used as a universal method for cleansing the body of everything from arthritis to tuberculosis, *klizma* therapy remains a mainstay of Soviet hospital care today. Every patient whose symptoms relate in any way to his gastrointestinal system—or who simply feels listless—receives an enema.

In Jim's case I know the use of enemas is unnecessary and even somewhat dangerous. Blood in the stomach or intestinal tract is an excellent cathartic, so I interpret Jim's lack of bowel movements as a sign that he has stopped bleeding and I am afraid the enemas might actually start new bleeding. But my protests are unable to reverse the blind faith that decades of use have given to *klizma* treatment. As the nurse brings the cold enamel bedpan, pitcher, and long rubber nozzle, I shake my head and leave the room.

I decide to wait until 8 P.M. to recheck Jim's blood level. That will give it enough time following the transfusions to reach a high level. At eight, the lab technician takes a blood sample and I pass an anxious thirty minutes waiting for the results. It is 13, the lowest yet! Instead of gaining, Jim is slipping dangerously. I cannot accept the results—it must be a mistake.

The Russians use an older method of determining hematocrits. It requires a thin glass tube to be filled with blood drawn from the tip of a finger. The tube is placed in a centrifuge for five minutes. The spinning forces the heavier red cells to the bottom while the plasma stays on the top of the tube. The hematocrit is the percent of the tube made up by red blood cells as opposed to plasma. This method, which has been largely replaced in the United States by electronic determinations, is not very accurate. You can often get a lower hematocrit value because tissue fluid from the fingertip is drawn into the tube along with the blood.

I convince myself that this is what the lab technician has done. I tell her I want to repeat the test myself. Jim understands and never moves as I take a small knife blade and open large incisions on two of his fingers. Although the blood flows freely, I have difficulty filling the tubes; they break with the slightest pressure.

"You think they could at least have good glass tubes in this country," I mutter. Jim, sensing my frustration and watching my hands shake, says "I think you're just clumsy." That settles me down and I fill the tubes to my satisfaction. But the results are the same. Jim's hematocrit is between 12 and 13.

Desperate, I take a sample of Jim's blood and examine it under the laboratory's microscope. Many of his red cells are no longer round but torn and fragmented; some look as if pieces have been bitten out of them. This pattern of destruction is frequently seen when a patient is given the wrong type of blood cells. The improperly matched cells, being recognized as foreign by the body's immune system, are attacked and eventually destroyed.

Is this why Jim's hematocrit has dropped from 20 to 13, despite the transfusions? Is his body rejecting the Russian blood?

I have watched the Soviets match each transfusion. The testing is crude, a simple mixing of the two blood types in a small dish, with microscopic observation to see if clumping or agglutination occurs. But it should have detected any major incompatibilities. Then I remember the problems Jim has had with fever every time he was given blood. The fever pattern is not specific for a transfusion reaction, but along with all the other clues, it makes rejection of the Russian blood a strong possibility.

I hurry back to the hotel. Regardless of why, Jim's blood level is now low enough to be a direct threat to his life and I have to tell someone.

We have scheduled a call to USIA headquarters for 9 P.M. With this new information there is no doubt we need a plane. I run the twelve blocks to the hotel and Don's room, arriving just as he hangs up the telephone. Before he can speak, I blurt out my worst fears, "Jim could die tonight. We need that plane now."

"Washington is aware of the situation and a plane is available, but it will take time." Don tries to reassure me. "Everything possible is being done."

On the way back to the hospital I try to calm down so Jim will not sense how scared I am. I have been sent to prevent the loss of American lives. And now, after months of treating sore throats and diarrhea, I have a complex emergency of enormous proportions and I am on the verge of failure. As I walk into Jim's room he moans softly. "I'm seeing bright colors and waves of light and I feel strange," he says. His heartbeat is irregular, his breathing is shallow, his eyes roll upward. Jim's brain is hallucinating from a lack of oxygen. He is dying.

Quickly I elevate Jim's legs with a couple of pillows and try to get more blood to his head. I kneel beside him, check his pulse, and pray the hallucinations will stop. My eyes fill with tears and I want to scream for help. A plane is coming but there is not enough time. Then, slowly and inexplicably, the hallucinations stop and Jim's heartbeat returns to a fast but regular rhythm.

The door opens and in walk three Russian doctors, the first assistant in Jim's surgery, the radiologist, and another woman doctor. Still bundled in coats and smelling of the cold night air, they have obviously been called in from home to see Jim. After briefly examining him, we hold a miniature middle-of-the-night consultation panel.

They say they are very concerned about this latest change in Jim's condition. They ask me what I would like to do. I want to tell them that all I need is a plane, but it would not help. We decide to give Jim another transfusion and agree on a meeting in the morning. Although I am still concerned about the possibility of blood rejection, I feel the situation is desperate enough to try another transfusion.

In the early morning I feel it is safe to leave Jim and return to the hotel. In my room I try to call Ksenia, but my telephone is not working. Nick Barsky walks into my room. A member of the exhibit staff, Nick has handled negotiations with the local officials and the embassy during the last few days.

"The embassy called," he says. "It will be seventy-two hours before the plane arrives." Even though we now have official confirmation of a plane, I am disappointed. "That's too long," I say slowly. "Tell them we need it sooner."

Tuesday, October 23

Back at the hospital I am told Jim's blood level has not risen, despite the overnight transfusion. I ask for a meeting. In the professor's office, I face my twelve associates, but the professor is cold and distant and takes little part in the discussion. He sits quietly, still in his pajamas, his white coat wrapped around his shoulders. "He is sick," one of the doctors whispers to me.

By this time the Russians are aware of my plans to evacuate Jim and it distresses them. Instead of the courtesy and respect that marked our other meetings, there is tension in the room. It is now "them" versus "me."

"Don't you know how ill he is?" one doctor argues. "You could seriously hurt your patient by moving him at this time." His colleagues agree. They demand that I reconsider my decision. Glancing about the room, at each of the twelve, I do question my medical judgment. Perhaps they are right and I am wrong. "You must not move him," another doctor insists. I agree to answer them within an hour.

I call Don and ask him to join me at the hospital. I want someone there to listen while I think out loud. He meets me in the lobby. "The plane will arrive sooner," he says. "Late Wednesday night or early Thursday morning." It is Tuesday noon.

I tell Don about the meeting and how I am considering delaying the evacuation. He objects. "If I were Jim," he says, "I would rather die in an American plane than in a Russian hospital."

"But I don't want him to die at all," I shout. My voice echoes through the lobby and many of the visitors stop their conversations to stare. Confused, I try to compromise my desire to leave with the Russian doctors' warning.

"Hold off the plane until Friday morning," I tell Don. That will give Jim one more day to stabilize and it will ensure that we leave the hospital in daylight. I do not want to make the trip to the airport, over the rough roads of Irkutsk, in the middle of the night.

A few minutes later I tell the consultation panel I will delay the evacuation. Then, as I am about to explain my blood-rejection theory, they drop a bombshell. They want to reoperate!

They insist that Jim's blood count is not rising because of continued bleeding. I disagree strongly and list my evidence for rejection. "No, you're wrong, Dr. Knaus," a physician responds. "We often have to operate two or three times in these cases to stop bleeding." I persist with my theory of repeated transfusion reactions. But I cannot get them to listen. I insist, however, that there be no further surgery. I withdraw my permission. My vehement reaction brings reluctant agreement.

Now the Russian attitude is clear. First they argued that Jim should remain, and only when I agreed did they insist on further surgery—a shrewd move. But further surgery on Jim is the last thing I want. We have to leave as soon as possible.

I will have to call Moscow with another change of plans. Through a massive effort of the embassy I have been granted a plane. Not satisfied, I had it speeded up by thirty-six hours. Then I delayed it one day. Now I want it immediately. Moscow will be rightly confused. Further, until now I had not realized the complexity of bringing an Air Force plane into the Soviet Union.

According to Nick Barsky, the nearest available plane is in Germany, eight thousand miles away. In an action the State Department calls "a historic first," the Soviets have given permission for the plane to fly to Moscow and pick up a Soviet Aeroflot navigator. The plane will then travel to Irkutsk, pick us up, and take off eastward. It will stop at Khabarovsk, on the east coast of the Soviet Union, drop the Soviet crew member, and then fly on to Japan. This means overflying the entire Soviet Union from west to east. An American plane has never been permitted to do this. At each point across the country the plane will have to be in constant radar contact with Russian observation posts, each one notified of the plane's fly-over time. Otherwise, an unidentified plane could create a serious incident, possibly leading to tragedy.

As further protection, the Soviets have also demanded that all numbers and insignias be painted out, except for a small American flag on the plane's tail. In addition, our Air Force needs information. Is JP-4 jet fuel available for refueling at Irkutsk? How large is the runway? Will there be an English-speaking controller in the tower? Taking care of all these details was difficult, and here I am demanding last-minute changes.

With the usual poor connection I reach the embassy officer. "Why another change of plans?" he asks.

"Things have changed with Jim," I answer. The details are too complicated.

"What exactly is available in Japan that you don't have in Irkutsk?" he demands. Now I know my judgment is still in doubt and I try to explain the problem with the blood. "Why can't we just send blood?" he responds.

I haven't considered that possibility and for a moment I hesitate. No, it is out, I decide. How can I convince the Soviets to give refrigerated American blood when they have fresh blood on hand?

"No, I need a plane," I insist.

Back at the hospital, I find the staff again having trouble with the intravenous line. They want to do a subclavian puncture to give Jim more blood. This means inserting a needle underneath his clavicle (collarbone) until it enters the large subclavian vein. It is an accepted and efficient method; unfortunately, it is also dangerous, running the risk of collapsing the lung which lies directly below the vein. Reluctantly, I agree. Fortunately, the procedure is done safely, but it exhausts Jim.

"When are we going to leave?" he asks. "When are they going to stop all this?" He is disgusted and frightened.

"I don't know yet," I answer. "The embassy will call as soon as they have an arrival time." I have not mentioned the possibility of a second operation nor have I informed him of the plane's delay. But I do explain the hazards of the evacuation.

"It's going to be extremely dangerous for you," I say, "both on the way to the airport and during the flight. Your blood level is low and we have no margin of safety. I think this is our only choice, but if you want to change your mind, I'll understand."

"I want to go, Bill," Jim answers, "I trust you." We sit there for a few minutes. I am holding his hand and he looks directly at me, "I might not make it, right?"

"You might not." I am amazed at how easily it comes out.

"Will you do something for me then?" He picks up a tape recorder from the nightstand. "I want to make a tape now for my wife and"—he fights back tears—"if I don't make it, please give it to her."

"Sure, Jim." Now I am the one trying not to cry. I hurry from the room and collapse in a chair near Jim's door. Vera brings me a glass of tea. She stands beside me for a moment, not speaking but with her hand on my shoulder. Just then, at the lowest point of the week, I look up. It is Nick Barsky. "The plane will arrive at nine in the morning," he says breathlessly. That is only twelve hours away.

I jump up and tell Jim. He brightens and jokes about the American nurses that might be on the plane. Vera smiles and wishes us luck.

When I tell Vladimir we will be leaving in the morning, he is surprised but calm. We decide to give Jim blood continuously overnight. I still believe he is rejecting it, but I am also concerned about the flight. Any small increase in his blood level might be lifesaving. I have felt especially close to Vladimir the past week and I tell him how grateful I am.

"There is no need for thanks," he says. "We are doctors and we do everything possible for our patients. You have made a difficult decision and I hope Jim makes it. He is important, not us."

Vladimir says he will make all arrangements for the morning and I decide to return to the hotel. As I am leaving, Jim presses the completed tape recording into my hand and says, "Try to get some rest tonight, Bill."

Back in my room, I feel exhausted and lie back on the bed to try to get a little sleep. Nick has told me there will be two nurses, two doctors, and a large supply of blood on the C-141 transport that will land tomorrow in Irkutsk. With that reasuring prospect I fall asleep immediately. Ten minutes later the phone rings.

It is the embassy. The Surgeon General of the United States wants additional information and he wants it now. An embassy officer reads me a list of his questions. "But I sent all that information to the State Department medical officer three days ago," I argue. "All you have to do is read him that cable."

"What cable?" he asks.

Now wide awake, I think about Ksenia and decide I must call her first thing in the morning. We are going to Japan and as soon as Jim is safe I will return. I try to think of a small gift I can bring her. It is a relief to think of such things again.

Wednesday, October 24

Morning comes and I reach Ksenia at home. The connection, as usual, is poor and we can barely hear each other. I explain that I am leaving for Japan, but will be back in a few days.

By her reply I can tell she does not understand. "Are you in trouble?" she asks. I think how strange it must be for Ksenia, who has been dreaming for years of ways to get out of the Soviet Union, to have me suddenly call and announce I am going to Japan "for a few days." There is no time to explain, however. My room is filling up with people. Through the static, I tell her I love her and will call on my return. I am not sure she hears me.

At the hospital it is obvious that word of our departure has spread. Routine is gone. Small groups of staff members stand expectantly about.

The professor and other doctors stop in to say goodbye. But mysteriously, something has happened to our close relationship. The professor is no longer the dominating figure he was on the night of surgery. He shakes my hand weakly and avoids my eyes. The staff asks for a final meeting.

I explain our plan for flying to Japan. They nod, and I sense their feeling of relief. Although they strongly disagree with my decision, our departure will permit their hospital to get back to normal. I promise to return with a report on Jim. They wish me well and I assume the meeting is over. But there is more on their minds.

They seem uneasy about bringing it up. Finally, one of the female surgeons presents me with a summary of Jim's hospital course. As I am thanking her, she interrupts. "I'm afraid we will have to ask you to sign a copy and leave it with us," she says timidly. "We have all agreed that Mr. Torrence should not be moved and we must ask you to assume full responsibility for this action."

Naturally I sign, but as I do, the fatigue of the last few days appears on my face. "We have made you unhappy, Dr. Knaus," she says apologetically. I assure them I understand fully. But for a split second I again doubt putting my wisdom against that of twelve other physicians. I shake off the thought and go out to prepare Jim. It is 10 A.M. The plane is an hour overdue.

By noon, the plane has finally arrived and the ambulance is on its way. We move Jim onto a stretcher. The Russians have already prepared him for the cold Siberian weather by bundling him in blankets and opening the window of his room.

We carry him gingerly down the steps and place him in the waiting ambulance. Nick, a Russian doctor, and I accompany Jim as the ambulance drives slowly over the rough roads. I keep my hand on Jim's wrist, noting an occasional irregular pulse beat. In fifteen minutes we are at the airport. There, I suddenly drop Jim's hand to look out the window. I see the huge gray tail of our plane with a small American flag painted on the uppermost part. The sight of that flag in the middle of Siberia, surrounded by Aeroflot jets, raises a lump in my throat. Our waiting is at an end.

The ambulance pulls up to the open rear doors and we lift Jim into the aircraft. As we secure him into position, one of the Air Force nurses asks me about his blood pressure.

"And what concentration of oxygen do you want him to have, Doctor?" she continues. She is detached, confident, precise.

"Fifty percent," I answer.

That short exchange puts me right back into American medicine. I tell the flight surgeon that Jim's hematocrit is 15.

"We don't like to put anyone in the air unless it is at least thirty," he says.

I look at him rather blankly and suggest we start giving blood. I say goodbye to Don. "I'll cable you from Japan."

Suddenly I realize Jim has been left alone. Although there is little I can do, after our week together I cannot leave him now. The pilot closes the rear doors and builds up pressure in the cabin. Only when a crew member asks me to take my seat for takeoff do I leave Jim's side.

A staff sergeant tells me of the tremendous excitement the landing of our Air Force jet has caused. It is the first American plane ever to land in Irkutsk and the Soviets have brought out two hundred cadets from a local air academy to watch. As soon as the plane landed, it was surrounded by Russian guards.

As we taxi to the end of the runway, a tremendous noise fills the cabin, reverberating off the bare metal skin of the interior. The sergeant, sitting next to me, explains, "A C-141 is not designed for a medical transport but for general transport. This plane's been converted for medical evacuations by sticking those canvas hammocks up." In one of these Jim is now strapped alone, in the middle of this huge raw-bellied plane.

"The takeoff will be the worst part of the trip for him," the flight surgeon says.

The takeoff is rough, and throughout the ascent Jim's hammock sways violently. When I see one of the nurses rise to attend Jim I join her. I have to lean over and shout in Jim's ear.

"How are you doing?"

"Dizzy, but I'm okay," he says.

We want to start giving him the blood they have brought from Germany, but the intravenous line has clotted during takeoff. I regret having criticized the Russians for the difficulties with Jim's veins. It takes two doctors and a nurse a half-dozen tries before we succeed in finding one. We use the light from a flashlight and I spill some of the blood over my shoes.

About three hours into the flight, color comes back to Jim's face. He grins widely and says he really feels stronger. His pulse rate decreases from the 120 to 130 of the past week to a more normal 95.

My theory is right! Jim's body is now accepting the American blood. Encouraged by such success, we start a second transfusion, during which Jim feels so improved he is able to sit up for the first time in a week.

"How does it feel?" I ask stupidly. I am so relieved that I can't stop looking at Jim and smiling.

"Fantastic," Jim says. "You have no idea how sore my back was."

The nurses are appalled at the circular bruises on Jim's back. I think of the night, which now seems long ago, when the hot glass cups were applied. I am so glad we left.

I visit the cockpit to talk with Yokota Air Base in Japan, advising them of our requirements on landing. From there, I can watch the tremendous white, frozen mountains of Siberia slip by. Back in the cabin, crew members are taking pictures through the windows. Exhilarated by Jim's improvement, I get out my camera too, and the flight surgeon suggests I shoot from the cockpit. As soon as I arrive in the cockpit the Soviet navigator glares at my camera. I suddenly remember why.

I have flown Aeroflot enough to know that no photographs may be taken while flying over Soviet territory. I put my camera back in its case, smile weakly at the Russian flyer, and return to the cabin. I tell the crew to stay out of the cockpit with their cameras and explain why. They look astonished. After months in the Soviet Union I have come to accept the many restrictions Russians place on visitors. The American flyers find it strange.

We took off from Irkutsk at 1:45 in the afternoon and at about 6 P.M. we land at Khabarovsk, on the Manchurian border, to drop off our Soviet navigator. Our brief stopover is quite an event locally. The Russian officials send out an official delegation, complete with caviar and champagne. They tell us the last American plane to land here was General Douglas MacArthur's personal plane, which ran out of fuel and made an emergency landing during World War II. We thank the delegation and the Russian navigator, clear ourselves through Soviet Customs, and take off for Japan.

Airborne again, the crew suggests I eat. I enjoy the first full meal I have had in three days. As Jim is receiving his second transfusion, he joins me with some bouillon.

"Don't look too good before we land in Japan," I joke, "or they'll think we're just out for a ride."

I settle back and try to sleep, but I am too excited. I call Japan and give the hospital a report on Jim's improvement. It is dark now, and the white landscape is replaced by a black curtain. I sit for a while between the two pilots, watching the softly lighted dials and feeling the plane surging forward. It is quiet here.

The last seven days have been the worst of my life. Although I am still anxious to get Jim into the hospital, I want these few hours in the quiet sky to last. Never before have I felt so complete a human being.

We land in Yokota at midnight. An MP boards and collects our orders and passports. I suddenly remember that, in the confusion of the evacuation, I have no written orders, nor do I have an entry visa for Japan. This disturbs the MP and he mutters something about stupid civilians, but I do not care. A beautiful Oldsmobile ambulance drives up and within minutes we are at the hospital.

We wheel Jim into the intensive care unit—clean, modern, and fully equipped. I talk briefly to the surgeon and outline Jim's case history of the last week. He reassures me there is little chance Jim is still bleeding.

Following the transfusions in flight Jim's hematocrit has risen to 26. The surgeon decides to give him two more pints of blood that night. This will put Jim at a safer level. I stay around the hospital, gazing around at American medicine and at Jim.

Thursday, October 25

At 3 A.M. the ambulance takes me to the visiting officers' quarters. I check in and go immediately to the telephone. Trying to call Moscow or Irkutsk is hopeless, so I phone USIA headquarters in Washington. The Japanese operator takes my order and within minutes I am talking with Washington.

I dictate a cable to the secretary and tell her to send it "top priority" to the American Embassy in Moscow. It reads:

> Arrived Yokota, Japan, eight hours after leaving Irkutsk. Evacuation successful. Torrence's condition markedly improved following transfusion of American blood.

I also ask the secretary to call Mrs. Torrence. Then I lie back on the bed and fall asleep.

At 7:30 A.M. the telephone rings. It is an Air Force corporal telling me I have to go to Japanese Customs immediately. My first night's sleep in four days and the Air Force is bothering me with details! He tells me to be ready in ten minutes. "I'll be dressed in an hour," I answer, slamming down the phone. I have had four hours of sleep— just enough so my body rebels at the thought of waking. In the shower for most of the hour, I rehearse what I am going to tell the Air Force.

But by the time I arrive at the office I am too happy just to be there to be angry. As I wait to be taken over to Japanese Customs, I hear an Air Force clerk complaining about having to type an emergency alert roster.

"And where did you come from?" he asks me, looking for someone with whom to share his troubles.

"Russia, Siberia, a little town called Irkutsk."

"Whew," he whistles softly. "It's lucky you left when you did. Nixon just declared a worldwide military alert because the Russians are threatening to send fifty thousand troops into the Middle East. You got out just in time."

I remember how I had planned to delay our departure one day, and say a silent prayer that we left sooner.

That afternoon I visit Jim at the hospital. He has been shaved and is sitting up in bed. "I've just talked to Rosemarie," he beams. "She and the kids are fine." His hematocrit has improved further and his full recovery seems certain. As I am about to leave, he asks, "Do you still have that tape I made in Irkutsk?"

"Yeah."

"Do you think I could have it now?"

I take it out of my pocket, remembering that terrible night in Irkutsk when neither of us was sure he would live, and place it on his bed.

Jim stayed at the Yokota hospital for a week and was then evacuated to a hospital close to his Virginia home. Despite an exhaustive diagnostic investigation at both Yokota and in Virginia, the details of the blood rejection problems encountered in Irkutsk remain a mystery.

There are four major blood groups, A, B, AB, and O. Everyone in the world has one of these four types of blood. In addition, there are a number of minor subgroups that are different in various parts of the world. Normally, these minor differences are not important and, if the blood is properly matched beforehand, there should be no reason why blood from persons of different ethnic backgrounds cannot be transfused.

Under certain circumstances, however, these normally insignificant variations among red blood cells can create problems. This is what I think occurred in Irkutsk. The testing that the Soviets performed prior to transfusion was only for the four major groups and not sensitive enough to detect other incompatibilities. Most of the

Russian blood Jim received, therefore, was interpreted by his body as foreign and destroyed. This destruction, combined with some minor blood loss after surgery, produced the dramatic and life-threatening fall in his hematocrit level. This would also explain why, when he was given his first blood transfusion on the plane, it was so successful. Unfortunately, to test this theory accurately it would be necessary to have a sample of the Russian blood, and in my rush to leave I did not think of bringing one. Nevertheless, while repeated transfusion reactions remain unproven, there is no doubt that when we reached Japan, Jim was critically ill.

In a news release issued seven months later, the Soviets suggested another explanation—a psychological crisis:

Official TASS News Release, Moscow, USSR, May 29, 1974.

> When Jim Torrence, a staff member of the U.S. Forest Service, came to Soviet Siberia, no one thought that the cordial invitation by Siberian children to show him around the mountains would end so tragically. Thirteen years ago, Torrence had an operation on his stomach and, as a result of an overstrain in the mountains, a long-forgotten disease made itself felt. Irkutsk physicians did everything possible, as Don Gayton, director of the exhibit, later pointed out in a letter to the Irkutsk medics, but following successful surgery Torrence, who did not, repeat not, know Russian, developed a psychological crisis which had a hard effect on his entire condition. It was decided to urgently evacuate the patient to the United States. . . .

I was unable to get a flight back to Irkutsk before the exhibit left, so I rejoined it in Moscow after a brief trip to Washington. There, although somewhat overshadowed by the Middle East crisis, the evacuation was the subject of much speculation and some hope in the diplomatic community. For the Soviets to allow such an unprecedented flight at a time when there was a possibility of conflict was remarkable and, to many Soviet experts, inexplicable. I would like to think the reason is simple. As Vladimir said, "Jim's life is important."

Jim completely recovered and is now the director of a large national park in the midwestern United States. I still hear from him. The last time he called, he was in Washington for a meeting. He complained he had a cold. I told him there was not a thing I could do for him.

During my remaining time in the USSR, as well as on my return trips and with the help of many other visitors, I have tried, unsuccessfully, to contact Ksenia.

A RUSSIAN MEDICAL FAMILY

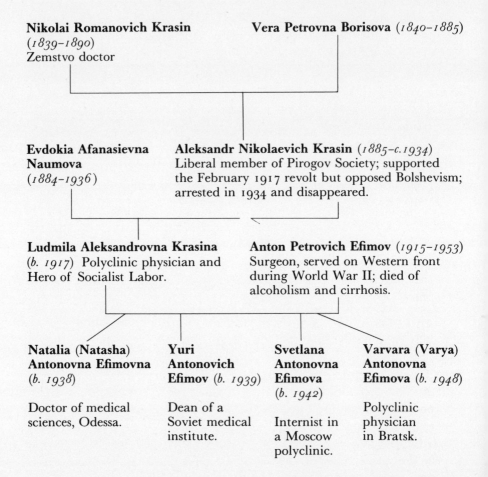

Nikolai Romanovich Krasin *(1839–1890)* Zemstvo doctor

Vera Petrovna Borisova *(1840–1885)*

Evdokia Afanasievna Naumova *(1884–1936)*

Aleksandr Nikolaevich Krasin *(1885–c. 1934)* Liberal member of Pirogov Society; supported the February 1917 revolt but opposed Bolshevism; arrested in 1934 and disappeared.

Ludmila Aleksandrovna Krasina *(b. 1917)* Polyclinic physician and Hero of Socialist Labor.

Anton Petrovich Efimov *(1915–1953)* Surgeon, served on Western front during World War II; died of alcoholism and cirrhosis.

Natalia (Natasha) Antonovna Efimovna *(b. 1938)*

Doctor of medical sciences, Odessa.

Yuri Antonovich Efimov *(b. 1939)*

Dean of a Soviet medical institute.

Svetlana Antonovna Efimova *(b. 1942)*

Internist in a Moscow polyclinic.

Varvara (Varya) Antonovna Efimova *(b. 1948)*

Polyclinic physician in Bratsk.

Other Persons Mentioned in Chapter

Dr. Nikolai Pirogov: St. Petersburg surgeon and early supporter of women in medicine.

Nadezhda Prokofievna Suslova: First Russian woman doctor to practice medicine in Russia.

Anton Chekhov: Noted Russian author and provincial doctor.

Natalia Petrovna Strassemann: Russian woman doctor, left shortly after October 1917, now lives in Washington, D.C.

Dr. W. Horsely Gantt: American doctor chosen to head American Relief Association efforts in Leningrad following World War II.

2

Vrach–The Soviet Doctor

A doctor should give part of his heart to each patient.
—OLD RUSSIAN SAYING

The great secret, known to internists and learned early in marriage by internists' wives, but still hidden from the general public, is that most things get better by themselves. Most things, in fact, are better by morning.
—LEWIS THOMAS IN *The Lives of a Cell*

Ludmila

When Ludmila Aleksandrovna Krasina decided to leave her job at the Cherniakhovsk Tractor Factory in 1936, she was nineteen years old. She had worked for three years, first at a foundry and later at the factory assembly line, producing heavy tractor axles. The dirty, repetitive, and tedious work had exhausted her. But it had also helped to dull the grief she felt over the unexpected loss of her father, Professor and Doctor of Medical Sciences Aleksandr Nikolaevich Krasin.

By the spring of 1936, the memories of that winter day two years before—her father's not coming home, the other professors saying they had seen him being forced into a black limousine, her mother's frantic, unanswered pleas to the police, and her classmates' sudden refusals to be seen with her—no longer occupied her thoughts. Ludmila had realized her life must go on, and she did not want to spend the rest of it as a factory worker.

Her decision to apply to the First Leningrad Medical Institute, where her father had taught, was motivated partly by her lifelong ambition to practice medicine and partly by a desire to clear her family's name. Although Ludmila had a "questionable" back-

53

ground, the Soviet government was so critically short of men and physicians in 1936 that she was accepted.

During her first year at the institute, Ludmila continued to work part-time to help support her mother, who had never completely recovered from the shock of her husband's sudden disappearance. In the winter, Ludmila found a job as a stoker for the Dzerzhinsky Hospital, filling one of its four large furnaces with coal during the long Leningrad nights. In the summer, she picked potatoes.

During her second year, Ludmila met and married Anton Petrovich Efimov, a medical student in the class ahead of her. Ten months later they had a daughter, Natalia, and the following year, a son, Yuri. While raising her family, Ludmila kept up with her class work. Anton, in fact, planned to delay his graduation for a year so that he and Ludmila could begin internship together at the Pushkin City Hospital. During the fourth year of Ludmila's study, she decided to become a *terapevt* (general internist) and Anton was well on his way toward training as a *khirurg* (surgeon). But their plans, along with those of millions of other Soviet citizens, were abruptly and drastically changed on June 22, 1941, when Adolf Hitler's German army invaded the USSR.

When I first arranged to meet Ludmila, that was everything I knew about her, all of it told to me by her second daughter, Svetlana, whom I had met in Moscow. Everything, that is, except what I'd learned from a small item in *Pravda:*

Moscow, USSR, February 20, 1974. Boris Petrovsky, Minister of Health, awarded Ludmila Aleksandrovna Efimova the Hero of Socialist Labor Medal today, upon her retirement after twenty-eight years as Visiting Physician and Administrator of Polyclinic No. 56, Frunze Region, City of Leningrad. Ludmila Aleksandrovna has distinguished herself as a physician for thirty-five years, including service during the second great fatherland war. In addition, she has contributed four children to the Soviet Union—all of whom are physicians. A daughter, Natalia Antonovna, is Professor of Medicine at the Odessa Medical Institute; a son, Yuri Antonovich, is Dean of the Kishinev Medical Institute; and two other daughters, Svetlana Antonovna and Varvara Antonovna, are *terapevty.* In bestowing the medal, Minister Petrovsky said that it is because of women like Ludmila Aleksandrovna that the Soviet medical system provides the people of the USSR with the best medical care in the world.

Initially, Ludmila refused to meet me. During most of her life it had been illegal and very dangerous for a Soviet citizen to become friends with a foreigner. In her lifetime Ludmila had never violated Soviet law. She was a grandmother and comfortable in her retirement. Why take chances? But Svetlana convinced her that things were different, better, and that I would be careful. Ludmila agreed.

Our first meeting was to be in a public place, a small café down the street from Polyclinic No. 56. At first I had trouble finding her in the steamy room. It was a typical winter day in Leningrad, with a strong northern wind whipping snow into whirlwinds. The small café was packed with people bundled in heavy, woolen coats, trying to escape the stinging cold. After a few minutes I recognized her from an old picture Svetlana had given me and by the anxious, worried expression on her face. She was sitting at a table against the window, a fur cap on her head, her hands clutching a large pocketbook.

As with many older Soviet women, the stressful years she had endured showed on Ludmila's face. Her hair, once dark brown, was dyed a rust color. The skin on her broad, flat cheekbones and large nose was heavily wrinkled, and her smile revealed a gold-capped front tooth. She squinted as I approached and the lines around her eyes deepened. I noticed she had a large circle of rouge on each cheek and, except for her wedding band, she wore no jewelry. The hand she extended was coarse, its palm rough with calluses from her many nonmedical duties. She smelled of cigarette smoke.

As I sat down I explained why I had wanted to meet her, how the newspaper article and my meeting with her daughter had convinced me she could tell me much about being a Soviet doctor.

"Chto mogu skazat?" (What is there to tell?) She began slowly lighting a cigarette. "In the past—for my father and grandfather—it was hard, terribly hard, being a doctor, but today it's a simple life. You go to work each day and try to help. But really there is not much you can do. Sometimes you can take away pain or convince someone to stop drinking. In the end, a doctor is not very powerful and a Russian doctor cannot do much more than a doctor in America."

"Of course," I agreed. "But you have been different—special. There is a long medical tradition in your family. You've been given many honors. You have had a proud career."

"Career?" Ludmila replied softly, raising her eyebrows. "I don't think you understand. I have had no time to worry about such luxuries. Life has been too difficult—too expensive—to think about careers. If you want to talk about such things, talk to my son, Yuri, or my oldest daughter, Natalia. They are modern physicians. They have careers. I have been a *srednii vrach* [average doctor], nothing more."

Medical School

There are over a million physicians today in the Soviet Union, a fourth of the world's total and twice the number working in the United States. In 1983, the Soviet Union is expected to reach a saturation point with 1,200,000 physicians. That's one doctor for every 220 of its citizens, compared to one for every 450 people in the United States. A few thousand of these physicians conduct research or teach, becoming *kandidaty* (doctors of medical science). Others become public health physicians (*sanitarnye vrachi*). Approximately 100,000 specialize in dentistry. But the vast majority, nearly 70 percent, become simple clinical doctors like Ludmila. These *srednie vrachi*—70 percent of whom are now women—form the backbone of the Soviet medical system.

Within the Soviet medical hierarchy a *vrach* is roughly equivalent to our general, or family, practitioner. But unlike the typical American graduate, who spends an average of ten to twelve years after high school becoming a physician, the Soviet student is finished in seven years. And while first-year medical students at Harvard and Iowa are memorizing the intricacies of the Krebs cycle or learning to recognize the microscopic differences between lung and liver tissue, students at First Moscow or Tashkent Medical Institute spend most of their time on physics, organic chemistry, and Latin, subjects normally taken during our four years of undergraduate college.

Anatomy, physiology, microbiology, pharmacology, pathology, and genetics, along with continued instruction in the history of Communism and theory of scientific Communism, are presented in the next two years. By the third year, specialization in general medicine, pediatrics, public health, dentistry, or pharmaceutics begins.

Despite this whirlwind exposure, which takes the Soviet teenager from high school physics and Latin to cardiology and gynecology in three years, the atmosphere is relaxed. To those who have witnessed the intensive drive for knowledge and the obsessive preoccupation with facts that characterize American medical students, the Soviet student appears strangely calm and unperturbed.

The lectures she attends for eight to ten hours a week with a hundred or so other students, combined with about twice as many hours in practical instruction, allow time for other jobs. Less time is spent studying after class than in the United States.

Examinations are oral. "You go to the instructor, answer a few questions, and he gives you a score from one to five. It's not very hard to get a five," Sophia, a third-year student, told me.

There are few dropouts as the large class of students (average size 550) breaks up into small groups for hospital training in the fourth and fifth years. The students look self-conscious in their newly acquired white coats and tall starched hats, waiting nervously for the professor to begin rounds. Here the emphasis is on patient care, and the Soviet student starts with the basics.

For the first four weeks of clinical instruction, a student is required to perform the duties of a nurse, making beds, bathing patients, and emptying bedpans. Then follow two years of practical instruction in physical diagnosis, radiology, surgery, obstetrics, gynecology, or pediatrics.

Following this "subinternship," the student sits for the state qualifying examination and receives a certificate as either a *terapevt* (general internist), a pediatrician, a public health physician, or, if they entered specialized faculties, a dentist or pharmacist.

Graduation, however, does not conclude with the new graduate running out to put an M.D. on the license plate of her new car. The *srednii vrach* is afforded few special privileges. She will live in the same crowded apartment houses, ride the same buses, and stand in the same lines as her patients. Despite her training and title, she is not an independent professional but a paid employee working for the world's largest employer of physicians—the Soviet government.

From Witchcraft to War

This intimate relationship between Russian doctors and their government began long before the 1917 Revolution. In the early 1700s, Tsar Peter the Great, the man responsible for raising St. Petersburg (now Leningrad) from the marshes of the Neva River, established in Moscow the first Russian hospitals and medical institutes, using German physicians as instructors. Life for these early medical students was difficult. They lived five or six to a room and, because of low stipends, were frequently forced to beg food from their patients' families. Because there was almost no secondary education, most students entering the institute were unsophisticated and ignorant peasants. They were frequently accused of drunkenness, vandalism, whoring, and "general debauchery." For punishment they were flogged and then shackled in chains.[1]

These early students had so little preliminary education that the course of instruction had to be long, often lasting seven or even ten years. Given the poor living conditions, harsh treatment, and the long course of study, it is little wonder that sixteen of the original fifty students (all male) in the Moscow Hospital School ran away. Eight others died as the result of the beatings.

Conditions improved later in the century, but for all of the eighteenth century the output of these early hospital schools totaled only a few hundred. The majority of Russia's doctors had to be imported. Unfortunately, most of these foreign physicians spoke no Russian and spent more time attending the imperial court or filling out reports for the government than they did treating sick peasants. By 1828, Russia had only one doctor for every 18,000 citizens (Italy had one for every 2,000, England one per 3,000). During his short lifespan, the average Russian never saw a physician.[2]

At this time in history, however, the lack of medical care was the least of the villagers' problems. Russia in the early nineteenth century was a backward, undeveloped country. The 95 percent of its 60 million population who lived in rural areas were struggling to survive, more concerned about having enough food than finding a doctor. They worked, as the writer Maxim Gorki recounted, "from sunrise to sunset for some bread and much misery."

Besides, the odds of benefiting from medical care were against them. The germ theory of disease, antiseptics, and anesthesia were yet to be discovered. Medicine was still in its "sympathetic" period,

---

[1] Efron Brokgauz, *Entsiklopedicheskii Slovar*, 1896 ed., s.v. "Meditsina v Rossii."
[2] Roderick E. McGrew, *Russia and the Cholera* (Milwaukee: University of Wisconsin Press, 1965), pp. 25–40.

when bloodletting, purges, and cathartics were used to recreate the proper balance of the body's "four humors." It was a time of desperate poverty, of geographic and cultural isolation—and of witchcraft.

"Many of my patients," Ludmila told me, "still go to women who prepare potions or who are supposed to *zagavarivat* [whisper] disease away." This modern-day belief in witchcraft dates back to the time when each Russian village had its own wise woman or witch healer (*znakharka*) to handle its medical needs. The *znakharka* wore a bag of charms around her neck. She used many herbal cures: poppyseed for earaches, root of geranium to stop intestinal bleeding, sage for toothaches, cabbage juice for ulcers.

She also served as a midwife, attending the mother throughout the pregnancy, frequently recommending that she lie in a bed of warmed sand and ashes during the final weeks. To hurry delivery, the pregnant woman might be rolled in the dust or forced to ride a horse for a quarter of a mile. After the baby was born, the umbilical cord was removed and tied around the mother's waist to control bleeding.

The *znakharka* approached the problem of sterility with the same mixture of superstition and rudimentary, often erroneous, medical knowledge. First, an investigation was conducted to make sure the husband had not been unfaithful to his wife, thereby wasting his potency on other women. If he was judged faithful, fault was thought to reside in the woman's large intestine. The *znakharka* believed an overdistended large intestine put pressure on the womb, making it difficult to become pregnant. Treatment consisted of vigorous enemas, using gallons of water to flush the colon. Anal intercourse was recommended.

From the sixteenth century and well into the nineteenth, practicing witchcraft was the major way a Russian woman could be associated with medicine. The situation improved in the 1850s, but it took a war to produce the change.

The Crimean War, a three-year conflict begun in 1853, was fought on a small peninsula, the Crimea, which protrudes into the Black Sea. There in the town of Sevastopol, during the fiercest battle of the war, the Tsar's army held out for eleven and a half months against repeated bombardments by the combined Turkish, British, and French forces before collapsing. The Russian defeat at Sevastopol was a landmark in Russian history, exposing the backward nation to the rest of the world and forcing a serious and widespread discussion of social and political issues.

Medicine was no exception. The Crimean conflict found the Russian soldier listless from a high-starch diet and too weak to withstand the epidemics of typhus and cholera which claimed more victims than the shelling. Even though they were fighting on their own soil, the Russians were not able to keep up with medical and other logistic needs as well as the British and French were. It was a brutal and shocking time for the empire. It demonstrated how far behind the European continent Russia was, both in terms of military preparedness and of public health. Compared to Great Britain and France, Russia was still in the dark ages.

One small ray of light appeared during the Crimean fighting—the introduction of nursing as an accepted profession. Late in 1854, at two English military hospitals, in Scutari (now in Istanbul, Turkey) and in Balaklava (now in Sevastopol), thirty-eight nurses, directed by Florence Nightingale, began treating British soldiers. A Russian contingent (which actually had begun to organize before the English) arrived on the scene and began work in Sevastopol about a month later.

The first group of twenty-eight Russian Sisters of Charity, formed by the Grand Duchess Elena Pavlovna, the Tsar's sister-in-law, was an unlikely lot, with illiterate peasant women working alongside members of the intelligentsia. Ekaterina M. Bakdavina, a Moscow society hostess whose father had once been governor of St. Petersburg, insisted on wearing a long formal dress while treating the soldiers.

Unlike the British nurses, who received double pay for serving in a war zone, the Sisters of Charity were all volunteers. Both groups had a hard time, initially, gaining acceptance. The Russian commander, General Menshikov, believed that "our soldiers will rape the sisters and the only contribution they will make will be an increase in the number of my syphilitics."

Of the original Russian twenty-eight, however, all (with the exception of a young peasant girl sent home because of sexual misconduct) were serious and talented women who, despite their lack of formal medical training, performed admirably under grim conditions.

In one two-month period, 8,484 Russian soldiers were either killed or wounded in Sevastopol. Bakdavina described the hospital scene in her letters to Moscow:

> The main room of the hospital had originally been a dance hall. The floor was white marble and huge red columns rose to the ceiling. In between were placed the beds, one right next to the other. With cannon shots and sounds of fighting coming in through the windows, the great mahogany and bronze doors would open and in would come the stretchers. Those with the most serious wounds were brought up front in the first use of a triage system for battle casualties. Hopeless cases were sent to the dread Gruschin house. The surgeons would operate on tables right in the middle of the floor, performing amputations and closing wounds. I admit I marvel at my coolness at the operating table. I hand them the operating silk and when I tie the knots the blood flows freely over my hands, my clothes.[3]

Many of the most important contributions of the sisters took place after the operation. They checked the patients for bleeding, calmed the frightened, and gave morphine to those in pain. As the number of sisters increased, they took over administration of the dispensary and supervised the finances of the injured soldiers. Members of the Tsar's army were paid for their battle wounds—fifty rubles for a leg, forty for an arm. While under the effects of chloroform or delirious from fever, the money could easily be stolen. At one time the sisters held a total of 60,000 rubles in payment for missing limbs.

By the end of the war, the value of the sisters was well established. The letters of Dr. Nikolai I. Pirogov, a distinguished St. Petersburg surgeon, were filled with admiration. In 1855 he wrote to the new Tsar, Alexander II: "I am delighted by the good results this women's organization gave. These results indicate that, up to now, we have completely ignored the marvelous healing gift of our women."[4]

After returning from the war, Pirogov continued to campaign for improved education and an expanded role for the Russian woman. His writing pioneered the idea of a female's right to an education and opened the way for the limited emancipation of Russian women in the 1800s.

[3] John Shelton Curtiss, "Russian Sisters of Mercy in the Crimea, 1854–1855," *Slavic Review* 25 (March 1966): 84–100.
[4] Richard Stites, *The Women's Liberation Movement in Russia* (Princeton: Princeton University Press, 1978), pp. 31–32.

The Great Reforms

The shock of the Crimean War brought many other far-reaching changes to Russia. Serfs were freed and the power and privilege of the few weatlhy families reduced. The previously rigid relations among the peasant, landowner, and nobility were relaxed, and in many ways the freedom enjoyed by the average Russian increased. The life of physicians also improved in the 1860s, during the period known as the Great Reforms. Up to this time, the social position of the Russian physician had been only slightly above the peasant's.

A medical statute of the 1850s, for example, decreed that a physician must treat the poor (meaning most Russians) without charge, write all prescriptions legibly, and appear "at the request of the sick." This made it a crime for a physician to ignore a patient's call for help. The first time he did so he would be fined a month's salary, and if it happened again his license could be revoked. Since no one could afford to pay for medical care, the doctor was forced to rely on government support. As a public employee, he was treated with disdain and condemnation by the more prestigious diplomatic and bureaucratic sections.

In 1864, however, seventeen years before he was killed by an extremist's bomb, Alexander II (known as "The Great Tsar Liberator") tried to make things better for the Russian doctor. In that year the *zemstvo* reforms made it possible for prerevolutionary physicians, among them Nikolai Romanovich Krasin, to obtain an element of freedom. Krasin, Ludmila's grandfather, had graduated from the Petersburg Medical Academy in 1864. "He was the first member of our family to practice medicine," Ludmila told me proudly. "At first he was going to be a university professor, a doctor of medicine, but when the *zemstvo* movement began, he decided to become a country doctor. I remember my father telling me that the 1860s were an exciting time in Russia. There was talk of freedom and a new awakening."

The *zemstvo* represented a return-to-the-land movement in Russia (*zemlia* means earth or soil) that divided the country into thirty-four provinces, each under the control of a local council. The council, which included peasants as well as wealthy landowners, was given power to tax real estate and business within its territory. In exchange, it was charged with the construction and maintenance of roads, bridges, primary schools, hospitals, clinics, orphanages, and other public services. The *zemstvo* hired teachers, doctors, Sisters of Charity, and other professionals.

The principles of the *zemstvo* reform, and the relative freeedom this form of employment offered, attracted many of the young idealistic graduates of Russia's medical institutes. A "peace corps mentality" sprang up in Russia among the *narodniki*, as they were known. But this group, which included painters, musicians, and lawyers as well as doctors, concentrated on the far reaches of their own land rather than on foreign countries. Three-fourths of the *zemstvo* physicians were under thirty-five years of age and almost all were Russian citizens. Each earned 1,215 rubles a year (about the same as a factory worker) for work in small rural clinics where, with the help of a *feldsher* (physician's assistant), they were responsible for the medical needs of four thousand people. Like most reforms, however, the *zemstvo* was incomplete.

Besides having too many patients, the typical *zemstvo* physician had too few resources and too many miles to travel each day. Dedicated as they were, physicians were unable to provide care to more than a fraction of Russia's peasants. Furthermore, some of the peasants they did reach were unwilling to accept them. The problems that Nikolai, Ludmila's grandfather, encountered were typical.

In 1866, Nikolai had moved with his wife to a small village sixty miles outside St. Petersburg. Nikolai Romanovich was a sullen, diminutive man who, by all accounts, felt more at home in a laboratory than in a clinic. But he felt it was his duty to help the peasants.

"They lived in a small house at the end of the village," Ludmila told me, recalling the description given her by her grandmother. "It was an old building, meant to be a storehouse. The roof leaked badly and the floor was mud. The villagers were supposed to supply my grandfather with food in exchange for his moving there, but few of them did and much of his salary went to buy bread."

The cool response Nikolai received from the villagers extended to his profession. "Most of the peasants still believed in witchcraft and didn't trust grandfather. They were sure he'd been sent by the tsar to make them sterile," Ludmila said. "Even members of the intelligentsia [intellectual elite] in St. Petersburg were skeptical. Some of his friends accused grandfather of going to the village so he could experiment on peasants."

After two miserable, lonely years and the birth of their first daughter, Nikolai and his wife moved back to St. Petersburg. He resumed his studies at the institute and four years later became a doctor of medical science. Two years later his first son, Ludmila's father Aleksandr, was born.

Not all *zemstvo* physicians had such dismal experiences. In fact, despite many problems, the *zemstvo* system achieved some important successes. Most of the accomplishments came not from crisis-oriented care but from public health measures. The *zemstvo* physicians supervised epidemic controls, performed medical statistical investigations, and gave vaccinations. By emphasizing the newly accepted theory of infection, the *zemstvo* began to dispel, for the first time, the villagers' long-held belief that curses, demons, and religious sins were the causes of all illnesses.

In the mid-1800s, for example, three-quarters of all children born to Russian peasants died before they were a year old. Investigation by a *zemstvo* physician revealed that infant illnesses and deaths increased sharply during harvest times. Working mothers were forced to leave their children in the care of the village *znakharka,* who insisted that each child drink potions from a supposedly magical container. This practice spread infection rapidly from one child to another. The *zemstvo* addressed the problem by establishing nurseries to care for the children during the harvest.

At about the same time, Vasilii Martinenko, a *zemstvo* physician working near Odessa, discovered that the peasants' habit of feeding their infants harsh black bread caused diarrhea, which in the hot summer months rapidly led to dehydration and, in many instances, death. Encouraging mothers to use more milk and less bread reduced the death rate dramatically.

Doctor Anton Chekhov

One of the lasting legacies of the *zemstvo* system was not its emphasis on public health but one of its physicians, a *srednii vrach* (average doctor) Anton Chekhov. The playwright and pioneer in development of the modern short story was a small child when the reforms started, his family having been serfs a few years prior to his birth. As a physician Chekhov was intimately involved with the reforms, and their incomplete success is a frequent theme throughout his writing.

In 1892 Chekhov and his family lived in Melikhovo, a rural estate a few hours by train from Moscow and close to the city of Serpukhov. By this time the reputation of the thirty-two-year-old writer was well established, his writing in great demand.

But in 1892 the area around Moscow was experiencing the beginnings of a severe cholera epidemic. The winter of 1890–1891 had been harder than usual and it was followed by a severe summer drought. The combination produced a famine, one of the worst in Russian history. There were at least 400,000 deaths with millions of others weakened, allowing cholera to spread rapidly. In a letter to Alexei Suvorin, a close friend and early publisher, Chekhov explained that,

> "I have become a district doctor for the Serpukhov *zemstvo* and am out chasing cholera by the tail and organizing a new district at top speed. My district consists of twenty-five villages, four factories and a monastery. I see patients in the morning and make rounds for the rest of the day. I ride, lecture the local rustics, treat patients and fume, and since the *zemstvo* hasn't given me a penny for organizing clinics I have to wheedle one thing after another from the rich. . . . I've turned out to be an excellent beggar. My soul is weary. I'm bored. Not being your own master, thinking only of diarrhea, being startled at night by dogs barking and a knock at the gate (have they come for me?), riding abominable horses over uncharted roads, and reading only about cholera, and waiting only for cholera . . ."[5]

In addition to his trouble with money, Chekhov's letters and writings also provide evidence that the great reforms had done little to improve the traditionally low social positon of Russian doctors. Later in the same letter to his confident Suvorin, Chekhov complains that,

> "My neighbor Count Orlov-Davydov, owner of the famous Otrada, is in Biarritz now to escape the cholera epidemic. All he gave his doctor to fight the cholera epidemic was five hundred rubles. His sister the Countess lives in my region, and when I visited her to discuss putting up a shelter for her workers, she treated me as if I had come to apply for a job. That hurt me . . ."[6]

[5] M. H. Heim, S. Karlinsky, *Letters of Anton Chekhov* (New York: Harper and Row, 1973) pp. 239–242.
[6] *Ibid.*, pp. 239–246.

In his play *Enemies,* Chekhov portrayed the life of a *vrach,* who, despite the reforms, was not respected. A wealthy landowner calls on the doctor in the middle of a winter night, asking him to drive fourteen *versts* (a *verst* is two-thirds of a mile) to visit his dying wife. At first the doctor refuses. He tells the landowner he has been up for the past three nights fighting for the life of his own son, who has just died. It is inhuman, the doctor argues, that he should be forced to leave his wife that night. But the landowner insists and when the doctor finally arrives, the "dying" wife has eloped with a lover.

"It is mean and contemptible," the *vrach* says, "to play with human beings this way. I am a doctor. You consider doctors . . . your lackeys, mere vulgarians. Do so if you wish, but you have no right to make a stage property of a suffering fellow creature."

Chekhov also complained in his personal letters about the persistence of outdated medical practices in many of the outlying provinces. "Bloodletting and blood-sucking jars are still used on a grand beastly scale," he said. "On the road I examined a Jew sick with cancer of the liver. The Jew is emaciated, barely breathing, but this does not prevent his *vrach* from placing twelve bloodsucking jars on him."

While working in Kharkov, Chekhov saw patients alongside one of the few prerevolutionary female *vrachi* in Russia. "When consulting we don't always agree," he wrote.

> "I appear as the bearer of good news, where she sees death and disease. At one time we received a young peasant girl with malignant glands on her neck. The infection had seized so many spots that any attempt at a cure was unthinkable. And so, because the *baba* [a pejorative name for young woman] does not feel any pain but will, in half a year, die in frightful suffering, the female doctor looked at her with such deep guilt, as though she wanted to apologize for her own good health—as though she was ashamed her medicine is so impotent."[7]

Despite this comment Chekhov encouraged the professional growth of women in Russia. The obstacles that Russian women had in gaining personal freedom and independence are frequent themes in Chekhov's writing.

[7] V. V. Hishniakov, *Anton Pavlovich Chekhov kak vrach* (Moscow: Megik, 1947). pp. 10–13.

In "The Bride," the last story he completed before dying of tuberculosis in 1904, Chekhov has Nagda, the main character, reject the traditional and subservient role for women then common in Russian society and strike out on her own.

Nadezhda Suslova

Unfortunately, Chekhov's attitude toward women was not shared by most other Russians. From the middle of the nineteenth century, after the Crimean War, Russian women, along with their British and American colleagues, were readily accepted as nurses but denied admission to medical institutes. The first woman to break the sexual barrier in Russia was Nadezhda Prokofievna Suslova, who like Chekhov was the child of a former serf.

In 1861, when Ludmila's grandfather was in his third year at the Medico-Surgical Academy in St. Petersburg, Suslova applied for admission. Although the sons of serfs had been permitted in the institution prior to 1861, Suslova's request was a first, and it created a stir within the academic and social circles of nineteenth-century Russia.

"I remember my father telling me how the students in my grandfather's class were angry that a woman had been admitted to the institute," Ludmila recalled. "They considered medicine an improper profession for females."

Nadezhd˙ ˙ ˍquest was not the only reason the name of Suslova was proﾑinent dinner time conversation in social circles around St. Petersburg. Nadezhda's sister, Polina, was at this same time mistress to one of Russia's greatest novelists, Fyodor Dostoevsky. The writer's long affair with Polina was, in fact, the basis of one of his better-known novels, *The Gambler*.

Both Polina and Nadezhda (whose name means hope) were part of an emerging class of intelligentsia in Russia who were challenging the established relationships between social classes. Nadezhda's father, a former serf who had obtained his freedom before the official emancipation, encouraged his daughters to get a higher education. Polina, while conducting a passionate and often turbulent love affair with Dostoevsky, studied at the University of St. Petersburg.

Nadezhda, who frequently acted as a go-between for the quarreling lovers, received encouragement from Dostoevsky to break with the female nursing tradition of the time and study medicine. As part of the Great Reforms, women had initially been permitted to attend and audit lectures at the universities and medical institutions, so Nadezhda began attending classes at the academy in 1861. Two years later, however, a carefully worded Ministry of Education directive was published specifically forbidding women to enroll as students. Nadezhda was expelled.

The motivation behind this temporary retreat on female education is central to understanding the attitude toward women that developed in nineteenth-century Russian medicine. This attitude of male superiority is still prevalent today and influences the way Ludmila, her daughters, and the thousands of other Soviet *vrachi* are treated.

One of the historical objections to women's entry into medicine was the claim by Russian men that Russian women were too emotional and physically incapable of withstanding the rigors of medical practice. An eighteenth-century Russian physician named Onatsevich, writing in the *St. Petersburg News,* questioned whether a female physician would be able to withstand the long hours of work and the hardships of traveling from village to village.

A study published in 1850 claimed that Russian women were characterized by sensitivity, love, and modesty, while men demonstrated honor, energy, and intellect. Because of these differences, women were best suited to provide comfort in times of suffering. Men, on the other hand, were expected to accomplish new works and deeds. These "scientific" conclusions supported the prevailing social attitude that women should be nurses and men, doctors.

This attitude infuriated Nadezhda Suslova and, upon being expelled from the medical institute, she immediately left for Switzerland and the University of Zurich. There she prepared and defended her dissertation on the physiology of the heart and in 1867 became Russia's first female physician. Upon returning to Russia, she persuaded the medical authorities to honor her degree and thus began a pattern that other liberated nineteenth-century Russian women could follow.

As the number of Russian women studying medicine in Switzerland increased, they became known as the Zurich Colony. The colony attracted some of Russia's most liberal and advanced women, who viewed science and medicine as a way to reach the people with their message of equal rights. Many of them organized political groups aimed at improving the lot of Russian women. By 1873, the Zurich Colony and its political activities had attracted the attention of the Tsar, who feared that the influence generated by the returning students with their radical ideas might be disruptive despite their small numbers (only 118 women studied in Zurich between 1867 and 1874). In 1873, Alexander II ordered all female students back to Russia, decreeing that those who remained would never be permitted to practice medicine in their home country.

So the promise of reform that had marked the early years of Alexander II's reign proved short-lived, especially in regard to women and medicine. True, women were again permitted to attend medical lectures, but only a few members of the intelligentsia did. The vast majority of women accepted the prejudice of their time and became Sisters of Charity.

When Alexander III took over in 1881, he made it even more difficult for women to become physicians. His minister of education, Dmitry Tolstoy, decided that the drive for emancipation of Russian women had gone far enough, and again closed all medical institutes to female students. His action met with protest from women's groups. After prolonged debate a new Women's Medical Institute in St. Petersburg was finally opened in 1897, and since then, Russian women have been permitted a medical education.

Initially, however, many old prejudices remained, and while these early female physicians enjoyed the same privileges as men, they did not get equal work. In the cities, most of their duties were limited. They served as doctors for maternity hospitals and girls' schools and as medical inspectors for prostitutes. They were at their best, according to a newspaper article of the day, "when providing compassionate understanding." Some of these early female physicians joined the zemstvo movement, where their medical expertise was more appreciated and less restricted than in the larger cities.

Regardless of problems, however, the movement Nadezhda Suslova started in 1861 was a success. By 1910, Russia had 1,500 female physicians, less than 10 percent of the total, but more than in any other country in Europe.

Natalia Strassemann

One of this small number of women who became physicians in prerevolutionary Russia was Natalia Petrovna Strassemann, the daughter of a wealthy landowner. In 1911, at the age of seventeen, she joined the Red Cross Sisters of Mercy, which in 1894 had absorbed the Sisters of Charity to become the largest nursing organization in Russia. It was another time of challenge and change for the country. The Russo-Japanese war, one of four major conflicts to be fought on Russian soil during the twentieth century, was almost forgotten, but the spirit, if not the deeds, of domestic revolution was in the air. The city of St. Petersburg would, within the next six years, change its name twice.

Dr. Strassemann now lives in the Georgetown section of Washington, D.C. Her small town house is crowded with icons and Russian paintings, along with her most treasured possession, a silver samovar smuggled out when she and her husband left Russia for Belgrade, shortly after the 1917 Revolution. Today it is difficult to imagine this tiny white-haired woman, who seems lost in her armchair, as a White Army sympathizer. Although eighty-seven years old, Strassemann remembers vividly the details of that time.

As a Sister of Mercy, Strassemann's first assignment was in a small hospital that was under the personal supervision of Empress Maria Fyodorovna, mother of the last Russian Tsar, Nicholas II. The hospital, like most private institutions, was supported by donations from wealthy landowners. At that time, hospital care in Russian cities was an unorganized affair. There were a few clinics and hospitals run by the government in addition to the privately sponsored free hospitals like the one in which Strassemann worked.

"There were thirty to forty beds to a room," she recalls, "and everything was plain and simple. The beds had iron frames with straw mattresses, but all was immaculately clean. The sheets were changed regularly and the halls scrubbed with a strong disinfectant. The sisters were very proud that their patients never had a bedsore. Never, no matter how long a person was sick. Sometimes we even used water beds to prevent bedsores, but mostly it was just good nursing care."

Every morning the head doctor would visit all the patients and Strassemann would walk behind him, carefully noting his orders.

After two years of this work, the young girl decided that she wanted to become a doctor and entered the special Women's Medical Institute in St. Petersburg.

"At that time it was difficult, but not impossible, for a woman to become a doctor," she recalls. "In fact, when I applied it was easier for a woman to get into medical school than it was for a Jew."[8]

Despite having their own medical institute, Strassemann is quick to point out that women were subject to discrimination. "There were no female medical professors and most patients still preferred to see a man for serious problems. For minor problems a woman was all right, but for complicated matters, a male *vrach* was always consulted."

Furthermore, although the social position of *vrachi* had improved from the early 1800s, it was, as Chekhov emphasized, still not considered prestigious to become a physician.

"None of the members of the aristocracy went to medical school." she told me. "They joined the diplomatic corps or became officers in the Tsar's army. Medicine was a career open to members of the intelligentsia who, like myself, wanted to help people. And it was open to the lower classes, who could improve their social standing through education."

The *vrach* living in a Russian city at this time could choose from a number of jobs. As a government *vrach,* he could make 1,500 rubles ($750) a year. He could teach in a university, where his basic salary would be lower but he could earn additional money seeing private patients, relying on the unwritten understanding about payment for services rendered.

"*Vrachi* never charged directly for their services," Strassemann recalls. "After treatment a patient would put in the doctor's hand whatever she felt the *vrach* deserved. Of course, it was different for the famous doctors," she explains. "For instance, Professor Serafimov, an important doctor from the institute, would make every person in his waiting room pay twenty-five rubles before he could be seen."

---

[8] Since 1887, the imperial government had established quotas for Jewish students in all institutions of higher education. In St. Petersburg, no more than 3 percent of the medical school class could be Jewish. Jewish physicians made up the majority in private practice, however, since they were prohibited from entering government or military service.

To gain the status and economic advantage of a professor, the prerevolutionary *vrach* had to return to the university, continue his studies for a number of years, write a dissertation, and pass a series of advanced examinations. In spite of this long course of study, many physicians chose to work toward an advanced degree. Research in Russian universities was among the best in the world.

At about this time the famous embryologist Ilya Metchnikoff discovered the way in which white blood cells help the body fight infection. Ivan Sechenov, a physiologist, was doing extremely detailed and advanced work on how oxygen and other gases are carried in our bloodstream. Another physiologist—and the most influential Russian scientist—Ivan Pavlov, gave modern science its first insights into the physiology of digestion.

Much of the political activity of these prerevolutionary physicians, both scientist and practitioner, was centered in the Pirogov Society, an organization named for the outstanding surgeon of the Crimean War. The Pirogovists were a natural outgrowth of the *zemstvo* reforms. A liberal physicians group, its members supported increased public health measures and improvements in the working conditions of the Russian population. They printed pamphlets describing how one could avoid contracting cholera by properly boiling water. In railway stations and in other public meeting places, they placed huge pictures of the number-one public health enemy of that time, the louse, urging people to visit a delousing station once a month. Partly because of the efforts of the Pirogov Society, a pioneer labor insurance law making employers responsible for accidents was passed in 1903.

The Pirogov Society was exclusively male. Female physicians who were politically active in prerevolutionary Russia were more concerned with woman suffrage than with medical issues. In fact, the tradition of the Zurich Colony extended to the early part of the twentieth century, with many female physicians providing leadership and inspiration to the small but active campaign for improved women's rights.

The Pirogovists, however, wanted nothing to do with the women's movement. They advocated increased government financing of medical and public health services but stopped short of accepting, as was first proposed in 1910, a unification of all Russian health services, including physicians, under government control. One of the major reasons the government wanted such control was to correct the unequal distribution of *vrachi*. At the turn of the century, when only 10 percent of the population lived in urban areas, 85 percent of the physicians were concentrated there.

Lenin and the Medical Profession

Following his return from the countryside, Ludmila's grandfather, Nikolai, had decided to establish a small private city practice. Like the *vrachi* Strassemann described, he would treat patients in exchange for fees based on their diseases and their ability to pay.

A typical morning found a cross-section of the intelligentsia of St. Petersburg in his office; a middle-ranking government bureaucrat with ulcer disease, for which Nikolai prescribed a combination of milk and honey; a philosophy professor with an advanced case of gout, to whom he gave a prescription for colchicine to be filled at the local *apteka* (pharmacy); and a retired army officer suffering from an advanced case of syphilis, who was now finding it increasingly difficult to walk. For him, Nikolai recommended hospitalization and treatment with arsenicals, but the old general refused.

Nikolai's was an isolated and protected existence, but after his experience with the *zemstvo* it was the kind of life he preferred, the kind he wanted to leave his son, Alexsandr.

Aleksandr Nikolaevich Krasin, Ludmila's father, had been born on November 14, 1885. From the time he was eight years old, everyone in the family was convinced that Sasha, as he was affectionately known, would become a doctor. As a child, Sasha's favorite pastime was sitting on the floor of his father's office, asking each of the patients about his illness and then writing out a prescription.

After his graduation from the medical institute in 1908, at twenty-three, Aleksandr Nikolaevich joined the Pirogov Society and, unlike his father, immediately became a social activist, urging reform of the antiquated and uncoordinated mixture of public and private hospitals in the cities and the lack of services to the countryside.

During the next eleven years he headed committees and organized meetings. In 1915 he helped prepare an article for the *Obshchestvennyi Vrach* (*Public Doctor*), the first official publication of the Pirogov Society. The article explained the health system in Germany and its implications for Russia. Germany under Premier Otto von Bismarck was, in the second half of the nineteenth century, a leader in social legislation. In 1883 it had passed the Sickness Insurance Act, the first law guaranteeing financing of medical care for all workers. This spirit of medical change spread east to Russia, and between 1912 and 1914 one out of every ten articles in *Moskovskie Vedomosti,* a Moscow newspaper, was about the reform of medicine.

"I recall how, as a small child, my father would talk about those days," Ludmila said. "How excited he was about the changes happening in Russia and how proud he was to be one of the leaders."

In February 1917, the Social Democrats took over the government and, in forcing the resignation of Nicholas II, ended a thousand years of tsarist rule. The new provisional government that moved into the Winter Palace acted quickly to organize medical services with the formation of a Central Medical Sanitary Commission. Aleksandr Krasin was chosen as a member of the new commission.

Unfortunately, the provisional government was not able to unite and lead the many groups that wanted to control the future of Russian medicine.

It was a frustrating time for Ludmila's father. He wanted the provisional government to succeed, but with the confusion, inefficiency, and dislocations created by the sudden takeover, progress was impossible. Six months after the removal of the Tsar, Bolsheviks, chanting "Land, Freedom, Bread," stormed the Winter Palace and removed the provisional government.

The successful revolutionaries immediately distrusted the Pirogovists, seeing them as a representative of the liberal bourgeois intelligentsia they wanted to destroy. The *zemstvo,* too, according to Vladimir Ilyich Lenin, the Bolsheviks' leader, was suspect, being known as "the fifth wheel of the tsarist regime." The Medical Sanitary Commission was abolished and replaced by a new medical council headed by a Bolshevik physician. A proletarian Red Cross was established to provide emergency care if physicians refused to aid the new regime.

In the days after the takeover there were disturbances, many of them violent, over essentials—food and shelter. Most Russian doctors, like the rest of the population, were fighting to stay alive and had little time to worry about what the new government had in store for their profession.

Krasin, however, was concerned that the Communist government would destroy the scientific strength of Russian medicine by foolish meddling. One day in November 1917, after Aleksandr Nikolaevich had retreated to the safety of university study, he went to hear the man who was to destroy his dream for leadership within the reorganized Russian health system.

Lenin's speech concerned his plan for change. Dressed in a torn black coat, the small, dark-haired man whose leadership had changed the course of history climbed up to the podium and began addressing the audience of doctors, nurses, and research workers in a calm, almost philosophical tone.

As he began speaking, Krasin recalled stories about Lenin's childhood and his exposure to medicine through his maternal grandfather, Dr. Alexandr Blank. Blank had graduated from the Petersburg Medical Academy in 1825. After his training, he objected to the bloodletting and purges and was possessed by a fanatical obsession with natural healing, or what he termed "spontaneous living." As part of his philosophy, he denied his children the "poison" of tea and coffee and made them drink only cold, clean water. He also believed in the healing power of cold water taken internally as enemas and douches. In the winter, to complement the hydrotherapy, his children were sent naked into the snow and wind. He recorded his philosophy in a book, *As Thou Livest, So Heal Thyself,* which he passed on to his daughter Maria, who used it in raising her son, Ulyanov, later known as Lenin.[9]

So the revolutionary, who as a boy had been forced to roll naked in the snow, told the group of physicians how terrible medical conditions in Russia were. Calmly he recited how thousands, even millions, of Russian workers were suffering and dying of cholera and smallpox and how the doctors were to blame. "You sit in your offices and laboratories," Lenin complained, "worrying about your salaries, your apartments, and where to go for an evening's entertainment." He quoted Veresayev, a nineteenth-century Russian doctor who had treated the nobility:

> Medicine is a science dealing with the treatment of the rich and free only. In relation to everyone else it is merely a theoretical sci-

[9] Robert Payne, *Life and Death of Lenin* (New York: Simon and Schuster, 1964), pp. 43–44.

ence dealing with how they could be cured if they were rich and free.[10]

Suddenly, Lenin's presentation changed. His face turned red, his neck veins protruded, he shook his fist in the air and shouted, "It is the workers that are the strength of our country and it is for them that we will take power from you, the doctors, and put it in the hands of the people. Soviet medicine will not be only for the rich."

The audience, many of whom were, like Krasin, Pirogovists or former Social Democrats, reacted with scattered applause, a few low whistles, and, afterward, much skepticism.

How did this fanatic with his small band of revolutionaries hope to control the entire Russian health system?, they wondered. Why, all the Russian physicians had to do was refuse to cooperate. Besides, most of them were aware that, despite the strong rhetoric, Lenin did not have a plan for his new health program. In fact, Krasin himself had heard rumors of infighting among the Bolshevik leaders over who should control the various departments. No, the doctors present agreed. Shout all he wanted, Lenin would be unable to change things.

Epidemic

On July 18, 1918, nine months after his takeover, Lenin signed a decree establishing the first nationalized health service of modern times. All branches of government having responsibility for various aspects of medical care were united under the first Soviet commissar of health, N. A. Semashko, a physician Lenin had met while they were both in exile in Geneva. The Soviets, at least on paper, had complete control.

The Russia that actually confronted the Bolsheviks, however, was in critical condition. Of its 130 million people, 5.5 million were infected with scabies and 3.5 million were feverish with malaria. And, according to a study done just before the Revolution, a fourth of all prostitutes in Leningrad had the rose-colored skin rash associated with the second stage of syphilis.

Infectious diseases accounted for most deaths, with tuberculosis

[10] V. Verersayev, *The Confessions of a Physician,* trans. Simeon Linden (London: Grant Richards, 1904), p. 9.

leading the list. Of the 1.3 million men registered for the World War I draft, about half received medical examinations. Thirty percent were found medically unfit.

Life expectancy in Russia was only thirty years. To find comparable statistics in other countries, it is necessary to go back to England of the 1750s or America at the time of our own revolution. Thus, at the time of its birth, the Soviet Union was 150 years behind the rest of the civilized world in regard to health care.

The influence that the epidemics, wars, and famine had on the new government's success in assuming responsibility for all medical care cannot be overstated. One of Commissar Semashko's first acts was to appropriate 25 million rubles to combat the cholera epidemic. It was the continued challenge of cholera, typhus, and smallpox that united the other ministers behind Semashko and enabled him to work with Lenin to build a unified health service that stressed prevention. The prevention emphasis came about naturally since the critical health problems facing the new nation could be solved with soap, clean water, and vaccines.

At first, however, things got worse. The social disorganization, malnutrition, cold, poor hygiene, and the massive migration of troops and refugees during the civil war created perfect conditions for disease to spread. Cholera appeared in mid-1918 and was soon joined by typhus, which rapidly became the leading health problem. More than 6 million cases of lice-spread typhus occurred between 1918 and 1920.

The March 14, 1920, *Pravda* reported:

> When the clothes of the soldiers of the Red Army were disinfected, a pile of what looked like grey sand two inches high remained on the floor of the disinfection room. On closer examination the sand was found to be lice.

It is little wonder that Lenin addressed the Seventh Congress of Soviets with the plea: "Either the lice will defeat socialism or socialism will defeat the lice." But to win, he needed a more organized, more efficient medical system. He needed control of Russia's physicians.

The epidemics, especially typhus, were particularly hard on the already inadequate ranks of physicians. Many of these *vrachi* did not have the immunity against infection acquired naturally by the peasants. During the postrevolutionary epidemic years, half of all Russian physicians contracted typhus. From November 1917 to August 1920, 46 percent of physicians in St. Petersburg died.

During this time, Dr. Strassemann worked in a small infirmary that had been transformed into a special clinic for typhus patients. "We were so infested," she recalls, "that when you walked through the clinic you could hear the lice crushing under your feet. It was strange how members of the upper classes were hit hardest by the disease. I was afraid to bring my father to live with me, afraid he would catch typhus."

While at this clinic Dr. Strassemann, along with the other *vrachi*, was drafted by the Red Army to treat soldiers wounded in the bitter civil war. "I refused to go," she told me. I had false documents made and my name attached to the X rays of a patient with tuberculosis so I could stay in Voronezh. When General Shkuro of the White Army occupied the town, he allowed me to help evacuate the sick and wounded. I was assigned to accompany two train cars filled with wounded soldiers. Another *vrach* had learned that the train engineer was a Red sympathizer, so on our way to Germany she sat next to him with a loaded revolver pointed at his brain. That's how I finally left Russia."

About eight thousand doctors were among the one million people who fled Russia in the first years after the Revolution. The exodus left the young government in 1920 with only 24,000 doctors—40 percent of whom were drafted into the Red Army. Most of these early Soviet *vrachi* found themselves working under conditions as poor or worse than those of the prerevolutionary days. The Bolsheviks had not had time to correct the vast internal destruction brought by the prolonged fighting of the civil and world wars. Concerned with maintaining their precarious balance of power, they were incapable of organizing the scattered and inefficient mixture of public and private hospitals and clinics that had existed under the Tsar.

Most buildings leaked and were unheated. Standard equipment such as thermometers and bedpans was absent. Suture materials were so scarce that surgeons used thread from old clothes to sew up wounds and made bandages from discarded newspapers. A report in 1920 by the labor commissar described the workers as "choking in the throes of hunger. The railroads barely crawl. The houses are crumbling and the towns are full of refuse." The Russian ruble, which in prerevolutionary days had been worth fifty cents, became almost valueless—it took 1,200 rubles to equal one dollar in 1920.

The effect of the 1917–1919 Civil War, coming on the heels of World War I, crippled the economy, halted food production, and toppled society. A tenth of the population became migrants, wandering hopelessly from city to city in search of a simple meal.

In 1922, U.S. President Herbert Hoover chose W. Horsely Gantt, a physician and researcher, to direct the American Relief Administration's (ARA) efforts in Petrograd (now Leningrad). During his year in the starving city Gantt witnessed widespread "calamity," as he described it in a 1937 book, "the intense suffering, indescribable horrors of severe famine, wholesale ravages of disease and beastial conditions to living."

A few months before his death in February 1980, at the age of eighty-seven, Gantt recalled to me the images of his assignment and of the worst famine in Russian history. "In the city," Gantt recalled, "dogs, cats, horses, rats, roots, earth, dung, and corpses were being sold for food. We heard reports of people killing sisters, brothers, parents, and even children for nourishment. I saw human meat pies for sale. One man hid his children under the floorboards at night for fear they would be stolen and sold in the local market."

In many cities, the population was reduced by a third to a half. Cholera and typhus spread like wildfire through the starving population. In some areas the local physicians reported to Gantt that 95 percent of the population was infected with syphilis. "But they didn't want to publish any statistics," Gantt told me. "They didn't want the rest of the world to know how bad things were."

Gradually, as the fighting stopped, things got better. Soap, small pieces of which had previously been used as money, became available (much of it supplied by the American Relief Administration). The number of typhus cases fell. Food supplies slowly increased. The use of uncontaminated water controlled cholera (which, unlike typhus, had been more concentrated among the peasants). Vaccination spread and smallpox, while not eradicated, became manageable. The final cost was 6 million dead, among them many of Russia's *vrachi*.

In a desperate effort to correct the deficit caused by war, famine, epidemics, and emigration—and in reaction to the quota system of the past—the Soviets opened the medical institutes to all comers.

Peasants who had not graduated from secondary school—and who frequently could not even write or read—became medical students. Final examinations were eliminated.

The individual grading system was replaced with collective or group instruction on the premise that strong students would help the weaker ones. It did not work. Most of the students were totally unprepared for higher education, much less medical training. Krasin, from his position at the university, objected to the relaxing of standards and criticized other professors for passing students who were unqualified.

Ludmila's father was also concerned about the deterioration in medical research that accompanied the Soviet takeover. Research could no longer be done for the sake of investigation; everything had to be aimed at a practical problem. Lenin wanted to spread medical knowledge throughout Russia. He was not concerned with new discoveries.

Other members of the Pirogov Society attacked the Soviets, charging them with "wrecking the country." The Pirogovists were convinced that the Soviets, by mandating free health care, would destroy the independence of physicians and extinguish the spark of private initiative that had characterized the *zemstvo* reforms. They accused the People's Commissar of Health of promoting veterinarians with Communist credentials over physicians with long and distinguished careers. In their journal, *Public Doctor,* they published a blacklist of all doctors loyal to the new regime.

Such violent opposition, however, was shortlived. As the Soviets consolidated their political victories, using *feldshers'*, nurses', and other medical workers' unions as their base, it became obvious that the new government would survive. Besides, Krasin and his fellow Pirogovists were in the minority. During the 1920s, most Russian physicians were detached from the political upheaval of the time. In fact, the lead article, a month after the Revolution, in *Vrachebnaya Gazeta (Doctor's Newspaper)* was not about the Revolution—it described the best way to stain microscope slides.

By 1922, the Pirogov Society was disbanded and the country settled down for seven years (1921–1928) under the New Economic Policy, which for physicians and the rest of Soviet society provided a brief respite from revolution.

During the New Economic Policy the severe shortages initiated by the Revolution continued. In an attempt at nationwide rationing, the financing of many government-sponsored services, such as medical care, were turned over to local, city, and regional governments, which set their own priorities. Because local governments could not afford to pay the salaries of most doctors, private practice was permitted. A few physicians were able to return to their prerevolutionary life-style. But it was an uneasy calm.

Although revolutionary authority and control were decentralized and factories were receiving priority for the limited funds, the Soviet takeover had caused irrevocable change in the Russian medical profession. Its objectives were no longer individual, but subordinate to the defense and political goals of the Soviet state.

Throughout the 1920s these goals meant diverting money from medicine to support other parts of the economy deemed more critical. This pattern was formalized in 1929 when official priority areas were established under the regime of Stalin, who rose to power shortly after Lenin's death in 1924.

Stalin

A former Georgian peasant who had been expelled from a seminary because of an erroneous diagnosis of tuberculosis, Stalin had a definite attitude toward medical care. In a way it was as cold and detached as that of Veresayev, the nineteenth-century doctor Lenin had ridiculed in his speech in 1917. Its philosophical basis, however, was entirely different. To Stalin, people were the most "valuable and decisive capital in the world." Doctors were instruments to keep the workers healthy so that they, in turn, could strengthen the Soviet Union's precarious economy.

Therefore, as he had done with tractors, bricks, cotton mills, and plows, Stalin made an increase in doctors one of his early goals. To accomplish this, his first commissar of health, M. S. Vladimirsky, turned to women, and to a practical no-frills approach to medical education. By 1930, the Soviet attitude toward medicine was quite different from that of prerevolutionary Russia—or the one developing in the United States.

In 1910, Abraham Flexner, an educator working for the Carnegie Foundation, rerouted the course of American medical education. Prior to his now famous report, American medical education had been a practical and largely informal arrangement. Almost anyone who cared to could establish a school of medicine. Instruction was uneven, done mostly for profit, and it was assumed that the new doctor would learn the skills needed for patient care when he served his apprenticeship with a practicing physician.

Flexner changed all that. He suggested a doctor needed to know not only what to do, but why. After the Flexner report, American physicians were expected to be both scientists and practicing doctors.

The Soviet Union, increasingly cut off from the rest of the world in the 1920s and 1930s, continued with its prerevolutionary educational system based on European models. Although this system had scientific instruction as its base, the emphasis in the Soviet classroom became more and more one of memorization and the use of protocols.[11] Medical care became a practical job, with emphasis on fundamental skills, not scientific knowledge.

Furthermore, the fighting had caused a severe manpower shortage. In response, the government set female quotas for certain industries where it was felt women could adequately replace men. Medicine became a high-quota industry and the medical institutes, closed to women for so long, suddenly became filled with female students.

This overnight reversal in the sexual orientation of medicine was motivated mainly by the desperate domestic and economic circumstances the country found itself in by 1930. Stalin's crude attempts at the collectivization of agriculture and rapid industrialization had created havoc.

According to Dr. Gantt, who after spending most of the 1920s working in Pavlov's laboratories was invited to Moscow in 1933 to visit his old teacher, there was another famine, this one caused by one man.

"Stalin had taken most of the grain," Gantt explained, "and sent it out of the country so he could buy heavy machinery. As a result there was widespread starvation and more epidemics. But no one

---

[11] In his book Professor Vincente Navarro emphasizes that despite the Revolution, the Soviet Union never entirely abandoned the scientific approach, but simply adapted it to its needs; see *Social Security and Medicine in the USSR* (Lexington, Mass.: Lexington Books, 1977).

talked about them. In fact," Gantt recalled, "to hide the amount of disease, names were changed."

"I remember going to the public health officer in Moscow in 1933. I asked him how many cases of typhus they had. At first he said none, but when I told him I'd seen patients myself, he said, 'Maybe fifteen cases in the last year.'

"But another doctor told me that last week alone, there'd been four hundred deaths from typhus. Then I learned that Stalin had issued an edict that typhus could no longer be called typhus but instead should be known as disease form No. 2. In that way there was no more typhus—Stalin had abolished it."

In view of the crisis, Stalin decided that what the country needed—and the only thing it could afford—was basic simple medical care, not scientific luxuries. The Soviet woman's ancient legacy as a folk doctor and her more recent success as a compassionate Sister of Mercy seemed to prepare her well for her new role as physician.

The thousands of women who were recruited into the medical profession in 1930 were different from the few dozen political activists like Nadezhda Suslova or the few hundred women from wealthy families, like Strassemann, who had characterized Russian medicine in the late 1800s. Medical institute classes were filled with women from working-class backgrounds. Women who had previously been Sisters of Mercy, or even orderlies, suddenly found themselves "promoted" to the status of *vrach*. Many had no ambitions beyond a weekly paycheck. The Soviet government responded in kind with a low wage scale and a social status for medicine that treated the new physician with no more respect than that given a factory worker. Professionalism was not rewarded nor even encouraged. Medicine became a job and women were the ones chosen to do it.

During a conversation in Moscow at her daughter's apartment, Ludmila told me about her first year as a medical student. "There were three hundred and fifty students in the class, and 80 percent of them were women. I was amazed at how easy the instruction was. All of the professors wanted the students to do well. They asked very simple questions and said that as long as we read each lecture [professors usually handed out copies of their lectures] we would pass. Many of my classmates had trouble with reading because their secondary school education had been so poor, so I helped them with the lessons.

"Many of my professors knew my father had been arrested, but no one ever mentioned it. You were afraid to talk, afraid to trust anyone."

The 1934 arrest and disappearance of Ludmila's father, although devastating to his family, was not unexpected. During the 1920s and into the early 1930s, Aleksandr Krasin continued to protest against the political, unsupervised admission of students to the medical institute and their uncritical promotion from one year to the next.

"Father was angry because his students were not getting a good education," Ludmila said. "He felt the government [which had taken control of all university medical institutes in 1930] was more interested in increasing the number of doctors than in how well they were trained. He protested to the faculty and demanded that his students take written instead of oral exams."

He was arrested two weeks later, on October 3, 1934. Ludmila and her mother heard about it through a friend who had seen him being pushed into a "black raven," the name given to the cars of Stalin's secret police.

"My mother tried desperately to find him," Ludmila recalled. "We went to all the police stations, all the prisons, but we weren't told where he was kept or what he was charged with. We just never saw him again."

The arrest shattered the Krasin family. Ludmila's brother moved to Moscow, and her mother went into a deep depression which lasted until her death four years later. Krasin was one of an estimated five thousand medical professors executed during the period of the thirties termed by author Robert Conquest "The Great Terror." It was the darkest time in Soviet history, when Stalin ordered 20 million Soviet citizens killed, tortured, or sent into exile in Siberian work camps.

Ludmila's memory of those days is protectively blurred. She recalls the grief and torment of the first months following her father's disappearance and the desperate search to find him, but she has forgotten most of the anger.

"Father was getting old," she said. "He probably shouldn't have still been teaching—and he had such strong opinions on everything.

But"—she stops, her nicotine-stained fingers wiping away tears— "they had no right to kill him."

The purges and political executions that took Krasin's life spread and grew during the thirties, further reducing the number of males and creating an atmosphere of fear. The effect of the purges on medical research was particularly chilling.

It was during the thirties that the Soviet government began its propaganda campaign to spread their interpretation of Pavlov's discoveries while discrediting classical genetics. The cornerstone of genetic theory is that inheritance of biological characteristics is linked to biochemical properties (genes) rather than to environment. But this conflicted with Soviet plans to improve the population through collective nurseries and other environmental manipulations. So genetics was dropped from the medical school curriculum for almost thirty years. Scientists and researchers in the field, such as Nikolai Vavilov, who had previously been internationally known, suddenly disappeared into prison camps. Stalin's policies toward medicine were similar to those used with his Red Army; for the sake of obedience, leadership was sacrificed.

This curtain of isolation brought an end not only to genetics, but to most Soviet medical and scientific progress. Foreign travel for scientists was prohibited. The Soviet government was suspicious of everything, fearful that any deviation from official policy would weaken their effort.

The new economic and political, as well as medical, goals were rigidly outlined through quotas and five-year plans. The first plan, launched in 1929, called for a fivefold increase in the number of doctors; by 1934 this goal had been met and even slightly exceeded. During the same period, the Soviets had also tripled the number of hospital beds and expanded the availability of TB sanatoriums and polyclinics. With the introduction of free medical services, however, the Soviets found that even this large increase in doctors was not enough to match demand. The available *vrachi* worked long hours trying to see a small fraction of the patients lined up each morning. The wait to get into hospitals was three to four weeks. Problems were not limited to medical care, however; every segment of daily life was a struggle.

Ludmila, her husband Anton, and their two children lived in an unheated two-room apartment which they shared with Ludmila's mother. In the winter, snow came in the windows and on the coldest nights Ludmila took her family to the hospital's furnace room where she had worked as a stoker. The government issued ration cards which, depending on one's occupation, permitted limited purchase of scarce items such as cheese, meat, and vegetables. There were lines for bread, and Ludmila frequently had trouble getting milk for her children. She heard stories about peasant uprisings and farmers' riots caused by the state plan of forced starvation through confiscation of their grain. It was rumored that the Red Army was massacring thousands of peasants to restore order. Between the political purges in the cities and the agricultural unrest in the countryside, it was a frightening time in which to live.

The Soviet Way

Nevertheless, for a nation that had long been without rudimentary medical services, the results of basic preventive measures, along with some improvement in living conditions, were impressive. The death rate decreased by half; infant mortality fell from 275 deaths per 1,000 in 1913 to 130 in 1930. Although the exact rate of reduction is difficult to document, the incidence of syphilis, gonorrhea, typhus, and cholera substantially declined. Patients with tuberculosis decreased until they no longer had to share beds in the sanatoriums.

This progress impressed the few visitors the Soviets permitted. One of them, Henry Sigerist, an American physician and historian, wrote upon his return:

> "From 1933 to 1937 the Soviet people began to reap the fruits of their labors. The new plants produced large amounts of consumer goods. Agriculture had been collectivized and food was plentiful. . . . The development of health facilities during those years was stupendous. The new hospitals, dispensaries and rural health centers had much higher standards than the old ones. The chief impression of the visitor in 1938 was that not only was there more of everything but that everything there had been greatly improved."[12]

[12] Henry E. Sigerist. *Medicine and Health in the Soviet Union* (New York: The Citadel Press, 1947), p. 32.

Sigerist's uncritical enthusiasm and acceptance of the early Soviet claims must be seen in the perspective of what was occurring in the United States. The 1930s saw an increasing commercial trend in American medicine. The image of the friendly, small-town family doctor was changing to that of physician as small businessman. In response to the increased scientific emphasis and need for technology, American physicians began to practice in large clinics. By this time, progress in scientific research had created the impression that medicine was too complicated for one person to master. Dr. William Mayo, one of the founding brothers of the Mayo Clinic (a model upon which many group practices were built), expressed the prevailing attitude when addressing the graduates of Rush Medical College: "The sum total of medical knowledge is now so great and widespreading that it would be futile for any one man . . . to assume that he has even a working knowledge of any large part of the whole."

The loss of the solo family doctor, however, was not without its critics. There was in 1930 (in what sounds remarkably like a complaint of the 1980s) the fear that group practice encouraged too many laboratory and X-ray investigations and that these tests unnecessarily increased the cost of medical care (a complete diagnostic evaluation in the 1920s at a leading clinic could cost $500). Furthermore, as specialization became more and more popular, new graduates refused to leave the safety of groups for isolated small towns. A survey done in thirty states during the 1920s found that 90 percent of rural physicians were not being replaced upon their retirement.

The increased emphasis on group practice was a signal to many older physicians that the close, warm, personal contact between the American doctor and his patient was coming to an end. Dr. James Herrick, writing in *The Journal of the American Medical Association* in 1929, argued that "A group diagnosis may be perfect in all its parts . . . but as a whole it is only assembled and machine made and may be a misfit. There is lacking the important feature of personal contact between physician and patient."

Despite these concerns, the 1932 report of the Committee on the Costs of Medical Care, a government-sponsored panel of physicians, lawyers, and social scientists who intensively studied American medical care for five years and whose report was influential in establishing future emphasis, encouraged the trend toward specialization and recommended that more hospitals be built so that physicians could have increased access to the machines needed to practice modern high-quality care.

These developments concerned Sigerist. He saw the important issue of disease prevention being ignored while the increasing cost of medicine made it less available to many Americans. The trends contrasted vividly with the Soviet plan Sigerist described. With basic services still in short supply, there was no talk in the USSR of specialization, of extensive medical technology, or of the need for closer doctor-patient relationships.

Neither Ludmila, her husband Anton, nor the other 2,000 students at the First Leningrad Medical Institute in 1936 were encouraged to become specialists. "We were told the country needed doctors and that everyone should go to work as quickly as possible," Ludmila recalls. The medical curriculum was shortened from six to five years, a move that proved unsuccessful and was subsequently rejected. The educational emphasis remained on the principles of public health, which had been so successful in reducing epidemics.

While the economic situation had greatly improved since the revolution, little money was available for vaccines, much less machines. Most of the new Soviet hospitals were simply large rooms filled with beds. Even simple X-ray machines were not obtainable. Drugs, scheduled to be produced by the state-run pharmaceutical industry, were also in short supply. A black market for vital substances such as digitalis rapidly developed and the use of herbal cures continued to flourish.

Ludmila kept a diary of her student days. One evening when I visited her cramped apartment in an old three-story building overlooking the Neva River, she took the journal down from the top shelf of her china closet. Sitting at the dining room table she read me excerpts, tracing the heavy black lines on the yellowed paper with her wrinkled index finger.

> October 24, 1937. Had our first cardiology lesson today. Professor Popov showed us his stethoscope and explained how it works. We were allowed to use it to listen to each other's heartbeat. Tanya's heart was going very fast and I had trouble telling the difference between the two sounds. . . . We went into a room to hear the heart of a young girl with stenosis of her aortic valve. The murmur

sounded hard, like her heart was angry. . . . Professor Popov told us that in a few years every *vrach* will have a stethoscope of her own. I wish I could have one now. It's difficult to learn about the diseases without hearing their sounds.

An entry in December of the same year described her first day in the hospital:

> I have three patients now . . . one is an old *babushka* from the village who has gangrene in her right foot. She injured it three weeks ago and now it will have to be amputated. I sat with her today and tried to calm her fears about the operation. She does not understand why it is necessary and she is frightened. . . . I learned how today to give *vnutrikozhnye* (injections).

Some of the pages, those where she had talked about her father, were missing. Ludmila had thrown them away, fearing that if they were discovered, she too would be arrested.

In 1938, hundreds of government officials were being arrested in Leningrad and thousands of ordinary citizens were pulled off the streets for questioning. It was a time of caution for the average citizen who, because of actions by the government, was increasingly deprived of personal freedoms. As a reaction to the official cruelty around him, the Soviet citizen turned more and more to close personal relationships with the few people he felt he could trust. So it was that the *srednii vrach* became a confidant to her patients, a person they could talk to without fear.

"I remember many of the patients I had as a student," Ludmila told me. "There was not much we could do for them, we were so short on drugs and supplies. But I would spend a lot of time talking to them, trying to make them less afraid. I suppose you could say we were more than nurses but less than doctors."

Ludmila's diary ends in June 1941, when the rumors of executions were replaced by conflicting stories about the German invasion. Could the Soviet army stop the Germans? Would fighting really reach Leningrad or, as some people predicted, would the war be over in a year?

The War and After

When it became obvious that the war would not be won quickly, Soviet physicians, along with the rest of the population, took up the battle against the German invaders. Ludmila's education was halted and she was sent to a base hospital thirty-five miles outside Leningrad where she treated some of the first casualties successfully evacuated from the western front. Her husband, Anton, was one of more than eight thousand young physicians who, after a brief three-month surgical training course, staffed advance hospitals. Only a few miles from the front, these surgeons performed initial examinations of the injured and handled emergency amputations. The system of advance, base, and long-term evacuation hospitals was modeled after the classification system developed by Pirogov during the Crimean War. According to Soviet statistics the system worked well, with seventy-three of every hundred battle casualties returned to active service, compared to only forty during World War I.

The reassuring statistics soften a much harsher reality: to survive the five years of World War II, the Soviets gave up more than any nation in history. Twenty million died. Another 10 million were crippled. More than a third of the Soviet Union's urban areas, including many newly built hospitals, were destroyed. During the early and darkest time of the war, when Leningrad was under siege and it seemed only a matter of time until Hitler would march into Moscow, Ludmila was sure that she, her family, and the life that they had just begun would be destroyed.

She sent Yuri and Natalia to live with Anton's parents in a rural village outside Moscow. "I didn't see Anton for over a year," Ludmila told me. "Svetlana, our third child, was born while I was at the base hospital. There was no way to tell Anton we had another daughter. By the time I went back to work at the hospital, we were terribly short of supplies. There was not enough cotton so we used moss, linden tree shavings, anything we could find to help the soldiers' wounds heal."

In response to the shortages, the Soviet government increased the use of medicinal herbs. Balsam, extracted from fir trees by the Botanical Institute in the Ukraine, was used to promote healing. Everything that could possibly be recycled was saved. Bandages, X rays, and splints were all reclaimed in a desperate attempt to stretch inadequate supplies, to help the increasing number of wounded.

By the time the fighting stopped, everything had been used and reused—there was nothing left. "We had run out of morphine six months before the war ended," Ludmila said. "I would sit with wounded soldiers, hold their hands, and pray for them to die quickly."

It is remarkable that during these five years of military, economic, political, and human challenges the country continued to educate and train more and more doctors. The Soviet Union entered World War II with one-sixth the number of physicians that the United States had. Ten years later the totals were equal.

After the war, Ludmila collected Anton, her daughters, and her son Yuri and found a small one-bedroom apartment in one of the Leningrad buildings not destroyed by the German bombing. Anton returned from the fighting sullen and despondent. Before the war, he had planned to return to the institute to complete formal residency (*ordinatura*) training in surgery. Instead, he took a minor administrative post at a small tuberculosis hospital. At night he would leave his family and go out to drink with old army comrades. Ludmila eventually took over all family responsibilities. When their fourth child, a daughter, Varya, was born in 1948, Anton was in a hospital recovering from alcoholic hepatitis.

Ludmila became a typical postwar Soviet wife. She raised the children, did the shopping, and worked. Her husband relived his years at war, a heavy dose of vodka softening the harsh memories. Because she had lived with shortages and suffering for so long, Ludmila accepted her fate with a dull, dogged determination. She would get up at six and make breakfast in the kitchen she shared with three other families. She made sure Natalia, Yuri, and Svetlana were properly dressed and off to school by eight. Before taking Varya to the *crèche* (nursery), she would carefully try to awaken Anton. On days when he got angry and began shouting, she would quietly shut the bedroom door. She arrived at the polyclinic by nine and saw patients for three hours. During lunch she tried to find fresh vegetables or some sausage for dinner; most often she failed. Finishing work at four, she picked up Varya and stood in line for bread and milk, careful not to get home later than six, her time in the communal kitchen. After dinner she helped her children with their lessons, having cleared the dinner dishes so that the apartment's one small table could be used as a desk.

According to a survey done at this time, the average Soviet housewife, like Ludmila, spent twenty-two to thirty hours a week doing shopping and household chores—in addition to her thirty-six-hour job. Shopping took so long because everything from meat to writing paper was in short supply. Ludmila was once given a small tin of canned American meat. She saved it for seven months to use as the main course at New Year's dinner in 1949.

The children prepared their lessons on small scraps of paper that Ludmila was given at the polyclinic for writing prescriptions. New clothes, obtainable only at black-market prices, were carefully repaired and handed down. Since Yuri was the only boy, he was forced to wear Natalia's old woolen coat. "How he hated that coat," Ludmila recalls. "Sometimes in the middle of winter he would go to school with only a sweater because he was ashamed to be seen in girl's clothing."

During these difficult years a strong bond of love and friendship developed between Ludmila and her children. Natalia, while still a young teenager, assumed responsibility for her two younger sisters. In reaction to his father's increased drinking, Yuri developed a strong, silent maturity greater than his years that would later bring him power and responsibility. "He was always telling me that he would take care of me," Ludmila says, "that he would not be like his father."

Anton's drinking increased. By 1952 he had an advanced case of cirrhosis and was no longer able to work. A year later he was dead. "Anton was a victim of the Germans," Ludmila maintains. "He came back from the war a changed man. He no longer wanted to be a doctor. He just didn't want to see any more suffering."

So Ludmila joined the third of Soviet households which, in the 1950s, were headed by women. There was never any thought in her mind of another husband. Her years of supporting Anton had reduced her enthusiasm for marriage and, besides, at that time there were no men Ludmila's age available. Like her family, the country was without male support, its daily needs dependent upon women.

Immediately after World War II, the Soviets had hoped that the large number of women in the medical system could be reduced. In 1946, the Ministry of Health announced plans to limit the size of medical school classes (the Soviet Union then had one doctor for every 700 persons) while increasing the proportion of male students. In 1946, however, there were not enough men left to meet the demand in the more critical areas of industrial production and agricultural recovery. Therefore, despite preference given male applicants, eight out of ten medical students were women. Only a minority of these women were interested in making medicine a full-time career, and it was during the postwar period that the character of Soviet medicine was firmly established.

It is often asked whether medicine is such a low-paying, low-prestige profession in the USSR because there are so many women employed or because the government considers medicine a low-priority service. The answer, from a historical perspective, is a little of both. Although politically liberated by the Bolshevik coup d'état and officially emancipated by the 1936 Constitution, the Soviet woman has never felt nor been treated as an equal where it matters most—in her day-to-day activities.

Although the average income of workers in the USSR was a state secret before 1964, Ludmila recalls that in 1950 she was paid sixty-two rubles a month—about half what she would have received as a construction worker.

When the government finally released wage figures in 1964, the average monthly salary in different industries correlated directly with the percentage of women employed. Industrial production, with less than 50 percent female workers, ranked first (112 rubles); medical care, with an 85 percent female majority, was near the bottom, with a monthly income of 82 rubles. At these low wages there was little incentive to do more than what was required. As a result, the optimistic 1946 estimate, that one physician for every 700 persons would be enough, had to be revised downward; the system was just too inefficient. Like Ludmila, the *srednii vrach* had to spend too much time taking care of her family and coping with daily living to devote her energies to medicine.

When economic and political realities made it necessary for her to provide medical care, she took on the responsibility, with no thoughts of improving her social position but, as in the case of her historical predecessors, the Sisters of Mercy, as a job to be done. The pay scale was set low both because women were involved and because, at that time, defense and industrial production were more important.

Because the typical female *vrach* did not always see medicine as a professional calling, she did not choose to become a specialist. For most of the 1950s and 1960s, Soviet medicine remained a profession characterized by a large number of *srednii vrachi*, working a few hours a day and providing simple medical care while they supported their husbands and children.

A survey reported in the 1960s revealed that male doctors in the Soviet Union worked an average of 270 days a year while female doctors put in 155 days, or 42 percent less time.

One of the women who entered the profession in the 1950s, and who illustrates the continued double burden of homemaker and *vrach* that Ludmila encountered, is her daughter born during World War II, Svetlana, whom I had met in Moscow and who first suggested I meet her mother.

Svetlana is a staff physician at a large city hospital in Moscow. She completed the First Moscow Medical Institute in 1965 and the day after graduation married a classmate, Vladimir. Although Svetlana had taken advanced training in cardiology after her *ordinatura* (residency), she did not complete her study and is considered a *terapevt*, a rough equivalent of our general practitioner.

As a hospital physician, Svetlana takes care of patients admitted to her floor or section, whether they are referred by their local polyclinic doctor or are brought in by ambulance. As is the practice in most European countries, Russian patients do not stay with the same doctor when they enter the hospital.

Although there is no billing system, and no insurance forms to be filled out (all hospital care is free), Svetlana still complains of the amount of paperwork she must do. "It seems I am constantly filling out reports for the labor unions, the factories, the Ministry of Health, or to send someone to a sanatorium, or to excuse someone from work." There are no dictating machines and Svetlana frequently types her own reports.

Nonetheless, her position would not be considered high-pressured by American standards. Svetlana sees fewer patients than the average U.S. physician, and since Soviet hospitals do not have the large number of laboratory tests and diagnostic equipment standard in America, the demands on her to keep up with advances are not great. And since Svetlana, like most of her colleagues, does not know a foreign language, she must wait for government translations of selected medical articles from other countries. Like her mother, Svetlana Antonovna sees medicine as a job, and at 150 rubles a month, she has reached her maximum income and position for her training.

"Our family has three rooms," Svetlana says, "three rooms for four people [they have two children]. My husband has a good salary, so we have enough money. But what I need is more time. This morning I stood in line for two hours to buy one chicken. By the time I get home at night there is barely time to cook dinner before it's time for the children to go to bed. In the morning it's the same, there is no time to talk. I can't ask Vladimir to help me, he has his job to worry about, so what can I do? Stop working? Then we would need more money."

We were talking in Svetlana's small office, off one of the main hospital corridors. Typical of most offices I had visited, it was empty, almost barren. A small desk, devoid of paper, and two chairs were the only furniture. The faded pink walls had none of the usual medical diplomas and certificates seen in the offices of American doctors, only a small portrait of Lenin. Svetlana got up to water some of the many plants on the window ledge. There were no books in the room.

The situation faced by Svetlana is not unique among Soviet women. The problem of how to combine a full-time job with raising a family in the many-papered and long-lined Soviet economy is considered an important contribution to the rising divorce rate and falling birthrate among urban women.

Natalia and Yuri

Of course, there are exceptions to this pattern of the Soviet woman as both worker and mother. Some Soviet women, unable to marry because of the shortage of males (in 1961 there were still 21 million more women than men in the USSR), have made medicine their life and developed careers as professors, scientists, or researchers. They are the ones whose pictures appear on the covers of Soviet magazines and are flashed on Moscow television as examples of female equality. One of the most successful women to follow this path was Natalia Antonovna, Ludmila's oldest daughter, who as a young teenager had assumed responsibility for her younger sisters.

Natalia Antonovna had entered the medical institute in 1954 and graduated six years later with an almost perfect record of 5s, the highest grade possible. She went on to become a candidate of science (a degree similar to our Ph.D.) in biochemistry and now, at forty-two, she is one of the youngest physicians to be granted the degree of doctor of medical sciences, a prestigious title given as recognition of professional accomplishment. Ludmila told me that I would find Natalia living in the Ukrainian portion of the Soviet Union, working as a professor of medicine at the Odessa Medical Institute.

Natalia's large, sun-filled office was on the top floor of the combined hospital and institute building. Plants were crowded around the windows, one wall was decorated with a handmade Armenian rug, and the obligatory portrait of Lenin hung behind her desk. The bookcase was stuffed with research reports, and a paper she was completing on the biochemical defect in Mediterranean, or Cooley's, anemia was spread over her large conference table. Natalia is a large-boned, bulky woman with plump, red hands and a warm smile. She wore a white lace blouse with a high, intricately designed collar. A large cameo hung from a thin gold chain around her neck. With her hair arranged carefully on the top of her head, she seemed a dignified, scholarly scientist—a strong contrast to her mother's rough appearance. Natalia poured two glasses of tea from a small silver teapot. Only the veins in her hands gave away her age.

"I was different from most of my women classmates," she began. "They were not interested in giving much time to their studies, assuming that the men would become professors and they would end up *vrachi.*" Natalia's break with that tradition was not difficult. Her high marks in medical school permitted her to begin advanced education as an *aspirant* working toward her *kandidat* degree, thus bypassing the required three years of government service. Since her dissertation involved a form of hereditary anemia found mainly in southern USSR, she moved to Odessa. There she quickly advanced through the local medical institute hierarchy to her position as professor and assistant administrator of the teaching hospital.

Unlike the situation in this country, where a physician on a medical school faculty will perform a combination of teaching, research, and medical-care activities, the Soviet scientist-physician seldom does more than one. Natalia, however, had been able to combine her research career with an interest in medical education, and was now responsible for lecturing second-year students on selected topics in biochemistry.

Natalia told me she had never felt discriminated against because of being a woman. She was a member of the Communist Party, belonged to the Ukrainian Academy of Medical Sciences, and had been allowed to attend an international research meeting in Bulgaria only six months before.

If there is no discrimination, I asked, why are there so few women leaders at the top? I pointed out that only once in the sixty-year history of Soviet medicine had a woman occupied the top position of minister of health (Dr. Kovrigina served from 1959 to 1964), and of the sixty deputy ministers of health, only 20 percent were female. Closer to her own career, I reminded Natalia that just 15 percent of professors are women and that the prestigious USSR Academy of Medical Sciences has nine male members for every one female.

Natalia smiled softly and reached over, touching my hand in a motherly gesture. "I'm not familiar with those statistics," she said. "I can only tell you that it has never been a problem for me, as a woman doctor, to practice medicine or, as a scientist, to do research."

As Natalia demonstrates, few Soviet female physicians are aware of, or even interested in, the political aspects of their profession. Moreover, in the minds of many Soviet men, a female physician like Natalia, who competes for power in the corridors of political arena, loses her femininity and is labeled an "Amazon." Liberation for a female physician, therefore, exists only if she sticks to the centuries-old Russian prejudice that women are well suited to treat suffering but not to make important decisions. This fundamental attitude toward male and female roles is no better illustrated than by the contrast between Natalia's career and that of her younger brother, Yuri.

Yuri Antonovich Efimov entered and completed the medical institute a year behind Natalia. He took further training as a *dotsent* (resident) in internal medicine, became a leader in his local Communist Party, and advanced quickly. At an age when most Soviet physicians are just completing their advanced training, Yuri had been appointed assistant dean at a medical institute in the southeastern region of the USSR. He performed well, and assumed the full deanship at age forty. By all Soviet standards, he is a fortunate man.

He has a car with a driver, a six-room apartment, and an almost unheard-of luxury—two bathrooms. Yuri and his wife have two children and they buy most of their clothes on the black market, where a coat made in the West (which may turn out to be Yugoslavia) can cost 500 rubles ($775).[13] The family also incurs large expenses because they must entertain many Communist officials, all of whom expect to be formally received.

As dean, Yuri admitted that he is frequently offered bribes of up to 2,000 rubles if he will give preferential admission and treatment to certain applicants. Although he denies accepting any such bribes, he acknowledges the pressure he is under.

"There are three to four applicants for every position," he told me. "There are also more men applying to school. In many ways there is much more competition than when I went to school."

Since I was staying in the city through the end of the year, Yuri invited me to spend New Year's Eve with him and his family. When I arrived, I could tell that his wife had been cooking for days. Starting dinner at seven o'clock, we ate and drank through five hours' worth of smoked fish, caviar, borsch, cheese, steak, chicken, wine, vodka, cognac, and tea until the time came for Soviet television to announce the *novyi god*. Instead of Times Square, we watched the crowd in Red Square. When the Spassky Tower Clock in the Kremlin struck twelve, the Soviet National anthem was played. Then, after midnight, Yuri's visitors began arriving.

No one stayed long, but a constant stream of Communist Party officials, fellow physicians, former students, and friends arrived and departed throughout the early hours of the New Year. By morning Yuri was exhausted, but as the last visitor offered his congratulations and said goodbye, he motioned me into a chair. "Mornings of new years," he began, "are good times to talk."

"Medicine—being a doctor—is a strange profession," he went on. "Patients think doctors are different, that all the emotions that affect them don't touch us. But they're wrong, they don't understand. A good doctor, the best doctor, is simple. He doesn't think about science and numbers and tests. He thinks about people—his people, his patients. We have a saying in Russia, 'A doctor should give part of his heart to his patient.'

"You don't have to be smart to know that; to know all people need someone to listen to them, to touch them. Books don't teach you that—no book teaches you *sostradanie* [co-suffering]. Like my

---

[13] In the winter of 1981, one ruble was equal to $1.55.

mother, the typical Russian doctor has suffered. She has buried sons, husbands, fathers. She has watched people starve to death—seen people beg for bread. She knows what is important.

"What's important is not prestige, not machines, not money—it's people. There is a lot of talk in the Soviet Union about changing the image of the doctor. We now have a professional oath to give Soviet doctors prestige. I disagree. A doctor does not need prestige. It only puts him above people."

Deciding how best to train doctors is a new problem for the Soviet Union, one that is causing a lot of discussion in their professional literature. For most of this century the USSR has concentrated on quantity, training enough doctors to staff the polyclinics, operate the hospitals, run the ambulance system, protect the health of the workers and the army; doctors to make their country strong. Today, after thirty years of relative peace—at least the absence of war—they have accomplished their goal. Now, faced with saturation (in 1980 there will be one doctor for every 265 Soviet citizens), they have different problems.

"The doctor graduating from the institute today," explains Yuri, "no longer wants to talk to his patient. He no longer feels with his heart. He doesn't understand *sostradanie*. They say it's an old-fashioned word—a throwback to religion. A good Communist, they tell me, doesn't have to suffer. They quote Gorki to me." Yuri explodes, his face becoming red, his fist pounding the table. "They quote Gorki to *me,* saying 'suffering is my enemy.' I argue with those who accept suffering.

"I know what Gorki said," Yuri goes on, calmer but still animated. "I was reading Gorki before they were born. I also know that the best doctor is a simple doctor who understands suffering. That must never change."

The personal anguish that Yuri expressed to me is not his alone. Over the past decade the Soviets have increasingly recognized and written about the deterioration in their doctor-patient relationships. Since the Soviets so seldom write anything negative concerning their system, the fact that such criticism appears at all probably means the problem is large and growing.

In 1969 the first conference on the deontology, or ethics, of the medical profession was held in Moscow. A main theme of that meeting was the growing number of Soviet doctors who ignore the feelings of their patients, treating them without respect. In response, the Hippocratic Oath was introduced into medical schools. Recent indications, however, make it appear that the problem is not improving. Dr. V. E. Rozhnov of the Moscow Institute of Medical Education wrote recently that "certain medical workers violate, at times, the laws of medical ethics in the most blatant manner, thus inflicting real damage to patients."

It appears that six decades of Soviet rule—with its emphasis on the institution instead of the individual—is now having a profound impact on the warm, human relationships that had previously existed between the Soviet doctor and her patient. The current minister of health, Dr. Boris Petrovsky, complains publicly that too many doctors are more interested in technology than in their patients. To persons in positions of authority like Petrovsky, this problem presents a dilemma similar to that encountered in this country in the 1930s. On the one hand, the Soviets want to upgrade their technologically deficient medical system and improve the scientific training of their physicians. In doing so, however, they are also changing the composition, character, and attitude of the *srednii vrach*.

To the man on the street the change is painfully evident. "Ten years ago I could go and talk to the doctor at my polyclinic," a middle-aged factory worker told me. "She would take time to listen. Today all the doctor wants to do is get finished, give you some medicine, and go to the next patient. Most of them don't even bother to ask your name."

It is tempting to link the problem between Soviet physicians and their patients, as Yuri and many Soviet citizens do, with the recent increase in the number of male physicians. Many institutes, such as the prestigious First Moscow Medical, now have more men in their entering classes than women. Upon graduation, most of these men are not satisfied with the standard hours, the low pay, and the routine patients seen by a *srednii vrach*. They are taking more training, becoming *dotsenty* in cardiology, *aspiranty* in physiology. They are staying closer to the research institutes and large city hospitals. They are less willing than their female counterparts to leave the big cities and work in the rural areas of the Soviet Union. Very few of the young male *vrachi* I met would be willing to do what Varya, Ludmila's youngest daughter, did.

Varya—Srednii Vrach

In many ways, meeting Varya was like confronting a young Ludmila. Varya has her mother's ruddy Russian features and, unlike her illustrious older sister and brother, she had no desire for a career.

Following her graduation from the medical institute in 1972, Varya was assigned to an internship in Bratsk, one of the Soviet Union's new towns in Eastern Siberia created to house workers who built and now run a huge hydroelectric dam. Many young graduates, when hearing of their assignment to such an isolated area, would have tried to bribe an important official or arrange an additional year of training in another city—anything to avoid Siberia. Varya, however, agreed readily to go.

"As a student, I was taught the four basic socialist rights—the right to work, the right to a free education, the right to free medical care, and the right to a pension following retirement. As a physician, my job involves all of these. First, it is a doctor's responsibility to keep all people healthy so they can work efficiently at their jobs. Second, schoolchildren need to be protected against childhood disease and taught good attitudes toward health that will allow them to enjoy retirement. Going to Bratsk is part of my responsibility. It is where I can make an important contribution."

Varya and her husband, Nikita, a former prizefighter who works as a laborer at one of Bratsk's large aluminum factories, live in a one-bedroom apartment on the fifth floor of a high-rise building. Bratsk was built in a previously undeveloped area so schools, shops, polyclinics, and hospitals had to be rapidly constructed. For efficiency and low cost, they all share the same drab concrete style. Little attention was paid to unnecessary comforts. Years after completion the roads remained unpaved and the resulting mud and dust gave Bratsk the appearance of a town unsure of its future.

"I see about fifteen patients a day," Varya explained one night as I sat at the table in their apartment. She was cleaning vegetables as she spoke, a newspaper spread on her lap to catch the trimmings.

"Most of them are not very ill." She continued smiling warmly at Nikita as he played on the floor with their daughter. "In fact, many times I simply sit and listen. My patients want someone to talk to— to reassure them that they are healthy. I don't use many drugs, sometimes an antibiotic or a mild tranquilizer. Mostly I prescribe a combination of herbs. We have some excellent herbal drugs."

I arranged to spend a day with Varya at her polyclinic. We arrived at nine-thirty in the morning, after she had left her daughter at the government-sponsored nursery. Five patients were waiting.

The first patient, Tanya Sokolova, was a short, muscular woman in her fifties who worked in the aluminum factory and whom Varya had treated in the past for hypertension. Tanya explained that, for the past few weeks, she had been bothered by pains in her chest.

"Where does it hurt?" Varya asked.

"Here." Tanya pointed to a spot directly beneath her breastbone. "It hurts especially after I eat and when I lie down at night, it's so bad I can hardly catch my breath."

Varya took out her stethoscope, a thin metal diaphragm attached to two rubber tubes, placed the ends of the tubes in her ears and listened to Tanya's chest and abdomen. Then, while her patient sat fully dressed in a chair, she put her hand over the right part of Tanya's abdomen and pushed. Tanya winced.

"*Zholochnye kamni* [gallstones]," Varya declared.

Varya then walked back to her desk and told Tanya it was her gallbladder that was causing the chest pain. It could become very serious, she explained, and it was necessary to follow her instructions carefully. First she should take a laxative, and then several deep enemas to clean out her colon. She would have to remain at home for the next week and drink ten glasses of hot water with juice a day. She should also drink a mixture of other fruit and vegetable juices, but no solid food. This treatment, Varya explained, would encourage urination and thereby help her body to pass out the offending stones. At the end of a week Tanya was to return, and if the pain and tenderness were not better, Varya would arrange an X ray of her gallbladder. At the end of the discussion Varya handed Tanya a slip that would permit her to miss six days of work, the maximum number Varya could excuse her from without getting the approval of her director.

Tanya remained in the office after the consultation, exchanging local gossip and, through anecdotes, gestures, and nods of the head, commenting on the problems of working and raising a family. Despite the seriousness of Tanya's visit and Varya's diagnosis, it was almost as if the doctor-patient relationship had been a prelude to the real purpose of the call, a visit between friends.

After Tanya left, I asked Varya about her diagnosis and the treatment, telling her that getting an X ray would have been an important part of the examination back home, as would an electrocardiogram, to rule out heart problems, and blood tests, to search for liver disease.

"*Da, da, ya znaiu* [yes, yes, I know]," she said, "but, here, a gallbladder disease is very common, and unless it's an emergency it takes two weeks to get an X ray and electrocardiogram scheduled. Meanwhile, it's more important for her to watch her diet, stop eating heavy foods."

About the diet, I told Varya I was unaware of any evidence that frequent urination would dissolve gallstones. We were testing drugs in the United States that might be able to dissolve gallstones, but a water diet?

"You're right," she said. "It probably won't do any good, but it won't hurt her, either, and it's a good way to get her to stop eating Don't worry," she smiled, "I know my patients. A little rest, a week away from the factory, and she'll be better. Wait and see."

The next two patients had "female" problems and Varya suggested they would be embarrassed to have me in the room, so I went out into the hallway and took a seat along the corridor. There on separate chairs sat about two dozen Soviet citizens, each with some form of paper in hand. For some, it was a copy of their medical record, which Soviets are permitted to take with them when referred from one doctor or clinic to another. Others held *spravki* (excuses), which permitted them to miss work. Many of them had expected to wait awhile and had brought books to read or small pieces of bread and cheese to eat.

After ten minutes Varya motioned me back into her office as a young woman carrying a pink slip left. "Abortion," she said simply, as I entered. "We do too many. It is not good for the women."

The next patient was a retired railroad engineer who came in dressed in a stained and torn blue suit with a half dozen medals dangling from his pocket. He was an old man and walked stooped over, holding onto his side, complaining of violent stomach cramps. Varya immediately left her chair, went up to the man, and put her short, plump arms around his shoulders, helping him over to the examining table. Gently easing him onto the table, she placed her hand on his forehead while slowly massaging his stomach—as one would calm a child.

"There, there, *golubchik* [an affectionate term], it will be all right." She called in one of her assistants and had her prepare a mixture of belladonna and ginger root for him to drink. After swallowing the brown, muddy liquid and emitting a few hearty belches, the old man said he felt better and shuffled slowly out of the office.

"Comes in all the time," Varya explained. "There is really nothing serious. His wife died recently and there is no one to take care of him, so he drinks too much vodka."

By this time it was noon, and Varya took an hour and a half for lunch, running to the market to buy three small cucumbers for her daughter at the equivalent of a dollar apiece. There were four patients in the afternoon. Two received prescriptions for antibiotics for cold symptoms, along with a strong recommendation to drink hot rosehip tea. One woman, who was having trouble sleeping because her daughter and son kept fighting all night in the living room of their shared one-bedroom apartment, received valerium, a mild tranquilizer. The fourth was excused from work because of low back pain. All of the visits had been friendly, extended affairs. Varya asked about their families (whom she often knew) and shared with them the availability of cucumbers at the market. When it was three-thirty she left, although there were still three patients sitting outside her office. I asked what would happen to them. "Someone else will take care of them, or if it's important they'll come back tomorrow. By morning, however, whatever they have will probably be better."

3

Soviet Hospitals—
Houses of Suffering

For a sick man even a golden bed won't help. —OLD RUSSIAN PROVERB

No system of medical care in the world is willing to provide as much care as people will use, and all such systems develop mechanisms that ration . . . services. —DAVID MECHANIC IN *The Growth of Bureaucratic Medicine*

Houses of Suffering

Officially, all Soviet hospitals are planned. They are not built because a church donates the property, or a citizens group decides the closest city hospital is inconvenient, or because a congressman gets a special bill passed authorizing construction. But this does not mean that Soviet hospitals are always built when and where the Moscow government decides.

Many Soviet hospitals are the result of building initiatives by labor unions, large factories, or trade organizations, such as the nationwide system of tuberculosis hospitals for railroad workers. As a result of these many pressures, there is an unexpected amount of chaos in Soviet hospital construction.

New hospitals spring up in Soviet republics where enough beds exist. Specialized hospitals duplicate general hospitals. The opening of a new hospital is seldom linked to the closing of an older one.

Since 1974, in an attempt to reduce some of this redundancy, the Ministry of Health has emphasized huge multidepartment hospitals: a 1,700-bed giant in Novosibirsk; a 1,660-bed tower to serve Rostov; and new facilities in Tyumen, Moscow, and Volzhsk.

Throughout its history, the Soviet government has steadily increased the total of hospital beds. From 185,374 beds in 1913, they rapidly expanded to 877,296 by 1941. Beginning in 1958, during

Nikita Khrushchev's period of industrialization, the Soviets concentrated on replacing most of the small *uchastok* (rural) hospitals with larger urban centers. Emphasis was on 1,000-bed hospitals and one 3,000-bed giant was constructed. The result today is a total of 3,142,-800 hospital beds nationwide, one for every eighty-two Soviet citizens, over twice as many as the United States' inflated and overbedded hospital system.

But unlike our infrequently filled institutions, most Soviet hospital wards remain crowded. The small metal-frame beds are jammed into every available corner and frequently spill out into the hallways. The mammoth 1,700-bed facility in Novosibirsk was needed because the waiting time for a hospital bed had been three weeks.

A major reason behind hospital overcrowding is the uniformly poor living conditions that most citizens suffer. Soviet apartments, like the hospital wards, are cramped, overcrowded spaces. Two, three, and sometimes even four generations live in two small rooms separated from their neighbors by thin, badly constructed walls. There is no privacy in Soviet living. Family discussions, arguments, and occasionally even lovemaking must take place in public.

When a family member becomes ill, the delicate balance of collective eating, cooking, and sleeping is disrupted. The bed that during the day served as a couch is no longer available. A sickroom can reduce the Soviet family's living space to half and severely strain already tense relationships.

As a result, every year one out of every four Soviet citizens is hospitalized, a figure much higher than in the United States. (Overall, there are 2.8 hospital days per person per year recorded in the USSR, compared to 1.2 in the United States). Patients are often admitted for cases of pneumonia, flu, and gastroenteritis, which would be treated at home by most American physicians. For as crowded as Soviet hospitals are, it is still easier to recuperate there than in a two-room apartment.

Once in the hospital, patients also stay longer. It is not unusual to find patients who've spent months undergoing treatment. In Yerevan, I met a woman who had been hospitalized for two years for treatment of ulcers. Every time she was ready to leave, her pain returned. During this time she had two operations, but for the last six months her only treatment was antacids and bed rest. There was no reason why she could not have gone home, except that after so long in the hospital it just seemed easier to stay.

Every disease a Soviet medical student learns about is associated with a standard number of hospital days permitted by Soviet regulations. Patients with a particular diagnosis almost always stays the maximum number of days. The allotted length of stay for an appendectomy is ten days. If the patient should recover from surgery in five days (as is common in the United States), he would still remain in the hospital for the full ten days, completing his norm. The Soviets keep women in the hospital nine days after childbirth and two weeks following a hysterectomy, double the U.S. stay.

Many of these long lengths of stay are old-fashioned and relate to a time when hospital practices were much different. Yet the Soviets give no indication that they plan to change. One reason may be that, despite medical and technological progress, Soviet hospitals are very inefficient.

A routine chest X ray can take a week to schedule and obtain. To order a radioisotope liver scan in Kishinev requires five separate forms, the approval of six persons, and a ten-day wait. Tests and X rays, once completed, often need to be repeated because of poor film production methods. In 1977, Soviet Minister of Health Boris Petrovsky, writing in *Trud,* a national workers newspaper, made the startling criticism that 75 percent of all Soviet X-ray film is uninterpretable because of its poor quality. When a patient is discharged, it takes twenty-four hours to prepare the bed for the next occupant, a procedure that takes only a few hours in the United States.

Confronted with this large, many-papered, inefficient, and impersonal bureaucracy, the typical Soviet patient has few pressure points. Seldom is an individual appeal successful. Soviet nurses and physicians are impotent and uninterested in changing rigidly determined protocol. Administrators are too concerned about meeting quotas for the current five-year plan to worry about consumer complaints.

Quotas are used by the Ministry of Health to determine whether a hospital is being used to capacity, and to project the need for more beds. Quotas exist for everything from the number of bandages to the ideal number of patients a hospital should have within various disease categories. A quota even sets a minimum number of opera-

tions a surgeon should perform each month. Another quota monitors the days-per-year that each hospital bed is unoccupied.

According to most hospital administrators and physicians I talked
with, these quotas are always met—at least on paper. If the number
of appendectomies falls below expectations, more cases are "in-
vented" to meet the quota. Similarly, the percentage of beds filled is
kept high. Otherwise, budget and supplies might be reduced.
Within the Soviet system such false reporting has never been considered dishonest. It is simply part of the well-established concept that
the easiest way to stay out of trouble is to do exactly what is expected.

Occasionally, however, the Soviet use of quotas produces a situation which cannot be altered or ignored. This occurred in Odessa in
November 1976, when the Ukrainian Republic Ministry of Health
noted a sudden increase in the death rate at one of its emergency
city hospitals.

Every Soviet hospital is permitted a specified number of deaths
per year, based on the size of the hospital and the types of patients it
treats. When a hospital's deaths exceeds the expected quota, an investigation is begun.

To reduce the number of deaths and avoid inquiry, a hospital
director occasionally will instruct his admitting physicians to refuse
ambulances with dead-on-arrival cases. Families of terminally ill
patients are encouraged to take them home so that death will occur
outside the hospital. Except for these minor manipulations, however, the number of deaths is closely followed and the death quota is
the most accurate of all hospital indicators. The Ministry of Health
uses the quota to follow the course of influenza and other epidemics,
as well as to monitor hospital performance.

The investigation that took place in Odessa was described to me
by a Soviet researcher traveling in the United States as part of the
U.S.-USSR health exchange. It was later confirmed by a high-
ranking official of the Ministry of Health. The hospital in question
did mostly emergency gallbladder and appendectomy surgery and
had reported a sudden increase in their postoperative deaths. It was
soon determined that all the dead patients had had their gallbladders removed by the same surgeon. The physician, an older member
of the staff, was known to be a heavy drinker and had been seen

operating while intoxicated. The investigation soon revealed that the surgeon was not remaining with his patients after surgery in order to check for blood loss. Unfortunately, some of the patients were bleeding internally; ten were found dead in their beds the morning after surgery. As a result, the surgeon was prohibited from operating. But none of the patients' families were told the reason behind the deaths. Even if they had known, there was little they could have done. American-style malpractice lawsuits are unheard-of in the government-controlled medical system. Soviet patients can bring legal action against a physician, but only in the hope of removing the physician's license, not for a monetary reward.

This example does show that the Soviets monitor and police the quality of their hospital care. A similar situation occurring in this country (and the use of this example is not meant to imply that similar situations have not occurred here) would probably be handled in much the same way. American physicians are extremely reluctant to criticize their colleagues publicly. Patients must be in substantial danger before action is taken against a physician. Then the censure is done quietly, frequently without acknowledging the true reason.

What is unique about this Soviet experience is the casual attitude the physicians and staff adopted to the growing problem. Although all the patients were operated on by a single surgeon, there were many other physicians available on the ward who, in theory, shared responsibility for any complications. Besides the allegiance to protocol, another distinction between American and Soviet medical education is the emphasis on the group or collective concept of decision making. No one Soviet physician is supposed to be directly responsible for such mistakes. But since no one physician is held directly responsible for any one patient, it often appears that no one is accountable. As the Soviets say, "In the USSR, everything belongs to no one."

The other major difference in approach to hospital care demonstrated by the Odessa experience is the lack of supporting technology.

All American patients, even those undergoing relatively simple operations, are closely observed in postoperative recovery rooms until their vital signs are stable and the possibility of bleeding is checked. Not so in the USSR. Patients having simple procedures are returned directly to their rooms, where only the most superficial checks are done. As a result, patients can and occasionally do unnecessarily die. How many is unknown.

Again, the main reason for this lack of attention to details—even life-threatening ones—is economic. Medicine has never enjoyed a high priority with Soviet economic planners. In 1918, the first minister of health, N. A. Semashko, complained that the minister of defense was continually getting more money for his budget than was being given to health. There is evidence that the same priorities exist today. In 1977, the current minister of health of the USSR, Boris Petrovsky, in the same newspaper article in which he criticized the quality of Soviet X-ray film, also complained that Soviet economic planners were cutting requests from medical institutes in half before final authorization.

Petrovsky, a cardiovascular surgeon, discussed the need for more artificial kidney machines; only a few dozen then served the entire country. He complained that many surgical instruments were unavailable. Supplies of imported rib retractors needed to perform surgery on the chest, for example, were inadequate to meet demand. Even simple, basic tools like thermometers were scarce. The 1975 plan had called for production of 30 million, but only 23 million had been completed.

Besides falling short on production, much of what is produced does not work very well. Take respirators, machines which take over when a person can no longer breathe because of disease or drugs. According to Soviet projections, there are only one-fourth as many respirators produced as are needed, and a third of these are broken. In building respirators, Soviet engineers used German and Swedish models. But unlike the precise, careful workmanship that went into those units, the Soviet version has bolts which do not fit and plastic knobs which, when broken off, cannot be replaced. Controls on these sensitive machines are often not calibrated properly, so that patients often receive too much or too little ventilation.

Even in Moscow, the showplace of Soviet government and the city where every citizen wants to go for treatment, there are serious hospital problems. In the March 5, 1976, issue of the *Biulleten*,[1] a lim-

---

[1] *Biulleten ispolnitelnogo komiteta Moskovskogo gorodskogo soveta deputatov trudiashchikhsia* Moscow (February 1976).

ited-circulation Soviet journal devoted to a discussion of problems within the government, medical technology came under fire. Botkin, No. 1 Pirogov, and a number of other city hospitals were criticized for improper and dangerous use of their anesthesia and X-ray equipment. These errors lead to frequent breakdowns and, according to the article, needless patient suffering. Many Moscow hospitals were experiencing severe shortages of equipment. The main health-care administration was accused of "indifference and laxity toward improving hospital conditions and failing to properly supervise the physician's treatment of the sick." The 1976 article, in calling for improvements, concluded that no progress had been made in improving hospital conditions since 1974, when the Fifth Moscow Soviet issued a resolution calling for improvement in medical care for the residents of Moscow.

Furthermore, the Soviets cannot claim, as can the Chinese, that their lack of medical technology is deliberate; that they purposely set out to deemphasize machines and develop a basic, no-frills approach. The truth is that the Soviet Ministry of Health has always had a *sputnik* mentality toward medical technology, the desire to get there first. For most of this century, however, they were denied the privilege of pursuing the dream. Defense spending got higher priority.

When given the money, Soviet doctors are just as susceptible to addiction to machines as their American colleagues. In some areas, in fact, Soviet medicine places more emphasis on technology than we do. Soviet citizens with varicose veins are not clinically examined prior to surgery but instead are given complicated radioisotope scans. Young children receive laser bombardments to shrink tonsils. Persons with head colds have a weak electric current applied across their noses. School children with bedwetting problems have electrodes attached to their heads and electrical impulses passed through their brains. In one of the few innovations likely to be adopted in this country, the Soviets have devised a unique method of shattering bladder stones by using high-frequency sound waves, thus avoiding surgery.

During a July 1979 interview with Dr. Gavrilov, deputy director of the prestigious Semashko Public Health Research Institute in Moscow, I asked him what he would do if suddenly given an extra 3 million rubles in next year's health budget.

"I would buy machines, laboratory equipment, and supplies for our hospitals," he answered without hesitation. At this point another physician in the room asked Gavrilov if he didn't want to qualify his remarks. Surely not *all* hospitals needed technology. "Of course," he admitted under pressure, "not *all* hospitals, but if I had extra money, I would spend it on medical machines."

Does the lack of such machines make a difference? The best way to tell would be to compare results. Do Soviet patients with the same diagnosis spend an equal amount of time in treatment? Do they recover as often and as quickly as their American counterparts? Is the quality of care, irrespective of surroundings, the same? In short, does the Soviet patient with a specific disease have the same chance of being cured as his American counterpart?

Unfortunately, differences make hard statistical comparisons impossible. We know that, as in other developed countries, the Soviets have traded epidemics of typhus and cholera for heart disease and cancer. But beyond the leading causes of death, the Soviets do not have precise statistical descriptions of why people die. Tables describing a particular hospital's mortality and morbidity rates are available, but aggregate national and regional summaries, in a format comparable to that available in the United States, do not exist.

Because of this problem, many Soviet leaders claim that the anecdotes, negative articles, and isolated descriptions, such as those given in this book, are useless. They also contend you cannot fairly compare the amount spent per bed by the United States and the USSR because of differences in financial structure and cost accounting. They label descriptions of cracking plaster and filthy bathrooms as superficial and unfair. There is more to hospital care, they argue, than clean bathrooms, electrically controlled beds, individual television sets, and computerized X-ray machines. These are simply external luxuries that reflect more about the American demand for profits than about good medical practices.

Soviet criticism of our dependence on medical technologies is, like most forms of propaganda, exaggerated but rooted in truth. Today the typical American physician owns or has access to $250,000 worth of diagnostic equipment. In 1979, they used their expanded "black bags" to do 5 billion laboratory tests for a total cost of $11 billion. This amounts to twenty-five tests for every man, woman, and child in the country—at an average cost of $55 per person. This $55 bill for laboratory tests is approximately half what the Soviet Union spent per person for all forms of medical care in 1978. But despite the large investment of the United States in technology, there is difficulty in linking the use of artificial kidneys, echo-cardiograms, computed tomography scanners, fetal monitors, and intensive care units with an improvement in our nation's health. Many other improvements (such as an improved diet and increased interest in exercise) have occurred at the same time. Thus, the recent advances in overall life expectancy in the United States, the decrease in infant mortality, and the reduction in deaths from cardiovascular disease may or may not be directly related to medical care.

Because of this dilemma, and the United States' current problems with galloping medical costs, the Soviets maintain that their more simple hospital system is better than the high-technology American approach. They emphasize that basic hospital care costs the Soviet citizen nothing, while a catastrophic illness can bankrupt an American family. In fact, propaganda about the cost of American medicine is one of the most frequently heard topics on Soviet radio, with quotes and statistics usually reported out of context.

"We've heard the speeches of your Senator Kennedy," finger-wagging Soviets would tell me. "In America, only the rich can afford doctors. Why, an ambulance will not take you to the hospital unless you give them money beforehand."

Or, "American hospitals make you pay your bill before they'll treat you." "Poor people have to beg for a doctor to see them." "Americans have to sell their homes and cars to pay for medicine."

The average Soviet citizen, who has never traveled outside the country, never seen a foreign magazine or newspaper, and never talked to an American citizen, has no way of knowing whether these statements of his government are true. He is not in a position to judge the authenticity of the often-heard claim that Soviet hospital care is the best, the most advanced, in the world.

Realistically, however, even without the opportunity to compare systems, the Soviet citizen reacts with skepticism to the portentous generalizations the government feels constrained to make about health care. He knows there are problems within Soviet hospitals. Rumors of the high infection rate, accidental deaths, inadequate testing procedures, and intricate gray market system are widespread. These problems are discussed and debated—in private.

When asked publicly to comment on medical care or to compare the Soviet and American systems, the average Soviet citizen, especially if he is talking to a foreign visitor, will spring to the defensive.

"U nas luchshe," I was told hundreds of times by dozens of Soviet citizens, *"u nas besplatno"* (Ours is better, ours is free of charge). To a Soviet, free hospital care is a source of pride—one of the few things he has that the Americans do not.

But even in the area of cost control, where the Soviets have been most successful, there are important qualifications. There is no evidence that the path to Soviet medical economy has been a deliberate, meticulous dissection of priorities. Within their professional literature and in texts of five-year plans, there is no debate and discussion over the value of one medical technology versus another. No attempt is made to evaluate a new operation or machine in terms of its cost-benefit ratio.

Rather, cost savings have been achieved by limiting the amount of money available for the purchase of machines. The USSR ranks at the top of developed nations in terms of number of physicians and total hospital beds, but at the bottom in medical technology investment. This means that not only are such high-technology services as artificial kidneys available to only a few high-ranking Communist officials, but also that the average patient is often denied more basic technological support.

According to the Ministry of Health, a third of Soviet hospitals do not have adequate laboratories for transfusing blood. The capability to culture bacteria from blood and urine is missing at a fifth of rural hospitals. When a laboratory exists, it is frequently closed nights and weekends.

In fairness to Soviet physicians and to a few of their political leaders, the country's problems with medical technology are readily acknowledged. Plans call for a two-and-a-half-times increase in the national budget for medical technology by 1985, along with an aggressive educational campaign aimed at improving the use of machines. Whether this effort will succeed where others, such as the 1974 Moscow initiative, failed, remains to be seen.

In a few areas of the USSR, however, where more money and freedom are available, the hospital situation is better. In 1977, Dr. Linas A. Sidrys, an American ophthalmologist, spent a three-month internship in Soviet Lithuania and reported that, despite bureaucratic obstacles, medical progress is being made.[2]

Lithuania is one of the Baltic republics annexed by the Soviet Union after World War II. The Lithuanians have accepted Soviet control reluctantly. They demonstrate a fierce independence and maintain a standard of living that is closer to that of Western Europe than to the USSR. The Kaunas Eye Hospital is an excellent example. Opened in 1977, the five-story, red brick building stands in sharp contrast to its gray, prefabricated neighbors. No white-on-red banners proclaiming the glory of Communism hang from its balconies.

Within the 240-bed institution the hallways are decorated with colorful art murals and modern art sculptures. The wards are bright, cheerful, and spotlessly clean. This very atypical Soviet hospital was financed entirely by a private institution, the Society for the Blind. In deference to the Lithuanian sense of independence, the society is permitted to keep profits from the goods manufactured by its members. It is one of the richest private organizations in Lithuania and is well known for its philanthropic activities.

Inside the hospital, according to Dr. Sidrys, the Lithuanians have some modern equipment, including a German-made slit-lamp ophthalmoscope (an instrument used for seeing the back of the eye). Nevertheless, even a year after opening they lacked necessities such as laser equipment, essential for the practice of modern ophthalmology.

The difference between the American and Soviet approaches is illustrated by how they remove cataracts. In the United States, a new technique is being increasingly adopted, using laser treatment of the cornea, with removal through a small pipette. This technique allows the operation to be done on outpatients with minimal discomfort and only a day or two off from work. In the USSR, the cataract is still cut and removed manually with tweezers. The incision is closed with rough catgut sutures instead of the delicate synthetic fibers we use for surgery on the eye. Following removal of his cataract, the Soviet patient is kept in the hospital with his eye patched for two weeks.

---

[2] Linas A. Sidrys, "International Comments," *Journal of the American Medical Association* 239 (May 19, 1978): 2181.

The high regard Lithuanians have for American medicine was demonstrated to Dr. Sidrys after he had completed his examination of a Soviet patient. As he turned to leave, he found the entire ward had lined up—for the privilege of being examined by the American ophthalmologist with an American ophthalmoscope.

The issue of quality of care, as opposed to quantity, is a central one when discussing the difference between Soviet and American hospitals. In the United States, much of what is done to the patient is directed at ensuring that all diagnoses, however remote, are excluded and that all forms of treatment, no matter how heroic, are offered. For the patient and his family, this aggressive and expensive approach provides some comfort, the feeling that "everything possible is being done." When any new technique is developed, we readily accept it.

For a few patients, this approach will backfire. The many X rays, biopsies, scannings, and probings will stimulate an unnecessary operation, lead to a harmful complication, or intrude on the person's dignity. The new technique may have unforeseen complications. The errors made in the modern American hospital, therefore, are most frequently caused by doing too much.

Under the Soviet system, the errors are more often those of doing too little. The condition of a patient's cardiovascular system is not fully evaluated prior to surgery, and he goes into shock on the operating table. A blood transfusion is not properly matched, and the recipient has a seizure. Blood tests monitoring white blood cells are not done frequently enough, and a life-threatening infection develops. All of these errors can, and do, occur in American hospitals, but from unofficial estimates, from a review of Soviet medical literature, and from conversations with Soviet physicians, they are more likely to happen in the USSR.

The human price paid as a result of these errors, while not impressive in terms of nationwide mortality figures, cannot be judged insignificant by the individual. The seriously ill Soviet patient is afraid. He fears that the doctors are not telling him the truth about his illness. He is afraid that if he needs anything out of the ordinary, a special drug, a specific surgeon, he may have to pay for it. He knows that the Soviet hospital system has the same problems as the factory where he works, the stores where he shops, the transportation system he uses. They are large, inefficient, and impersonal bureau-cracies.

"This is why," an old man who was recovering from a heart at-tack told me, "We still call them *bolnitsy* [houses of suffering]."

An American in Botkin

Slowly lengthening fingers of morning sunlight crept down the wall, along the floor, and over the rungs of the white-enameled bed, until they reached David's closed eyes. He awoke slowly, squinting and blinking while trying to remember where he was. The room was a high-ceilinged, large white rectangle with a tall window at one end and a single doorway at the other. It was filled with sixteen beds, seven along each wall and two in the middle. The aisles were just wide enough for a person to pass.

The beds were all occupied by men who, as evidenced by their snoring, were sleeping soundly. The other thing that David noticed immediately was the smell, a musky, sweet, slightly nauseating odor of old urine and damp sheets. Propping himself on one elbow, David slowly recalled the events of the last few weeks that had put him in the general surgery ward of Moscow's Botkin Hospital.

Two months before, in January 1978, David had completed his third year of study at a U.S. medical school. Restless after seven continuous years of study, many of his classmates had decided to take part of their senior year away from the university. It would be their last opportunity to travel until after internship and residency.

Armed with a college background in Russian and taking advan-tage of a government student exchange program, David arranged to spend his six-month elective time in Moscow. His project was to study the Soviet Union's approach to controlling environmental carcinogens, and he was excited about going.

Before leaving, he spent a few days in Washington and we talked about the differences in the two countries' approaches to medicine. From what he had read, David saw the Soviet medical system, with its strong central planning authority, lack of sophisticated technol-ogy, and emphasis on primary medical care, as more efficient than that of the United States, with its unorganized, duplicative, expen-sive, crisis-oriented, high-technology approach.

In many ways David's simple, friendly, unassuming, and enthusiastic embrace of the Soviet system reminded me of accounts I had read of Americans who immigrated to Russia shortly after the 1917 Revolution. Some of these Americans, anxious to build a true workers' democracy, found jobs in the many new Soviet factories, married, raised families, and were absorbed into the population. In fact, in many Soviet towns it is not unusual to find people whose grandfathers came from Detroit, Cleveland, or New York City. Other immigrants, however, finding living conditions harsh and working standards primitive, became disillusioned with the Soviet dream and returned home.

Initially, things went well for David. The students at the Moscow University dormitory where he stayed were friendly, constantly pumping him for information about life in America. He spent hours answering questions about the number of hippies in American cities, why former president Richard Nixon was treated so badly by the press, and whether President Jimmy Carter was as wealthy as he appeared. The only thing wrong in those first few days was David's stomach. Like many foreign visitors, David found the typical Soviet diet edible but fat-filled, greasy, and hard to digest.

To add to his discomfort, David found that, unlike his personal friendships, negotiations with the Soviet medical bureaucracy were not doing well. Despite letters of recommendation and a Soviet-signed agreement permitting him to work in the environmental field, two weeks of effort had produced no contacts. Each office he visited at the Ministry of Health referred him to another, but no one wanted responsibility for assigning David to a particular physician or institute.

Finally, after a week of being handed down the Soviet bureaucratic ladder, David arrived at the bottom rung. He met his ministry-appointed advisor, an elderly, semiactive professor who was totally unaware of David's identity or project. It was obvious the professor had no use for an aggressive American exchange student. After ten minutes of futile conversation, he showed David the door.

David applied to the science attaché at the American Embassy for help. But since he was a student, there was little the embassy officer could do. The Soviet bureaucracy, in addition to being enormously inefficient, slow-moving, and suspicious when dealing with foreigners, is also very status conscious. In matters involving science and diplomacy, official titles and degrees are very important and, lacking both, David had no clout. It soon became apparent that the Soviets were planning, as they frequently do, to ignore David entirely. They knew his visa would expire in a few months and their problem would be solved.

Perhaps it was the frustration of knowing that he was being ignored and being unable to do anything about it, perhaps it was the greasy diet, or the Georgian cognac that he was always urged to drink; most likely it was a combination of all three that turned David's upset stomach into a burning inferno. With a familiar, frightening regularity the pain began in the front of his stomach, spread under both ribs, and then stabbed into his back. He had had the pain before. It came from chronic gastritis, an inflammation of the stomach lining. In the past, the pain had always gone away with rest and a bland diet—neither of which he had been able to find in Moscow.

One morning when the attacks came one after another, David noticed his stools had turned black. He went to the embassy physician who confirmed that David was bleeding internally—not rapidly, but bleeding nevertheless.

Frightened by this new problem, David for the next five days lived on Vikalin, the only available Soviet antacid preparation. Unlike the many American varieties of mint-flavored and buffered antacids, Vikalin is a brown, extremely bitter tablet, swallowed whole. While he was in the *apteka* purchasing Vikalin, David looked over the many *travy* (herbal preparations) that are routinely stocked at one end of Soviet pharmacies.

There were small red packets containing anise seeds that, when mixed with honey and water, were supposed to relieve gas. Dill seeds, in green envelopes, were for heartburn; camomile tea was for ulcers. Some of David's Russian friends recommended that he try *kumiss*, fermented mares' milk, which is widely used for many kinds of stomach disorders. Unfortunately, *kumiss* was not available in Moscow that winter. There were also rumors of a mythical herb that healed all stomach ulcers and even "cured" early stomach cancer. But the miraculous drug was said to be sold only at the Kremlin's polyclinic and was reserved for high-ranking members of the Communist Party.

So, despite Vikalin and camomile tea, the black stools and the pain continued. David tried to relax but he became more and more concerned that his attempts at self-treatment might be dangerous. He had to decide then either to leave the country—something he was not prepared to do after only three weeks—or seek help from the Soviets.

Like Soviet citizens, David had a number of places he could go for medical care. There were the Ministry of Health polyclinic (he was their official, although unwelcomed, guest), the clinic associated with Moscow State University, and the Moscow polyclinic for foreigners.

Polyclinics are places where most Soviet outpatient care is performed. They range in size from a few examining rooms with a staff of three or four *vrachi* in rural areas to large urban centers with hundreds of physicians.

Although all polyclinics are staffed by Soviet doctors, they are sponsored by various organizations. Most large factories (over 4,000 workers or over 2,000 if the occupation is dangerous, such as mining) maintain an individual polyclinic for their workers, as do the police, the military, government bureaucracies, and the Communist Party.

In the larger cities, in addition to the many polyclinics, there are specialized dispensaries that treat only one part of the body, such as the heart, or one disease, such as tuberculosis.

The Saturday afternoon David decided to get help, the polyclinic at the Ministry of Health was closed, so he chose the polyclinic for foreigners which, according to his Soviet friends, was one of the best in the city. When he told the secretary at the main reception desk about his problem, she decided he needed to see the gastroenterologist.

Since it was a Saturday, the gastroenterologist on duty had already gone home, so David saw a *terapevt* (internist), an extremely pleasant woman in her early fifties. She asked him a few basic questions: How long had he been having black stools? Was his pain relieved by eating? Was his head spinning? Then she took his blood pressure and handed him two laboratory slips, one for a blood test and another for a stool exam. When David arrived at the laboratory, he found it closed for the weekend.

Returning to the *terapevt*, David was told to try again on Monday. Frightened, David suggested that something be done immediately. The *vrach* shrugged her shoulders and sent David down the hall to a surgeon. The female surgeon told David to pull down his pants. She put a finger in his rectum and then concluded from its dark color that David was bleeding internally and should be hospitalized for nine days.

This unexpected demand made the pain in David's stomach worse and he tried to delay his admission, explaining that his problem wasn't really that bad. It could wait a few days.

"Nyet." The surgeon shook her head firmly. The ambulance was already on its way. David balked at the need for an ambulance, but she explained that since he was ill, he would have to go to the hospital by ambulance. There was simply no other way to do it.

The ambulance arrived forty-five minutes later. Like most cars used for routine calls, it came staffed by another female *vrach* who asked David the same questions as the first doctor at the polyclinic. After learning that he was an American, she took David to Botkin, the only Moscow hospital with a special section for foreigners.

Botkin, named after a famous nineteenth-century Russian physician who performed some of the original observations on infectious hepatitis (a disease which in the Soviet Union still bears his name), is an old, sprawling hospital of loosely connected two-story buildings. Despite an ambitious building program begun in the 1960s which now gives the Soviet Union twice as many hospital beds as the United States, many older Russian hospitals are still being used. Botkin was completed before the 1917 Revolution. The many separate buildings, with their high ceilings, long, wide hallways, and large windowed rooms, would have made a fine museum but, as David would soon discover, were not designed for modern hospital care.

Upon his arrival in the Botkin emergency ward, a fourth medical history was performed by an emergency room physician assigned to interviewing new patients. He was quick and to the point, inquiring about all the tests that would be done in the United States in a case like this. The *vrach* then made an initial diagnosis of *iazva*, ulcer disease. This on-the-spot diagnosis, really an initial impression since it was unsupported by any testing, is extremely important for both the hospital and the patient.

In the Soviet Union, all these diagnoses are entered into the *bolnichnyi* (sick list), which is used by the hospital to justify its budget and by other branches of the Ministry of Health to decide on the need for different kinds of hospital treatment. The *bolnichnyi* list is also used to decide whether the changing environment, with its increasing industrialization and chemical pollution, is damaging to the people's health. Soviet reliance on this informal and untested *bolnichnyi* list in rigorous population studies is one reason Western experts believe that the conclusions reached are not very accurate.

For the patient, the diagnosis he is given on entry is also vital, for both economic and medical reasons. Every Soviet citizen is permitted a standard number of sick days according to the diagnosis. This is the only way to get excused officially. At the end of the illness the "list," as it is known, must be presented at the workplace.

Soviet medical students are taught the number of days permitted for each illness as part of their basic education. Since a person is paid his normal salary while sick (either in the hospital or at home), the choice of initial diagnosis can mean the difference between two weeks away from the factory, or four.

From a medical perspective, Soviet *vrachi,* unlike their American counterparts, do not spend a lot of time ordering many tests, searching for rare diseases. They assume that common diseases occur commonly, and in most cases are willing to begin hospital treatment based on the initial impression of the admitting doctor.

In David's case, the emergency room *vrach* concentrated on questions related to ulcers. Did different foods have any effect on the pain? Was it worse in the fall or spring? Had he ever bled from the stomach before? Had he ever had ulcers before?

With the exception of his problem with fatty foods, David said no to all these questions. Nevertheless, in a twenty-four-year-old with stomach pain a duodenal ulcer is the most likely diagnosis, and it was the one written on the front of David's chart. Had he been a Soviet citizen the diagnosis would have allowed him twenty-one days off work.

Official excuses were the last thing on David's mind as he was directed into the next room for processing. He was told to remove all his clothing and to place identification and money in a paper bag. In exchange, he was later given a thin white chemise and a pair of drawstring trousers, along with thick flannel pajamas.

For the moment, however, David was given only a sheet and ordered onto a stretcher for the trip to X ray for a chest film and, later, to his room. He protested, saying he was quite capable of walking.

But, hospital regulations required all patients entering the hospital to be carried in on stretchers; the Soviet Union does not manufacture wheelchairs.

Once in the sixteen-bed ward, David was on his own. His bed, second from the window along the wall, had a single mattress and a small pillow. Besides a scarred metal nightstand, the only equipment was a radio earphone on the wall which broadcast the main Moscow station. No curtains separated the patients.

Despite the large number of beds, Soviet hospitals are always crowded. One reason is that a great many of the 3 million beds are in small rural (*uchastok*) hospitals, which are the bottom line in Soviet hospital organization. These rural hospitals provide only simple basic services. Any patient developing complications must be transferred to larger and better-equipped city hospitals.

Another reason for the crowding is that no incentive exists for discharge. The Soviet citizen is not charged for his basic hospital stay; he is, in effect, being paid for his time. Nor is the Soviet doctor pressured to discharge patients early. In fact, the paternalistic attitude of most Soviet hospital *vrachi* toward their patients (they assume the patient does not know how to take care of himself) encourages continued hospitalization even after treatment is completed. Finally, enforced bed rest is a long accepted part of Soviet medical care and, with crowded housing conditions, hospitals are the only place to rest.

As a result, the average length of stay in Soviet hospitals is long—fifteen days in 1980, a full ten days longer than the American average.[3]

The patients in David's ward were typical. Most of them had been in the hospital at least a week. One, a forty-year-old accountant with recurrent kidney stones, had been receiving treatment for three months. In the bed across from David's a retired schoolteacher with congestive heart failure was beginning his second month's stay. His heart problem had initially responded, but he continued to lose weight and was too weak to leave.

Three of the patients were recovering from appendectomies (average stay ten days), one man had recently had his gallbladder re-

---

[3] The length of hospital stay is generally longer in Eastern Europe. The USSR's averages are similar to those of Hungary and other neighboring countries.

moved, and another had to have his spleen excised when it began bleeding after an automobile accident. One man had been waiting for two weeks for a free operating room to have his varicose veins stripped. David learned all of this within his first hour; word spreads rapidly when there is a new arrival in the ward. Diagnoses, recent experiences, and opinions on which doctor is the most friendly are all exchanged. A collective camaraderie is quickly established which makes the lack of communication between doctor and patient less frightening. Soviet patients, even when they are American medical students, are not told much about their diseases, nor are upcoming treatment plans discussed. After David had been in the ward for an hour he was taken, without explanation, to one of Botkin's operating rooms. A surgeon and anesthesiologist were waiting. Stories he had heard about the Soviets' rush to operate flashed through David's mind.

What the Soviets were after, however, was not David's stomach—at least not this time. He was placed on the operating table and an intravenous solution of glucose and water begun. When he asked whether the treatment was given to expand the volume of his blood, the answer was no, the solution was for nutrition. Since the glucose solution contained only a few hundred calories, which could easily have been acquired by drinking a cup of fruit juice, there seemed to be little purpose in the exercise. When he persisted in discovering the reason behind the treatment, David was told that they were simply following routine—all patients with his diagnosis received an infusion.

This strict attention to protocol is a direct descendant of the rigid, programmed approach to medical education fostered during the early history of the Soviet Union medical institutes. According to the Ministry of Health, there are plans to reduce this emphasis on protocol, but, as David discovered, remnants of it are still a significant part of Soviet hospital practice.

On the way back to his ward David surveyed the rest of the floor. There were three other sixteen-bed wards as well as four smaller rooms with eight beds. Separated by a corridor was the women's wards where the atmosphere was more cheerful. Flowers were on many nightstands and the women were wearing colorful robes. There was a TV viewing area. Even the bathrooms were newer and cleaner than the men's.

In Botkin, as in most older Soviet hospitals, toilet facilities are primitive. On David's floor there were three toilets for seventy-six men. These had no seats and, unless one brought a morning copy of *Pravda,* no toilet paper. Making the problem even worse, the Soviets dispense enemas as readily as American hospitals give back rubs. The toilets are always in use and frequently overflow, constantly covering the bathroom floor with a sticky mixture of urine and feces.

Near the end of his hospital stay, David was given a total of five enemas in preparation for an X ray of his colon. The Soviets use enemas both for treatment and in preparation for tests. David, along with the other men, lay on a couch in the bathroom. A matronly woman used a single kit for all patients that morning, simply rinsing the nozzle in soapy water between patients.

For his first few days in Botkin, however, David was left alone. Although the official schedule, posted in the hallway, called for visits three times a day by the surgical staff, rounds were actually conducted only once, by the ward's chief surgeon, Anna Petrovna Belikova, a woman in her late twenties who had just completed two years of *ordinatura* (residency) in surgery. Anna Petrovna would spend one to two minutes each morning with every patient, ordering tests, writing notes, and prescribing drugs. In the afternoon, along with other staff surgeons, she performed simple operations, removing appendixes, sewing over ulcers, or stripping varicose veins. She was hardworking and efficient.

There were other surgeons assigned to David's ward (official Soviet statistics claim one surgeon for every nine hospital patients), but none of them was as intimately involved in day-to-day patient care as Belikova. But even her workload was limited by the strict attention to the six-and-a-half-hour day observed in all Soviet hospitals. Precisely at 3 P.M., Anna Petrovna took off her tall, white starched cap, removed her lab coat, and went home to her daughter and husband. A small staff remained on call for any emergencies that might occur.

The relationship between Soviet hospital physicians and their patients is different from that found in the polyclinics or other outpatient settings. All Soviet medicine suffers from the long lines, endless paper transfers, and bureaucratic malaise that pervade the Soviet economy. The physician is simply another employee, responsible more to the system than to the patient.

Polyclinic physicians, however, do pay more attention to patient demands than hospital *vrachi*. One reason is that the polyclinic doctor is likely to see the patient repeatedly over the years and an informal rapport may develop between patient and physician. Not so in Soviet hospitals. The hospital doctors in charge of the ward assume all responsibility for diagnosis and treatment. It is a one-time relationship since, given the size and complexity of the Soviet medical bureaucracy, it's unlikely a patient would encounter the same hospital physician twice. This contributes to a brusqueness between patient and physician that is remarkable even to a Western observer used to the hit-and-run conversation of some American physicians.[4]

In David's case, try as he might, he was unable to determine what was in store for him. Each morning he questioned Anna Petrovna regarding what other diagnostic tests were planned and how much longer he would have to stay in the hospital. She dismissed his questions with a motherly pat on his arm, telling him to be patient or explaining that a new test was planned. When David asked why more frequent blood tests or additional stool samples were not being taken to monitor his bleeding, she thrust out her ample chest, informed him that he had no right to question those decisions, turned sharply on her heel, and marched away.

The other patients in David's ward were puzzled by his actions and a few were visibly upset over his brazenness. They considered it *ne kulturno* (in poor taste) to question the physician's judgment or choice of treatment. The attitude expressed by the engineer with the kidney stones was typical: "There is no reason to question what the doctor says," he admonished David. "She works hard and tries to do a good job. Besides, everything's free, don't complain."

Soviet doctors are taught that telling a patient the exact details of his disease will reduce his chance for recovery. Thus, a patient who has suffered a heart attack and, as a result, has had a sudden, temporary disruption in its activity, is never told that his heart stopped. In the mind of the Soviets this knowledge could precipitate a recurrence of ventricular fibrillation. In the same way, the old man in the bed across from David was told not that he had stomach cancer (which was the established diagnosis) but that the ulcer was "pre-

---

[4] The Soviets also rotate physicians between hospitals and polyclinics, either on a half-day basis (*dvukhdnevnaia sistema*) or every-other-day system (*cheredovanie*). Even under these systems, however, the polyclinic atmosphere is more relaxed.

malignant" and that, if surgery was not immediately done, it would become cancerous. It is also characteristic of Soviet medicine that the old man was told directly, loudly, and quite abruptly—in full view and hearing of the rest of the ward—that his stomach would have to be removed. There was no further explanation, no alternatives were given, and when the frightened old man began crying, no effort was made to console him.

The prospect of surgery was also beginning to concern David. Since being admitted to the hospital three days before, he had received no treatment. He was supposedly scheduled to have his blood level checked every other day, but it had only been done once. In fact, the only routine check David had had performed was the recording of his armpit temperature every eight hours.

He had heard from Anna Petrovna that he was scheduled for an endoscopy so that a direct look at his stomach and a possible biopsy could be done. On the fourth day he was told no endoscopy would be done for a week. But the next day he was told not to eat breakfast and to put on one of the three robes allocated for his ward. Following a nurse, David left the building and walked out into the cold March air. He shivered at the unexpected cold and felt the wet snow working its way through his thin slippers.

Unfortunately, the building where all endoscopies were done was a quarter-of-a-mile walk from the main hospital. Since most endoscopic procedures are done on outpatients, and since Botkin had only one instrument, it was kept in the clinic.

Shivering and wet after his walk, David entered the building and stood in line waiting his turn. After an hour he was instructed to lie down on the table and open his mouth—wide. A nurse grabbed both of his arms and held them to his sides. Another held his head in a tight lock. Because he had seen an endoscopy done as a medical student, David knew that the long, black tube (about the thickness of a small garden hose) would be placed into his mouth, down his esophagus, and then into his stomach. At the other end, a physician would use a lens and light source to look at his stomach's interior and, if necessary, take biopsies of any suspicious areas. None of this had been explained to David beforehand, and from the muffled screams and sounds of struggle that had come from the room, it was obvious that few of the Soviet patients had been properly prepared for the uncomfortable and disconcerting invasion.

David cooperated as best he could, trying to swallow the black tube without gagging, wishing that some sort of mild sedation had been given. But soon the tube was in his stomach and, after ten minutes of looking, the surgeon, whom he had never met before, withdrew it. As soon as David regained his voice, he asked his examiner what he had seen.

"Nothing," was the curt reply. "Your doctor will tell you." Later David secretly read the doctor's note in his chart. It described some minor bleeding in his duodenum, the first part of the small intestine where it joins the stomach.

Relieved, David found his own way back to his ward and waited. Each day on rounds Anna Petrovna came by and told him his treatment would start "tomorrow." One time he was told that he would have to take a mixture of antacids and atropinelike drugs to reduce the acidity and spasm in his duodenum; another day, that an analysis of his stomach acids would be necessary before treatment. On yet another morning, the recommendation was that he should rest for a week before any further therapy be done.

The reason behind the confusion was partly David's disease and partly the Soviet system. First, duodenal inflammation is an unusual diagnosis and a difficult one to treat. There is often, as in David's case, a relationship between the pain and a period of emotional upheaval. Antacids and drug treatment, while occasionally reducing some of the symptoms, seldom treat the real cause of the problem. Second, and probably more important in David's case, Anna Petrovna was limited in her actions by what was available.

She admitted to David that she had wanted an upper gastrointestinal X ray on him before his endoscopy. The schedule had been full, however, and she was not able to have the exam done. She had also decided to start David on a treatment program using antispasmodics, but the hospital pharmacy was temporarily out of the drug.

Most medications given to Soviet hospital patients are free. The selection, however, is far smaller than in American hospitals. The pharmacy at George Washington University Hospital, for example, lists sixty-seven different antibiotic preparations. Botkin lists eight, of which only four are routinely available.

The main reason for this is the absence of commercial pharmaceutical manufacturers in the USSR. Since the state is responsible for all production, only one type of each major drug is manufactured. Even lifesaving preparations such as antibiotics are subject to the vagaries of Soviet industrial distribution. Streptomycin, for example, will be on every shelf one week and then suddenly disappear the next. The reason is not only that the basic supply is inadequate, but that hoarding encourages shortages.

Shortages are extremely common within the Soviet economy. One week the stores will be out of shoelaces, the next week pencils. Most often these shortfalls are the result of poor planning and insufficient production methods. The Soviet citizen has learned to live with this uncertainty by purchasing large quantities of limited goods as soon as they are displayed. In 1978, there was a shortage of lipstick and when it finally became available, women stuffed dozens of tubes in their handbags as insurance against a future deficit.

A hospital administrator in Ufa told me that since these shortages are also found in the medical industry, he always orders twice as many antibiotics as he needs, with the knowledge that he will not always have his order filled. When I asked him what effect such a philosophy would have on the national supply of antibiotics, he answered simply that the nation was not his responsibility. His only concern was getting enough medicine for his hospital, and some extra to trade.

This trading of scarce supplies among Soviet medical institutions is an accepted means of maintaining the inventory. By chance, one hospital will obtain its entire requisition of suture materials and thereby have an excess. The administrator will then contact a neighboring institution and agree to trade sutures for syringes. Some of the excess items obtained in this way make their way into the black market. It is common for a patient's family to be approached about purchasing a drug, currently unavailable at the hospital, for three to five times its normal price.

So David spent ten days in Botkin after his endoscopy without being given any drugs. Removed from the frustration of fighting with the Ministry of Health, his pain decreased on its own, his nausea improved, and he stopped bleeding. During the days before his discharge David found he was actually able to eat the three hospital meals a day and was, in fact, still hungry.

David ate together with the other patients in a small dining room. Although there were supposed to be special menus available for different patients, the actual food was identical and did not vary from day to day. David made friends with some of the other patients' families, however, and got extra helpings from the food they kept in special refrigerators on each floor. Better nutrition in hospitals was a major goal in the 1971–75 Soviet health plan and appeared again in the 1976–80 document.

But David's real frustration—after he had accepted the fact that the Soviets had nothing to offer him therapeutically—was the nurse in charge of his floor.

Nina Andreevna had orangish-red hair and a short, powerful body that strained at the seams of her clothing. She had been a nurse at Botkin for ten years, and since most of the other nurses were younger, she demanded acknowledgment of her seniority with public displays of rudeness. With a few exceptions, Soviet hospital nurses are a disagreeable lot. Receiving only the most basic medical training, their duties are limited to starting intravenous therapy, giving injections, and supervising the work of the matrons. Like other Soviet women who occupy minor roles, such as elevator operators, store clerks, and hotel floor managers, Soviet nurses assume an attitude of officiousness which is out of proportion to their responsibilities.

For Nina, her symbol of power was the hallway chair. The chair and a small desk were the only pieces of furniture in the wide hallway. From her perspective behind the desk, Nina could watch all visitors, make sure no isolation patient left his room, and see that the doors were always closed. On spotting any of these violations, or any other behavior she judged inappropriate, Nina Andreevna would point her finger at the guilty party and shout so that everyone would hear:

"Young man, young man, what are you doing with that coat on? No coats allowed on this floor.

"Pytor Grigorievich, what are you doing in the hallway without your slippers. It is not permitted. Go back to your room.

"Quiet there! Where do you think you are, hooligans? Keep your voice down in the hospital. Loud talking is not allowed."

What Nina hated more than loud voices, dirty overcoats, or loud talking was someone sitting in her chair. Despite the chair's being the only seat in the corridor, no one was permitted near it. Once David unknowingly sat in the chair while waiting for the bathroom to become vacant. He had no more touched bottom when Nina flew out of a side room to pull the chair out from under him.

"This is not permitted, not permitted," she screamed. "No one may sit here but the nurse in charge."

David observed that the nurses' attention to rules is not accompanied by a similar interest in their patients. There is little in the way of direct contact between nurse and patient. Pulse, blood pressure, and other vital signs are never checked, except in critical cases. Medications are infrequently given. Beds are changed once a week and traditional nursing responsibilities, such as baths and back rubs, are rarely done.

What David observed in Botkin is not an isolated problem. Hospital nursing in the USSR is not a respected job. In the past, many young women like Nina used nursing as a stepping stone toward a better position as a *feldsher* (physician's assistant). With the increasing tendency for Soviets to pick men and the more successful female students for their medical institutes, however, nurses are finding it harder to transfer out. Like many citizens, these nurses use what little authority they have to try to find the feeling of personal importance and identity that is so elusive in Soviet life.

An article in the April 1978 issue of *Meditsinskaya gazeta* criticized the nursing profession for lacking compassion, tenderness, and warmth for their patients. The article contrasted current care with that given by the prerevolutionary Sisters of Mercy and concluded that nursing was much better when nurses thought of their patients first and the rules second.

Isolation

Most Soviet citizens I met were afraid of going into the hospital. Like reluctant patients in every country, their fears centered around being alone and losing control over their lives. The USSR, with its strong emphasis on central planning, increases these concerns. The country's recently completed massive hospital building program replaced many of the smaller rural hospitals with 600- to 1,000-bed institutions in or near major cities. This means that the hospitalized Soviet villager is often hundreds of miles from home, isolated from family and friends. In fact, surveys have shown that anywhere from 10 to 25 percent of a city's hospital beds are filled with people from the countryside.

But even for urban dwellers the hospital is seldom geographically convenient. Hospitals are chosen by the patient's diagnosis, so it is not uncommon for a patient with a heart problem to be sent a dozen miles across town rather than to a hospital nearby. Once admitted to the hospital, a person is quickly stripped of the personal possessions every Russian uses to insulate himself from the dreariness of Soviet life.

This geographic and emotional isolation is one reason that such strong bonds develop among Soviet patients. Without these bonds, the patient becomes a nonperson. He is a faceless body in a bed, in a ward, within a hospital, inside a system where individuals seldom matter. Banding together with others in his ward, he becomes part of a group, and however informal, groups are where a Soviet citizen feels most at home.

But the hospital group, unlike other official Soviet organizations, is informal, dynamic, and surprisingly democratic. Its members include the patients admitted to a ward, those receiving treatment for a particular disease, or persons recovering from the same operation. Since hospitals house a broad cross-section of Soviet society (only a small number of powerful citizens are entitled to treatment in the special Communist hospitals), it is possible that a steelworker from the Urals will find himself next to a Moscow economics professor, with a Ukrainian peasant across the aisle.

Despite their different backgrounds, they now all share certain feelings in common. They are frightened and confused. In becoming patients, they have given up small markers of daily life that, however simple, gave them a feeling of individuality: a bright scarf that made the universal dark-grey overcoat and black hat appear almost fashionable, or too-red lipstick that encouraged someone to look up in a crowd. For others, it might be a collection of books back in the crowded apartment—some of them officially forbidden—or a small room where, after the children were asleep, the parents could be alone.

To the hospital patient, all of these things are suddenly unavailable. They are replaced by white underwear, flannel pajamas, a brown robe for men and a blue one for women. Reading material must never be placed on the bed. As a patient, you are really not even sure of the bed. You can be moved at any time without warning or explanation, depending on your condition and the needs of the hospital.

In such a situation no one else, not even your family or friends, can understand how you feel, and so you make friends with people you normally would not speak to if you were well. Sometimes the group's leader is the patient with the most seniority. Often it is the person who talks the loudest. Women's groups tend to be less formally structured than men's and a single leader seldom emerges.

Regardless of leadership, every hospital group protects its weak. An old peasant from Tula, his heart weakened by age, is helped down the hall to the toilet. Two men hold each arm while he squats, a third cleans him when he is done. At meals, the patients in his ward take turns bringing him back plates of food.

But the group makes a distinction between weakness and being weak. If the old man vomits in the middle of the night (perhaps the dose of digitalis the doctors have given him is too strong), he will be shouted at, called a pig; his roommates will demand to know why he had not warned them he was ill. Moaning or constantly complaining of pain is never tolerated from anyone, regardless of age. It is considered childish, embarrassing, and the patient who persists is moved into the hall.

The group's main function is gathering intelligence. Shortly after a new patient is checked in he is quizzed concerning his medical background, what hospitals he has been in before, the operations he has had, and what treatment he expects to get. There are rapid dissemination and analysis of this experience. His facts are compared to those of other patients. So he has had his gallbladder out. What hospital? Do you remember the surgeon? How long did it take? Did they put you to sleep?

"Sleep? For a gallbladder?" someone will laugh. "Gas is too expensive to waste on such a minor operation. Why, when I had my appendix out, they spent two hours looking for it, pulling on my guts till I vomited. Sleep? They save that for *rak* [cancer] operations."

Once the newcomer is thoroughly questioned, he is given a standard indoctrination: the best hour to go to the toilet, what to do when it is time for the weekly bath. "A hundred men through three tubs in two hours. You feel dirtier than when you went in." He is told which matron can be talked into giving a back rub without the usual three-ruble fee, and the best day to try to get clean sheets. "Once every ten days, whether you need them or not," someone smirks.

If his disease involves surgery, there will be a discussion of who the best surgeon is and how much it will cost to have him operate. Regardless of the diagnosis, however, there will undoubtedly be someone in the ward who, through his own experience or that of a relative, is an expert on the subject.

All this is necessary because most Soviet doctors seldom talk to their patients. Soviet physicians consider their patients ignorant of basic health information and incapable of understanding the complexities of modern medical practice.

"Patients are their own worst enemy," was a phrase repeated by many Soviet doctors. "They don't understand how different drugs and treatments work. They're suspicious about everything you do. The less you tell them, the better."

Another factor encouraging this philosophy of silence is the long-held belief that too intimate a knowledge of disease may delay or even prevent recovery. Just as persons with heart attacks or cancer are seldom told their diagnosis, it is not unusual to find Soviet citizens with surgical scars who are unaware of what type of operation they had or of what might be missing.

"I think they cut out part of my stomach," a woman in Ufa told me, "but I'm not sure. The doctor never told me."

There was a time in recent Soviet history when such an approach was understandable, even defensible. A short four decades ago most of the Soviet population were illiterate peasants who believed in the mystical powers of witches and the healing ability of spirits and demons. To them, hospitals were places the rich went to die and if a poor person was admitted, it was only for experimentation. Within the records of these early hospitals there was a column labeled: "Patients who ran away." It has taken the Soviet government most of the 1900s to revise this centuries-old fear. In doing so, it provided little in the way of personal health education, concentrating instead on broad public health campaigns in which people were simply told what they should and should not do. With epidemics raging throughout the country, the why was not considered important.

Today, with most mass infections controlled, the Soviet government has not switched to a more sophisticated educational approach. Detailed information on most common diseases is not available to the average Soviet, so rumors and traditional beliefs persist. Most Soviet physicians, unused to sharing information, evade questions.

For the hospitalized patient, who is no longer an ignorant peasant, the desire to know what may happen to him tomorrow is becoming increasingly important. Because Soviet patients are frequently grouped by diagnosis (patients needing appendectomies and other emergency operations in one hospital, cancer patients or those with chronic problems in another), elaborate discussions and even debates concerning proper diagnosis and treatment frequently take place.

Patients hospitalized for kidney stones, especially common in some of the southern regions of the USSR, discuss when is the right time to operate versus the conservative approach of fluids and *narkoz* (anesthetic). One man is convinced he has found the best position to minimize the ripping pain associated with passing a small stone. Another says that a strict diet of mineral water prevents a stone's recurrence. One patient I spoke to suggested a home remedy for passing kidney stones—three glasses of beer followed by a high-speed motorcycle trip down a bumpy dirt road.

Patients recovering from the more traditional surgical approach warn those awaiting an operation that the first few postoperative days are the worst. Pain from the wide surgical incisions, along with the constant leaking of urine, reduces a person to a childlike dependence on others. If your wife is not able to stay with you, they advise, then be sure you have money to pay the nurse or orderlies to change your dressings, bring your food, and help you to the bathroom. An extra ten rubles for the narcotics nurse—so she will bring your pain injection on time—is also necessary.

This unofficial but widely practiced system of payments for routine hospital services is part of a vast gray market that exists throughout the Soviet economy. As opposed to a traditional black-market system, where illegal goods are bought and sold, payment for some basic hospital services is more like an indirect subsidy. The monthly wage for nurses and orderlies is set so low (forty to sixty rubles a month) that unless they earn extra money they may starve.

The total costs incurred in this way are not large—two or three rubles for attention during an eight-hour shift—but they make the much-publicized Soviet claim of *besplatno* (free of charge) and inexpensive hospital care less absolute.

In addition to the informal service charge, there is also the occasional practice of large direct payments to physicians. Most often this involves contracting with a well-known institute surgeon to guarantee that he, rather than one of his colleagues, will perform the operation. The prevalence of contracting (with payments often running from two hundred to four hundred rubles) varies, depending on where in the USSR the patient lives.

In the large Russian Republic, payments are relatively common, as they are in Soviet Georgia or Armenia. Within the Baltic republics, such as Estonia, Latvia, or Lithuania, however, direct payments are considered in poor taste and are only infrequently made.

Some families I talked with complained bitterly about the practice, claiming they felt forced to pay large sums so that their father or mother "would not be butchered by some amateur." Others I met said payment was unusual and limited to those areas of the Soviet Union—like Georgia or Armenia—where everything from French sweaters to American cigarettes is bought and sold illegally.

Vladimir, a young man who had formerly lived with his parents in Moscow, explained how his father's illness cost the family most of their savings.

"First it was 100 rubles to get him admitted to a small room in Botkin. Twenty rubles a day for the nurses—my father was old and couldn't control his bowels very well. Then 350 rubles so that a certain professor performed the surgery. It was a difficult operation and my father had a weak heart. The antibiotics were another two or three hundred rubles. In the end, however, all of it was wasted. Father developed an infection and died."

For most Soviet citizens such costs would be considered unusual. The average patient enters the hospital, pays a few rubles to the nurse and orderly, and nothing more. Patients never request a better room. The surgeon who operates is the one on duty that day. No "special" drugs are given; whatever is available is used. There is one problem, however, that every patient has in common with Vladimir's father—the threat of infection.

Infection

Russian citizens have long had a distrust and fear of surgery. For most of the eighteenth and well into the nineteenth century, persons were advised never to *idti pod nozh* (go under the knife) for fear they would suffer a painful death. As operating conditions and medical practices improved, most of the pain and some of the fear were relieved. But even today, Soviet citizens, acting from superstition, try home remedies, traditional cures, and denial in an attempt to delay or avoid an operation. Most of them have heard too many stories, known too many families where surgery was the final and fatal treatment.

Postoperative and other hospital-acquired infections are a major problem in the Soviet medical system. The exact size of the problem is difficult to determine since hospital and communitywide infection statistics are not available. According to medical journals and conversations with Soviet physicians, infection rates are much higher in USSR hospitals than in the United States. In fact, most Soviet physicians with whom I discussed the infection problem preferred comparing their incidence of postoperative infections with that found in developing countries, such as Afghanistan, rather than with the United States or other developed countries.

Wound infections are especially common. A Moscow heart surgeon confided to me that a third of his patients become infected postoperatively and, in many cases, their deaths are directly related to the infection.

One obvious reason behind this problem is the relaxed, open-door policy the Soviets have in their operating rooms. With few exceptions, anyone associated with the hospital is permitted in and out of the room while surgery is going on. Minor operations, such as dilation and curettage (a common method of abortion), are performed with little attention to sterile precautions.

How this can lead to problems is illustrated by the June 1977 experience of a young Englishwoman who had a spontaneous miscarriage while traveling in Kiev, USSR. The details of her case were provided by a British physician, G. A. Hobbs, who was traveling with her. Although a foreigner, the treatment she received was exactly the same as described to me by dozens of Soviet women. Her case is unique, however, because she was reevaluated at the end of her treatment and the complications documented—something that rarely occurs in the Soviet system.[5]

While in Kiev, the young woman, who was in the early months of pregnancy, began having cramps and noticed vaginal bleeding. Dr. Hobbs was called to examine her. Normally, the combination of cramps and bleeding mean that the pregnancy is threatened but danger to the mother is small. In this case, however, Dr. Hobbs found that the miscarriage was incomplete. Parts of the fetus remained in the uterus, causing heavy bleeding and threatening to put the woman into shock. When her blood pressure decreased dangerously to 80/60, Dr. Hobbs dialed 03, the nationwide telephone number for emergency medical assistance, and asked for an ambulance.

It arrived with a driver, a young male *vrach* (doctor), and a *feldsher* (assistant). To Hobbs, the ambulance service doctor appeared remarkably disinterested. He briefly felt the pulse rate of the thoroughly frightened woman and measured her blood pressure. He ordered the *feldsher* to give a small intravenous injection of glucose and vitamins. Then he demanded, despite Hobbs's objections, that the patient be dressed. When she sat up, her blood pressure was so low she fainted. There was no stretcher available, so Hobbs and the patient's husband carried her down to the ambulance in one of the hotel's chairs.

When they arrived at the October Hospital in Kiev, the bleeding woman was kept waiting while her name and diagnosis were entered into the hospital's *bolnichnyi* list for the day. An orderly removed the woman's clothes, put a hospital gown on her, and shaved between her legs. A short, perfunctory history was done and she was taken to the evacuation suite.

The room contained two operating chairs, a water basin, and a table filled with instruments. The woman was placed in one of the chairs where she sat at a 45-degree angle, her legs spread apart, with a space beneath her buttocks into which the blood and the products of conception could fall.

Without warning, a female *vrach* thrust a gloved hand into the patient's vagina and indicated that she would have to scrape the

[5] G. A. Hobbs, "Personal View," *British Medical Journal* (November 1977): 1413.

uterus. She picked up the curette with her bare hand. Anesthesia was a few small injections of Novocain drawn from an open bottle. They didn't relieve the pain of the scraping. When the young woman nearly fainted from pain, the *vrach* told her to be quiet. There were no masks, hats, gowns, or sterile towels used.

Throughout the scraping the patient's blood pressure remained dangerously low at 70/40, but no attempt to give fluids or blood was begun. It was only after she had been removed from the operating chair and taken to a small crowded room that a blood test was performed and an intravenous solution begun.

As usual, this was done using a blunt needle, crude red rubber tubing, and an open glass bottle with a broken top, into which fluid was poured from a large jug.

Because her pulse rate was still high and blood pressure low, Dr. Hobbs asked for a second bottle of fluid. He was told one was enough and that she was given it only because she would be on a plane in the morning.

"But she may need a blood transfusion," Dr. Hobbs argued.

"We never give blood for this condition," was the quick reply.

Dr. Hobbs was able to get his patient released from the hospital the next morning, even though she had developed a fever. Three days later, when they both arrived back in the United Kingdom, she required two pints of blood and a four-week course of antibiotics for the pelvic infection contracted during the unsanitary operation.

In the USSR (where abortions outnumber births four to one), the problem of such infections is more than a medical curiosity. Soviet gynecologists I spoke to acknowledged that their rate of infection is much greater than it should be—and that some of these infections leave a woman unable to become pregnant again. But when asked about solutions, most simply shrugged their shoulders. What can they do?

Why does a country capable of open-heart surgery, complex chemical and radiation treatments, and sophisticated computer analysis of electrocardiograms have trouble accepting and enforcing well-known standards of hospital sterility?

Part of the problem is that the rubles spent on elaborate medical research institutes are not representative of the overall priorities the Soviet government has for medical care. In 1980, the government spent approximately 18 billion rubles for "health protection." This amounts to $105 for every man, woman, and child in the USSR. For the typical hospital bed, the Ministry of Health allocates four to ten rubles a day (approximately $6.20 to $15.00).[6]

There are many results of this economy. One is that hospital care has remained a basic, simple, no-frills undertaking. The millions of pieces of our "throwaway" hospital technology, such as plastic syringes, disposable needles, once-used glass tubes, and paper drapes, are unheard of in the USSR. All of these items, while increasing the cost of medical care, also make it easier to protect the patient from hospital-acquired infection. In the United States, almost everything that touches a patient today is immediately thrown away. In the Soviet Union, nothing is.

All Soviet needles are saved and resterilized. The thick rubber tubing used in transfusions is washed out after each use, wrapped in gray cloths, and baked in an oven. After repeated sterilizations, it becomes sticky, difficult to hold, and impossible to properly disinfect. Instead of sterile intravenous bottles, packaged and shipped from a factory, the Soviets pour solutions into an open bottle, much as you would fill the radiator of your car. For protection, the bottle is covered with a thin piece of cotton gauze. Such practices lead to infection. They allow bacteria to enter the bloodstream, creating shaking chills and fever which, if not detected and treated, can promptly lead to serious complications and even death.

The dull needles sometimes break off in patients' arms and surgical removal is necessary.

The lack of disposable equipment was a direct contributor to a severe epidemic of staphylococcal infection that in early 1978 spread rapidly through four Moscow maternity hospitals. The epidemic was directly responsible for the deaths of twelve children and kept many other infants hospitalized and under treatment for weeks. Many of these children finally left the hospital alive, but the deep scars on their faces would be a lifelong reminder of Soviet medical economy.

The infection problem, however, is caused by more than a lack of money. The age of plastics and disposables, after all, is a recent phe-

---

[6] Comparable figures for the United States are $943 per person and $200 per hospital bed per day. The USSR totals include rubles spent for physical cultures and other non-medically related items.

nomenon even in our country. Before plastic, plain boiling water and careful attention to hand washing and sterile procedures worked quite well. The Soviets fail to obey many of these simple rules because of a traditional belief that infection is usually brought into a hospital, rather than contracted from within.

This belief began during the early 1930s, when hospital construction was just beginning in the USSR. The devastating epidemics of cholera, typhus, and other infectious diseases were still not entirely controlled at that time, and the majority of the population were illiterate peasants, ignorant of even the simplest rules of hygiene. Most still believed that typhus came directly from God.

It took a concentrated, mass education effort over several decades to redirect their suspicion from devils to dirty, lice-infested clothes. Until this could be accomplished, it was necessary to prevent peasants from entering the hospital and contaminating the patients with lice.

A strict protocol was established. Patients were stripped of all clothing before admission. Visitors were required to take off their coats, cover their shoes with rags, and put on a gown over their street clothes. Items such as sweaters or woolen jackets were forbidden, since they were especially likely to contain lice-infested dust.

Reminders of this strict hospital policy are still evident today. Any visitor to a Soviet hospital will get only a few steps beyond the door wearing a coat. A militant nurse or officious secretary will call out, *"Tovarishch, tovarishch* [comrade, comrade], coats are not permitted in the hospital."

Similarly, no one is allowed to sit on a hospital bed or—a serious violation—place a magazine or newspaper on its sheets. Never mind that those sheets have not been changed for a week—infection comes into a hospital, not vice versa. This same old-fashioned belief is the reason recent mothers are prevented from any outside contact for two weeks after delivery. Visits by husbands and family take place only through glass. It is not unusual to see new Soviet mothers surreptitiously hanging out of windows, waving to their husbands on the street below.

Unlike the historical epidemics of cholera, typhus, malaria, and yellow fever, however, the infectious diseases of today cannot be stopped at the hospital door. Modern hospital bacteria no longer just travel from person to person, but are also spread by dirty needles, doctors' hands, improperly sterilized instruments, and open intravenous solutions.

The Soviets are not ignorant of these facts. It is just that their teaching and protocols, carefully formulated and established for other problems, have not adapted to the times. Change comes slowly in Soviet Russia. The *babushka*'s fear of the woolen coat or heavy sweater has been passed down to her granddaughter the nurse. The more important prohibition, that sterile instruments should not be touched, although officially taught, lacks this historical emphasis and is frequently ignored.

Pyotor Grigorievich's Cancer

At sixty-five Pyotor Grigorievich had been a pensioner for five years and had hated every day of his retirement. For all of his forty-year working career he had been active. Beginning as a construction worker, he was promoted to foreman by the time he was thirty. During the war he served as a supply commander at the western front. For the last ten years he had been the assistant director of a large truck repair factory. He and his wife, Anna, had raised four children.

When Pyotor first retired, he planned to improve their small *dacha* (summer house). He wanted to plant a garden, knowing that his 120-ruble monthly pension would not buy many fresh vegetables. He also looked forward to spending more time working on his car. It was a 1954 Muscovite and had not run in eight years. Pyotor kept it locked in a small garage where it was carefully wrapped in plastic and surrounded by old boxes. Stealing cars for parts is a well-established and lucrative crime. Pyotor himself had been trying to buy a carburetor, stolen or otherwise, for five years. Then he and Anna could drive to the country instead of taking the train.

But all of Pyotor's plans changed when Anna suddenly and unexpectedly died. After the funeral his eldest son, his wife, and their two children moved in with him. The son, a schoolteacher, spent most of his free time drinking and took no interest in his father. Pyotor's daughter-in-law, forced to work and raise the family, resented the old man's presence in the cramped apartment. Under Soviet law, however, the apartment belonged to Pyotor. So she grudgingly accepted the fifth chair at the dinner table and waited for its occupant to die. Even Pyotor's grandchildren were irritated by his insistence on keeping his private bedroom.

Alone, he stopped visiting the *dacha*. He lost interest in repairing his car. Pyotor spent most of his time sitting in the small, muddy park outside the apartment building.

It was there that the pain first began gnawing at his stomach. He blamed his daughter-in-law's cooking. She didn't understand the need of an old man for simple foods. Every night she cooked a highly seasoned, Armenian-style meal. It was simply another reason, Pyotor thought, why his son should have married a Russian instead of this dark-skinned girl with no hips. He began eating only bread, potatoes, and cheese. But the pain became worse and he was unable to sleep. Finally, Pyotor went to the polyclinic at the factory where he had last worked.

The *vrach* waited while Pyotor removed his blue suit coat, took off his heavy woolen sweater, unbuttoned his shirt, and pulled off his old pair of cotton underwear. As each layer came off, it became obvious that the pain was more than indigestion.

"You've lost a lot of weight, Pyotor Grigorievich," the *vrach* told him.

"It's my daughter-in-law's cooking," he complained. "I can't eat it without pain."

"No, it's not the food. You need to go into the hospital for tests."

"Never," Pyotor replied. "I have never been sick in my seventy years and I will not go to a hospital now."

"You are a fool, Pyotor Grigorievich. But in the end you will go when the pain becomes worse."

The pain did increase, and Pyotor began vomiting after the smallest meal. Soon he was able to drink only tea and eat a little cheese. He made arrangements to travel to Moscow. Although there was a large district hospital near his apartment, Pyotor felt, as do many Russians, that everything—hotels, restaurants, food, and medical care—is better in Moscow. And Pyotor, twice awarded the Hero of Socialist Labor, decorated during the great fatherland war, an early supporter of Communism, felt he deserved the best.

On Pyotor's admission to Moscow City Hospital No. 68, the examining physician felt his now sagging abdomen. Two inches below the sternum he palpated a hard mass the size of a small green apple.

"Is it cancer?" Pyotor asked when the examiner called another physician over to confirm his discovery.

"Of course not, old man," the doctor assured him. "It's nothing."

As part of the routine hospital tests, Pyotor had an electrocardio-gram and chest X ray, along with a determination of his hematocrit level and a urinalysis. During his first two days in the hospital, he received intravenous injections of glucose because he was unable to eat without vomiting.

On the third day, he was taken to endoscopy. He was placed on his side on the heavy metal table while a nurse and a nurse's aide held his arms down. The surgeon, without explanation and without any medication or local anesthetic, forced a long, black rubber tube down Pyotor's esophagus and into his stomach. Using a small pair of forceps that fit through one of the channels in the gastroscope, he took a piece of Pyotor's tumor to examine under the microscope.

For the next week, Pyotor walked the hallways of Hospital No. 68. The patients usually walked close to the wall, moving slowly and keeping their hands in the pockets of their robes. The center was kept clear for physicians, nurses, and visitors who walked quickly, arms swinging freely, talking loudly.

During this week, Pyotor had no further tests. Although he still could not eat, there were no injections. Each morning he looked up expectantly as the doctors made their rounds, but they simply nod-ded and passed on. Finally, on the eighth day, they stopped at his bed.

"Your stomach must come out, Pyotor Grigorievich."

The words could not apply to him, he thought. They must have confused him with another patient. Perhaps the next bed or the one across the room.

"Do you hear me, Pyotor Grigorievich? We have to operate and remove your stomach. You have a tumor."

"*Rak* [cancer]?" Pyotor looked bewildered and frightened.

"No one said that, old man. If you don't have surgery, then it will be *rak*. An operation is your only chance."

Pyotor's case illustrates the direct approach that Soviet medicine takes to a problem. Pyotor arrived at the hospital with abdominal pain, vomiting, and weight loss. A stomach mass was felt and cancer was the presumptive diagnosis. The tumor was biopsied, determined to be malignant, and removal recommended.

Contrast this with what probably would have occurred to a similar patient in an American hospital. Large automated chemical analyzers, which run from six to eighteen tests on a single sample of blood, would have checked the level of minerals, chemicals, proteins, and waste products in his blood. The results would have indicated how well his kidneys were functioning, and whether, as a result of his protracted vomiting, there were electrolyte abnormalities in his system. Following this, a sixty-five-year-old American patient would have been closely questioned regarding other symptoms to determine whether he was a good surgical risk.

Then, after confirming that the mass was actually cancer (which could have been done with the same technique the Soviets used), extensive preoperative testing would be performed. This evaluation would have included X rays of his upper and lower gastrointestinal systems, along with a radioisotope scan of his liver and spleen. If the patient was in a large private or university-related hospital, a test on a million-dollar machine called a Computerized Axial Tomographic Scanner (CAT) might be ordered. The CAT scan would produce a detailed cross-section of his abdomen, giving the exact location of his tumor in relation to the rest of his internal anatomy.

From a combination of these results, the American physician would decide if surgery was needed. If all the tests were negative, indicating that the tumor had not spread beyond the stomach, and if the patient were otherwise in good health, then an operation aimed at removing the tumor would be scheduled. If, however, there was indication of distant spread, surgery would be deferred in favor of chemical or radiation treatment.

The patient and his family would be presented with the results of all tests and the alternatives for treatment. They might be given statistical estimates of the chance of surviving the initial treatment and what might be the long-term prognosis. The risks of surgery and the possible complications would be explained. If the patient asked directly whether the tumor were malignant, most American physicians would answer yes, but quickly add that cancer is no longer an incurable disease. There is hope.

No attempt was made in Pyotor's case to test for tumor spread, or secondaries, as the Soviets call them. Since the outlet from his stomach was blocked by the cancer, some type of surgery had to be done.

Frightened and alone, Pyotor dissolved into tears after being told of the operation. The reaction by the collective of five doctors who were making rounds was to move on to the next case. A nurse, following behind, yelled at him to stop being a child. If he needed an operation, he needed an operation, and that was all there was to it. Nothing was to be done.

Pyotor sobbed softly through the rest of the day and into the night. The other patients in the ward ignored him until it was time for bed. His muffled whimpers kept them awake.

"Quiet, old man," they shouted, "there are other sick people here. You're not the only one, other people have it bad, too."

For the next two days Pyotor lay quietly in his bed, ignored by staff and patients alike. The next morning the chief surgeon stopped by his bed.

"So, Pyotor Grigorievich, what will it be? Do we operate?"

Pyotor turned his head on the pillow and, looking down at her shoes, mumbled his weak consent.

Two days later they came and gave him an injection. An hour later they carried his loose, sleeping body to the operating theater. They brought him back three hours later, a large bandage covering his belly, blood soaking through the top. He was moaning softly.

When the chief surgeon looked in on him that evening, she whispered softly to the man in the next bed, *"Rak* everywhere, he's filled with tumor. There is nothing we could do."

But the next morning, when Pyotor asked her what she had found, she said, "It was as I told you—premalignant. But the ulcer was larger than we thought. You will have to have radiation treatments." Before he could ask more questions, she turned on her heel and left. Pyotor's eyes followed her out the door. He knew she was lying.

According to many Soviet surgeons I spoke with, operations like Pyotor's are performed frequently because surgery is the most direct, accessible, and least expensive diagnostic test available.

The hospital, the operating room, the surgeons, are all inexpensive resources. Having a surgeon take a direct look at Pyotor's tumor costs the government less than investing in the scanning, X-ray, and other diagnostic machines and the trained personnel to operate them. Although this leads to many more cancer operations, it does not often change the outcome.

In the United States, the extent of Pyotor's cancer would have shown up on one of the preoperative tests and he would have been sent directly for radiation. Regardless of where the evaluation took place, however, the prognosis would be the same—death within a year.

4

Medical Research

In the course of its development science has known but a few courageous men who were able to break down the old and create the new, despite all obstacles, despite everything. —J. V. Stalin, discussing the work of I. P. Pavlov

Pavlov and Paraplegics

Spartak Oganessyan is a scientist at the Institute of Cardiology in Yerevan, Armenia, USSR. His field is myocardial metabolism, the care and feeding of the body's most important muscle, the heart.

He works on the third floor of the six-story institute. It is a gray building in the outskirts of Yerevan, a city of half a million people situated in the shadow of Mount Ararat, the mountain where Noah's Ark is believed to have landed. Surrounded by mountains, the research institute is frequently blanketed by a wet, low-hanging mist that covers the window outside Spartak's office.

The office is reached by passing through an outer room crowded with glassware, tubing, centrifuges, and spectrophotometers. Inside is a small paper-cluttered desk, positioned to take advantage of the infrequent light. Over the desk is a large, torn, plastic copy of the Mendeleev periodic table of the elements.

Spartak's research concentrates on microscopic portions of heart muscle removed from animals and humans at different stages of heart failure. These biopsy specimens are minced, chopped, homogenized, washed, and then painstakingly analyzed for minute differences in their concentration and type of proteins.

Spartak's goal is to describe in exacting biochemical detail what happens when this muscle fails. The work is important, he believes, because a better understanding of the molecular changes taking place in a failing heart could lead to improved drugs for treatment and, perhaps, even prevention of this life-threatening problem.

Myocardial metabolism is a specialized field. Worldwide, there are only two or three hundred researchers speaking its unique language. They communicate in an internationally understood jargon of protein absorption curves, ATPase enzyme activity, optical characteristics, intrinsic viscosity, and reaction velocity. They publish their work in a few small-circulation scientific journals, one of which, the *Journal of Molecular and Cellular Cardiology,* has Spartak Oganessyan on its editorial board.

Over the years, from reading and critizing each other's papers and from meeting at annual conferences (Spartak has been permitted to attend only those meetings held in Eastern European countries such as Czechoslovakia), a casual familiarity pervades the scientific exchange.

The scientists refer to each other by their first names. They talk of Peter's obsession with a certain theory, or the Hungarian's insistence that he has found the final solution to why heart muscle reacts differently under stress from muscle cells in the arm or leg.

Spartak knows all of the principal participants in his field, if not by face, then by reputation. He eagerly awaits the arrival of the latest journal or announcement of an upcoming symposium. When I visited his laboratory, he proudly handed me a copy of his latest article, and halfheartedly tried to clear a small area of his cluttered desk. He sat down for a moment, but immediately jumped up to illustrate a point on a blackboard crowded with figures and notations, the random clutter that frequently accompanies scientific accomplishment.

Throughout our two-hour meeting, Spartak talked continuously. He explained his latest theory about how heart failure develops and how he had adapted a German-manufactured analyzer to the peculiar plumbing of his laboratory. Knowing that I was not a specialist in his field, Spartak tried to relate the results of his work to clinical problems, explaining how he hoped his experiments would eventually help patients.

Realistically, though, Spartak is more motivated by his natural scientific curiosity than by a practical desire to design new cardiac drugs. He knows that, at best, his research effort can only solve a small piece of a much larger puzzle. Spartak's obsession is aimed not at a dramatic, prize-winning breakthrough but toward a methodical search for truth.

As a result, Spartak has, scientifically speaking, made it. He has overcome problems of language, funding, and politics to carve out a place for himself in the competitive world of international science. In the Soviet Union, Spartak is a remarkable man.

He is remarkable because, for most of this century, Soviet medical researchers existed in a politically and scientifically controlled vacuum. Scientists were isolated from the rest of the scientific world by the paranoia and random terror of Stalin, disrupted by the advancement of Communist Party officials over knowledgeable researchers, and separated from their proud Russian traditions by the demand that all research conform to the findings of one man—Ivan Petrovich Pavlov.

By the 1917 Revolution, Pavlov's reputation as a world scientific leader was firmly established. In 1904 he received the Nobel Prize for his work describing the digestive process. Three years later he was made a full member of the Academy of Sciences. Since 1891 he had directed the Institute of Experimental Medicine in what is now Leningrad.

According to Pavlov's biographer and former associate, E. A. Asratyan, when the new revolutionary government seized power, they rushed to embrace the work of the great physiologist. Lenin took the time in the early and dangerous days of his leadership to issue a special decree proclaiming the "outstanding scientific contributions of Academician I. P. Pavlov which are of enormous significance to the working people of the whole world." The revolutionary writer Maxim Gorki headed a commission aimed at "creating in the shortest time the most favorable conditions for the scientific work of Academician Pavlov."[1]

A major reason behind Pavlov's popularity with the Soviets was that his discoveries linking changes in behavior to physiological principles could be closely related to the Bolshevik philosophy which said that environment could determine the individual.

Actually Pavlov's concentration on the physiological as opposed to the philosophical origins of human emotions and mental illness was an elaboration of work that had begun in Russia years before

[1] E. A. Asratyan, *I. P. Pavlov, His Life and Work* (Moscow: Foreign Language Publishing House, 1953).

Pavlov was born. A 19th century Russian physiologist, Ivan Sechenov, wrote a book called *Reflexes of the Brain* which stimulated Pavlov to begin his scientific studies.

Pavlov's experiments led him from discoveries outlining the control of digestion, to his now classical description of the conditioned reflex. Because many of Pavlov's discoveries could, on a superficial level, be used to support the political philosophy that nurture was more important than nature, Lenin was an immediate Pavlov supporter. For him and other Marxist proponents, it was a short step from the scientific theory of mechanical materialism advocated by Pavlov to their political dogma of dialectical materialism.

In order to further strengthen this association, the Soviet government created a public image of Pavlov as a dedicated Communist. The following quotation, taken from N. C. Mansurov's book *Pavlov and the Struggle for Materialism in the Natural Sciences,* is typical of what Soviet scientists and the general public have been reading for forty years. According to Mansurov, "Pavlov was convinced of the rightness of the peace-loving politics enacted by the Communist Party and the Soviet government. He hotly expressed his full agreement with them."

But while Pavlov's salivating dogs might have appeared superficially similar to Marxist philosophy, and the image of the white-bearded scientist as a good Communist was useful for political purposes, the new Soviet government took liberties with Pavlov's carefully controlled laboratory experiments that he never intended. As a result, Pavlov quickly came to despise the very leaders that honored him.

"Pavlov was the commanding figure in Soviet science in the twenties and thirties," recalled W. Horsely Gantt, former professor of psychology at the Johns Hopkins University and, until his death in 1980, one of only two persons alive who had worked with the Soviet Union's best-known scientist. "Everything circled around him. Stalin made it a crime to disagree with Pavlov. All new scientific discoveries, no matter in what field, had to agree with Pavlov's writing. These requirements had the effect of retarding, rather than stimulating, discoveries, and as a result Soviet science became very stagnant."

When I first met Dr. Gantt in 1978, he was eighty-six, a white-haired, vigorous man who seldom wore a coat, regardless of the cold. He went to Russia in 1922 to head the medical division of the American Relief Administration (ARA) in Petrograd (now Leningrad). Gantt told me of his surprise when he encountered Pavlov still working. The 1916 *Encyclopaedia Britannica* recorded that Pavlov had died.

Finding the great scientist alive, Gantt, upon completing his ARA work in 1923, arranged to return to Russia and from 1925 to 1929 he worked in Pavlov's shadow. "I would spend the day in his laboratory, learning his research techniques. At night, I'd go over to Pavlov's apartment. He loved to listen to classical music and since records were so hard to find in Russia, I'd bring him mine."

I talked with Gantt in his Baltimore home, an English-style cottage overflowing with books. Letters from famous Russian composers and ballerinas whom Gantt had befriended while living in Leningrad and photographs of Pavlov in his laboratory adorned the walls.

"Pavlov distrusted the new government and what they'd done to the Russia he'd known," the tall, white-haired scientist related. "I remember we'd talk about his work. Pavlov resented the way government leaders tried to make him out to be a good Communist. He hated Communism. He used to say—to anyone who would listen—that Marxism was founded on three things—fraud, deception, and violence.

"Pavlov would never even let Gorki into his apartment. He called Gorki a 'dog' and he would often say that Lenin had suffered from syphilis.

"In 1927, Pavlov wrote a letter to Stalin, a copy of which I have. He complained to Stalin about the things that had been done to destroy the intelligentsia—that as a result of Stalin's actions he, Pavlov, was ashamed of being a Russian," Gantt told me. (Stalin's private secretary did not want to give the letter to Stalin, fearing that the emotional leader would have Pavlov killed.) "But when Stalin read it, he simply laughed. 'Let Pavlov say what he wants,' he said. 'We can still use him.'

"Pavlov once did some experiments on the inheritance of acquired characteristics with mice," Gantt recalled. "The experiments suggested that conditioned behavior might be passed on from one generation to the next. He reported only two paragraphs of that work. But the government made a great deal of those paragraphs, claiming that it proved socialist theory, that the proper environment would determine the individual. But," Gantt went on, "Pavlov went back and tried to repeat the same experiments. He found the results didn't hold up. Pavlov told me the whole thing was the biggest mistake of his scientific career."

The Soviet government used Pavlov's work to support their belief that through education, you could change certain Russian characteristics. It formed the basis for T. D. Lysensko's pseudoscience of vernalization in agriculture, which, by suggesting that environment could improve wheat yields, brought disaster to many Soviet farms. This politicization of scientific theory also had a detrimental effect on the structure of Soviet research, a phenomenon Gantt observed in the 1930s when he returned to visit old colleagues.

"The research institutes had become small dictatorships. Everyone, all the other scientists, tried to please the head scientist by producing experiments that supported his theories. I remember being intrigued by the work of Professor Beikov. At the time, Beikov had results showing that you could condition a kidney to produce certain types of urine. It was fascinating work. When I returned to Johns Hopkins I tried to duplicate his studies, isolating a dog's kidney in his neck with and without nervous connections. I worked for several years but I couldn't produce any evidence to substantiate Beikov's findings.

"That doesn't mean that Beikov was dishonest," Gantt explained. "It's just that the Soviets concentrated on protocols. If you do enough protocols you'll eventually get one to work out the way you want it to. Since the people working with Beikov knew what he wanted, they did the experiments over and over again until they once got the right results. They didn't bother to do any analysis."

Unfortunately, the destruction of true science, prominent during Stalin's years in power, left a legacy that, in certain areas, persists today.

In the first joint Soviet-American meeting on psychobiology, held in California in April 1978, American scientists noticed that while the Soviet presentations emphasized the neurochemical changes that might be linked to differences in human behavior, they presented no chemical or objective data. According to one observer, "The difference [in psychobiology] is that the Americans have small theories and lots of data. The Russians have large theories and much less data."[2]

The influence that Pavlov's discoveries, combined with Stalin's sponsorship, had on Soviet medical research is illustrated by a book published in the Soviet Union in the 1950s entitled *The Achievements of Soviet Medicine*. The volume stresses the importance of Pavlovian theory, not just on psychology and behavior but on heart disease, surgery, aging, hypertension, and cancer. According to the book, without Pavlov there would be no modern medicine.

Stalin's death brought some relief. Charlatans like Lysensko still flourished, but Nikita Khrushchev did stop the killing of scientists who disagreed with the government. The new premier also recognized the need for Soviet science to become part of the world. He supported better communications between Soviet scientists and their foreign counterparts.

Unfortunately, Khrushchev approached science with a series of sporadic and uncoordinated reforms similar to those that brought him agricultural disaster. He went on a shopping spree, buying Western technology and permitting selected foreign scientific reports to be imported. But many of the modern machines were out of place in the old-fashioned Soviet laboratories. The few scientists having access to them did not understand how they worked, and when they required adjustment, there were no technicians. Covered with canvas, they became expensive countertops. Since so few scientists knew foreign languages, many reports went unread.

Most important, Khrushchev's reforms did not extend into the leadership positions of the medical research institutes. Directorships remained in the hands of scientists who had proven their Communist loyalties. To them, progress outside of conventional channels—the innovation of which true science is made—was viewed as dangerous. The massive Soviet research bureaucracy carefully constructed under Stalin adapted to Khrushchev, but did not change.

The current minister of health of the USSR, Boris Petrovsky, who

---

[2] Constance Holden, "Russians and Americans Gather to Talk Psychobiology," *Science* 200 (May 1978): 1115.

has held his leadership position since 1964, is trying to improve the level of medical research by strengthening these institutes. He has established and improved research in cardiovascular disease, cancer, and environmental problems.

According to Houston surgeon Michael DeBakey, a close friend and professional colleague of the minister, Petrovsky would like to emulate in Moscow what DeBakey has achieved in the Texas Medical Center, a world-famous collection of hospitals and research institutes.

"When Petrovsky visited Houston," DeBakey told me, "he said how he'd like to have the same things in Moscow, how he wants to modernize the system. A great many of the practices and traditions now in use in Soviet research are holdovers from an older, now out-of-date European attitude. You have to remember, though," DeBakey cautioned, "that from what I've seen, the Soviets have a huge, unyielding medical bureaucracy. Any progress, no matter how small, is difficult, takes an enormously long time, and much of the research effort is politically controlled."

Today all the directors of the large Moscow medical research institutes are high-ranking Communist officials. The same is true of most smaller regional institutes located in the other Soviet republics. This political domination, with the top directors enjoying large apartments, special shopping privileges, and vacations in Sochi, a resort on the Black Sea, produces resentment on the part of other lower-ranking scientists.

In July 1970 the Soviet newspaper *Literaturnaya gazeta* published an extensive opinion survey of Soviet scientists. Prominent among their complaints was the lack of stimulation and understanding from their administrative superiors.

"Most research directors," a scientist at the First Moscow Medical Research Institute told me, "are out of touch with the work of their scientists. They are too busy watching out for their own careers. Most are afraid to sponsor or encourage new work for fear it will not be successful and will anger ministry officials. They spend their small budget on standard, safe experiments. They make sure the institute publishes enough papers to meet its quota."

Dr. Y. Sheinin, senior associate of the Institute of World Economics and International Relations in Moscow, compared the position of Soviet and American scientists in his 1978 book, *Soviet Science Pol-*

icy.[3] Soviet scientists, according to Sheinin, enjoy the advantages of national planning and centralized priorities, thus eliminating wasteful duplication. The American scientists, on the other hand, are permitted the advantages of greater innovation, responsiveness to consumer demands, and decentralized decision making. In a remarkably candid summary, Sheinin suggests that the Soviet scientist would benefit from similar freedoms.

Finding money for new projects is a serious problem for the individual Soviet scientist. The country's research priorities are set in five- and ten-year cycles. Since all support comes from the government, there is little flexibility to follow new areas. Unlike the United States, there are no private foundations or other sources of support for unconventional ideas or development of new techniques. This rigidity leads to a cynical attitude among many Soviet researchers. "Our newspapers," one scientist explained, "are constantly talking about a new research technique or invention being developed for the first time in the Soviet Union. What they fail to say is that the same technique has been in use in the United States for ten years."[4]

In addition to money, another important difference between American and Soviet researchers is where they work. In the United States, most major research centers are geographically and administratively linked to medical schools and teaching hospitals. Research scientists frequently have teaching assignments at the medical school and, when they are not in the laboratory, spend time with

[3] Y. Sheinin, *Science Policy: Problems and Trends* (Moscow: Progress Publishers, 1978).

[4] Determining exactly how much the Soviet Union spends on biomedical research is difficult. The figures do not appear in their official budgets. Ministry of Health officials, when asked about the totals, explain that the government supports all forms of medical research but that the exact numbers are not available. According to intelligence analysis in this country, the Soviet research investment is estimated at 3 percent (approximately $837 million) of their total 18 billion ruble health budget. In comparison, the U.S. federal government spent approximately $7 billion on biomedical research in 1979.

Although the Soviets have a smaller budget, the total number of medical scientists working in the USSR is approximately twice what it is in the U.S. According to a recent analysis performed by Louvan Nolting and Murray Feshbach of the Foreign Demographic Analysis Division of the U.S. Census, there are 43,000 Soviet specialists with advanced degrees in medical and pharmaceutical sciences compared to 18,164 in the U.S.

Because of a large increase in the number of Soviet scientists in technical fields like engineering and physics, the percent of Soviet scientists working in medicine, as compared to other fields, has actually decreased from 13 percent in 1950 to 4.9 percent in 1974; see e.g. "R & D Employment in the USSR," *Science* 207 (February 1, 1980):493-503.

medical students, interns, and residents. Thus, by example and by lecture, an American medical student is introduced to the techniques of medical research and how laboratory work relates to the clinical needs of the patient in the hospital. It has been a mutually beneficial relationship. Many of the answers provided by American medical research laboratories have begun as questions asked at a patient's bedside.

The Soviet approach is different. The sixty-seven scientific medical research laboratories in the USSR are administratively and physically separate from the medical institutes. Researchers seldom teach and the clinicians who care for patients do not perform research. The emphasis in Soviet medical institutes is on memorization of treatment protocols. The vast majority of medical students are never exposed to scientists.

If a medical graduate decides to pursue research, he has to go back to school for an additional three to five years of training. Breaking the links among teaching, patient care, and research made sense to the Soviet Union when they were first developing their medical system. At that time, they needed doctors, lots of them, quickly. Today, they realize that maintaining two separate systems leads to the stagnation of both. Medical research is frequently out of touch with the needs of practicing physicians. For their part, the clinical doctors remain unaware of recent discoveries.

One example of the practical problems this arrangement can produce is found in the Soviet pharmaceutical industry. The Soviets have problems with their drug industry. Supply of essential products never seems to meet demand. Even when the amounts produced are adequate, distribution difficulties seem to prevent the medicine from getting where it is needed. A report from the National Committee of People's Control published in *Izvestia,* on August 20, 1970, typifies the problems:

> The inspection established that serious shortcomings exist in the provision of the population with medical drugs. A significant number of pharmacy stores lacked the most necessary and simple drugs [such as] iodine. Many hospitals do not receive the needed drugs on time. As a consequence, we receive many complaints from organizations and individual citizens.

According to Dr. V. A. Yakovlev, head of the Council of Scientists of the USSR Ministry of Medical Industries, which is responsible for production of most drugs, research institutes spend too much time on "unpromising research projects, conducted frequently out of tradition alone or prompted by vague subjective factors." There is a need "to more closely link the searches for new drugs to a medical basis."

Reasons for this lack of original research activity, according to Yakovlev, are the technical and scientific isolation of research institutes and the existing incentives which encourage directors to fill their yearly quotas with old compounds repeating the past year's work over and over again.

Furthermore, once new drugs are developed, there is a problem getting information on their use to pharmacists and physicians. Writing in the *Meditsinskaya gazeta* in December 1971, the head of the Lithuanian pharmaceutical industry complained that physicians did not know the properties of the medications they used. In January 1972, the editors of the scientific journal *Farmatsiya* listed as a top priority the need to inform physicians of available preparations.

In response to these criticisms, the Soviets have made changes. In the drug industry, they have introduced limited advertising of new compounds within their medical journals, thus reducing reliance on the mimeographed sheets that pharmacists were supposed to circulate to hospitals and physicians. They have also begun to provide incentives for the discovery of new compounds and to link the initial research with production and distribution.

The situation in regard to Soviet medical journals is, in itself, a rough index of the current involvement and interest in research on the part of the average Soviet physician. Although the USSR has a million physicians and dentists, the circulation of their two major monthly journals, *Soviet Medicine* and *Clinical Medicine,* is 70,000, or seven percent of the possible readership.

By contrast in the United States, the combined circulation of *The New England Journal of Medicine* and *The Journal of the American Medical Association,* which are both issued weekly, is 400,000.

On a more general level, the necessity of linking medical research with practice was discussed at a 1973 Moscow meeting when two prominent speakers, N. A. Preobrazhenskii, director of the First Moscow Medical Institute, and J. F. Isakov, chief of the medical education department of the Ministry of Health, both stressed the need for better integration of medical research and teaching. In 1976, many Moscow and Leningrad medical students began instruction in research techniques as part of their standard training.

Another way the Soviets have chosen to improve the quality of their medical research is through the increased exchange of scientists. Although informal exchanges had gone on since World War II, in 1972 the United States and the Soviet Union signed the first formal Health Exchange Agreement.

This agreement, which was reviewed in 1977 for a second five years, provided for the exchange of scientists and the completion of joint research in six major areas of medicine and public health.[5]

Since most of the scientists exchanged, and all of the formal plans, came from the National Institutes of Health (NIH), the exchange agreement led to what is now known as the Bethesda-Moscow shuttle.

In the first three years of the exchange, hundreds of Soviet scientists made the trip, filling the Ramada Inn on Wisconsin Avenue, a block from the NIH Bethesda, Maryland, campus. They toured major research centers from New York to San Francisco and attended luncheons, dinners, receptions, and scientific meetings. It was as if the terror of Stalin had been replaced by the warmth of international cooperation.

Unfortunately, however, the political dogma that was necessary to avoid imprisonment under Stalin was still necessary to get a visa. Initially the Soviets sent only those scientists considered safe: institute directors, high-ranking Communist Party officials, persons used to foreign travel and who were likely to return to the USSR.

The results of this medical tourism were thousands of pieces of paper, proposals calling for more exchange, more cooperation. The Soviets, still reluctant to relax a fifty-year-old tradition of secrecy, limited discussion to procedures, not actual experiments.

Gradually, the diplomacy and the political posturing began to frustrate pragmatic American scientists who, while initially intrigued by trips to exotic Russia, began to view the exchange as a gigantic waste of time.

---

[5] The six areas are cardiovascular diseases, cancer, environmental health, arthritis, influenza and acute respiratory disease, and the organic basis of schizophrenia. A separate agreement in the field of artificial heart research and development was also signed.

In response to these criticisms and the threatened withdrawal of cooperation by some American workers, the Soviet government liberalized their visiting-scientist policy. Younger scientists with first-hand research experience began arriving at Dulles Airport. A few Soviet researchers were even sent for training at U.S. institutions. These scientists developed personal relationships with their American counterparts, and the exchange of scientific ideas, initiated by Khrushchev a quarter of a century before, finally began.

This exchange revealed the picture we now have of Soviet biomedical research—a complex out of step with the rest of the scientific world. Talking one-on-one with Soviet researchers demonstrated the damage done by decades of isolation.

There were, of course, exceptions. Scientists like Spartak, who balanced their scientific and political responsibilities so that they could pursue the former, developed immediate rapport with their American counterparts. It was what they had always been waiting for.

Moreover, Soviet research did provide important new information. Soviet scientists were the first to discover the cancer-causing properties of Red Dye No. 2. Using an ingenious application of high-frequency sound waves (ultrasound), Soviet researchers developed a method of shattering stones in a patient's bladder without surgery.

Mark Ravitch, professor of surgery at the University of Pittsburgh and a frequent Soviet traveler, found Soviet surgeons using a new technique for repairing lung tissue during operations—wire staples.

"I found the device, a small staple gun, for sale in a surgical supply store in Leningrad," he told me. "I brought it home and an American company, after making some minor changes in its design, is planning to market it soon."

Another recent example of Soviet innovation that may soon have value for American patients is a new approach to treating severe myopia, or nearsightedness, with surgery rather than eyeglasses. I first learned of this unorthodox approach in 1979 when I was invited to a press conference at the Soviet Embassy in Washington, D.C. There, in an ornate second floor reception room, I met Syvatoslav N. Fyodorov, Director of Moscow's Research Laboratory for Experimental and Clinical Problems of Eye Surgery. Dr. Fyodorov, a small intense man dressed in a black leather jacket, spoke rapidly to a large group of Soviet journalists and a few American reporters. He explained how he made sixteen small incisions around the cornea of the eye. These sixteen incisions or cuts enlarged the eyeball thereby correcting the abnormality in myopia and immediately improving vision.

After the conference Fyodorov told me he had performed this operation on over 2,000 patients with 97 percent success. He claimed that widespread use of radial keratotomy, as he called the surgery, could reduce and almost eliminate the need for millions of eyeglasses.

Although I was initially skeptical of Dr. Fyodorov's claims I followed the progress of radial keratotomy. By the end of 1980 the operation had won some converts in the United States. Ophthalmologists in twenty-three American hospitals had operated on over 1,000 patients. Continued evaluation is essential, however, before the technique becomes widespread.[6]

To a great extent Dr. Fyodorov's success is attributable to the efforts of Minister of Health Petrovsky to create super research institutes in the major Soviet cities of Moscow, Leningrad, and Kiev. These coupled with the solid traditions of medical research in the Baltic republics, is providing a small but reliable base for future improvement. The increased interaction of Soviet and American scientists is also helping to clear some of the long-standing political dogma from Soviet research techniques.

But because of its overall one-sided nature, the exchange program has its detractors. Some American scientists contend that the exchanges should be linked to human rights. A few exchanges have been canceled because of the USSR's failure to permit free emigration of Jewish scientists. Other critics complain that we're giving the Soviets more than we're getting. A Library of Congress report completed in late 1978 for Representative Benjamin Rosenthal (D., N.Y.) charged that while we were granting their Soviet counterparts complete and unlimited access to information, studies, and equipment, American scientists visiting the Soviet Union were subjected to restrictions and often were not permitted to see scientists on request. The Soviets were accused of hiding discoveries.

---

[6] Since Fyodorov's "pinwheel surgery" is not the first attempt to change the shape of the cornea, further evaluation is needed. Previous such efforts have led to serious deterioration in vision after time; see e.g. *The Medical Letter* 22 (November 14, 1980): 23.

An American medical scientist quoted in the report said, "During my visit to the Soviet Union, things were quite formal. Visits with various scientists were brief and consisted of formal presentation of already published data.... The United States is gaining nothing that I can detect from this program."

On balance, the Soviets are probably gaining more from the medical exchange. In one area, development of an artificial heart, the exchange program may actually enable Soviet scientists to surpass their American colleagues.

In 1972, Michael DeBakey, through his friendship with Minister of Health Petrovsky, helped establish a U.S.–USSR research program concentrating on the artificial heart. Artificial heart research is an area that DeBakey has been involved in for many years, as one of the technology's main clinical supporters.

At the beginning of the exchange, the Soviets were far behind in development of the device. Initially, American scientists provided their counterparts with expertise regarding the types of materials that would be most compatible with the human body. The Soviets, according to DeBakey, combined this information with computer programs designed to regulate the artificial heart's pumping action.

Since 1972, according to DeBakey, the Soviets have devoted much more effort to the project than the Americans have. A 1974 U.S. report on the artificial heart, prepared by a special NIH panel, concluded that while further research should be done, questions over demand, cost, and safety might turn development of such a device into a moral and ethical dilemma. The controversial report put a damper on research funding. The same considerations did not seem to trouble the Soviets.

"They have thirty or forty scientists working full-time on the artificial heart program," DeBakey explains, "far more than anything we have going. It's simply a matter of these numbers and time. I think the Soviets may put it all together and come out with the first prototype. I know it's very important for them. They view the project as a medical sputnik."

If the Soviets are first with the artificial heart, it is doubtful, considering their experience with other medical technologies such as artificial kidneys and pacemakers, that they will use the device widely.

"They'd probably only do a hundred or so operations a year," DeBakey predicts, "maybe set up a model laboratory in Moscow.

For them it would be the challenge of doing it that would be the most important. They'd like to be the first."

Being first in such a complex and dramatic area as artificial heart research would provide much desired prestige for the Soviet Union. Recently, premature announcements by the Soviets of scientific breakthroughs, such as the case of Levon A. Martinian, have proved an international embarrassment to their research program.

Martinian's story begins a few years ago when the physiologist from the Orbeli Research Institute in Yerevan published a report claiming he had discovered how to regenerate spinal cords of rats, using a unique combination of enzymes.

To be able to do so would mean new life for thousands of people paralyzed from spinal cord injuries. For years, various surgical and medical treatments have been tried. All have failed. Some scientists believe that, once interrupted, human nervous pathways can never be fully restored.

Others, such as Dr. Lloyd Guth, chairman of the Department of Anatomy at the University of Maryland and a leader in the field of neurobiology, believe that we are just beginning to discover the how and why of nerve regeneration. Guth points out that the recent isolation of nerve growth factor, a sort of insulin for nervous tissue, along with other new insights, provides the basis for slow but steady progress toward a final solution. An October 1979 symposium at the Smithsonian Institution concluded that significant progress toward understanding nerve regeneration had occurred and that, at some time in the future, paralysis might be reversible.

Many desperate paraplegics, however, find it difficult to wait for science. They seize any opportunity, no matter how premature, that might result in their walking again.

When the Soviets published Martinian's monograph and announced that his enzyme therapy was being tested on paraplegics at the Palenov Institute in Leningrad, many American paraplegics and their supporters traveled to the Soviet Union to become part of the initial group of patients. Palenov Institute in Leningrad, tried to discourage the visits. But pressure from patients and their families continued. Senators and congressmen petitioned the Soviet government. By 1975, six Americans had made the trip.

One, a young man from California, returned walking with the assistance of a walker. But at home and away from the intense physical therapy the Soviets used, he regressed. Still, armed with this one temporary success, the pressure continued, and six more Americans made the trip.

In December 1978, a thirteenth patient, Kent Waldrep, a former Texas Christian University football player who had become paralyzed in a game against Alabama in 1974, returned from the USSR able to walk with mechanical assistance. Although Waldrep admitted that most of his progress was due to the physical therapy, the twenty-five-year-old from Grand Prairie, Texas, did bring home a supply of the special enzyme, "just in case."

But by the time Waldrep returned from his forty-five-day enzyme treatment in Leningrad's Palenov Neurological Institute, the National Institute of Neurological and Communicative Disorders and Strokes (NINCDS) had already made its decision regarding the validity of the enzyme treatment. Two years before, Dr. Murray Goldstein, director of the NIH institute, had persuaded the Soviets to let Dr. Martinian come to Bethesda and review his work with NIH scientists.

"When he arrived," recalls Dr. Goldstein, "we found the technology used in his microscopic sections were pre-World War II. There was no way for us to judge his experiments as they existed."

Because of the intense public interest, the NINCDS felt they needed more proof one way or the other. They issued a contract to Dr. Guth's laboratory to independently test the Soviet work. The University of Maryland researcher hired five scientists and three technicians and spent two years attempting to duplicate Martinian's results.

"We used Martinian's enzyme technique on 120 injured animals." Guth told me in late 1978. "None walked."

What was the reason behind Martinian's success?

"It appears that he didn't really succeed in cutting the animals' spinal cords in the first place," Guth explained. "He used an old, blind technique of cord transection that's been invalid for twenty years. The experiments were scientifically inadequate and, furthermore, from what I can tell, the Soviets don't yet understand basic neurobiology."

Dr. E. Shannon Stauffer, chairman of orthopedics and rehabilitation at Southern Illinois University, believes that Waldrep's improvement was due solely to the intense physical therapy, and that it is temporary. "The Russians are thirty years behind us in facilities and thinking," he told a news reporter in 1979. "We used to do the same thing—get people into walkers. But we found that people have to stay in constant therapy to keep it up."

Waldrep disagrees. In a 1979 interview with Dennis Breo, a reporter for the American Medical Association's national newspaper, *American Medical News,* the ex-tailback said:

"The Russians offered me hope. Of course, all the American neurosurgeons and rehab people want to label it a false hope. But let me tell you, it's not a false hope. I don't think our doctors realize how important hope is for any human being in any situation, but especially in a situation like this."

Cancer—A Missed Opportunity

Rak. The word is harsh, rough, abrupt. Formed deep in the back of the throat and then rolled over the tongue, it is a sound feared by all Soviets. When the word *rak* is spoken, heads will nod and eyes will look down in sympathy. Every Russian knows that with *rak,* there is no hope.

"Just listen in on the talk in the courtyard outside your apartment building or in the office corridor during the smoking break," Dr. Guldzhan Bakhmetova wrote in the March 20, 1974, issue of *Literaturnaya Gazeta.* "You are likely to hear that cancer has been rejuvenated, that it has become more virulent, that prevention and, all the more, cure have become virtually impossible."

As the Soviet Union pulled itself into modern medical times it, like other developing countries, exchanged epidemics of typhus and cholera for cancer and heart disease. Today, cancer is a major health problem in the USSR. Similar to the U.S. experience, one of every four Soviet citizens will develop cancer and one of every five will die from it. Next to heart disease, cancer is the major disease killing American and Soviet citizens.

But the types of cancer occurring in the Soviet Union remain distinct from those found in the United States. Breast cancer, for example, is less common in the Soviet Union than in the United States. For every 1,000 Soviet women screened, an average of 2.7 cases are detected, compared to 3.4 for this country. Furthermore, the incidence of breast cancer is higher in Estonia, one of the Soviet Union's recently annexed Baltic republics, which, when compared to the rest of the Soviet Union, enjoys a higher standard of living.

Stomach cancer, a tumor often associated with a diet high in smoked, salted food, is the most common type of cancer in the USSR; in the United States it ranks seventh.

Analyzing why these differences in cancer incidence occur could provide important new insights into how environmental pollution, drugs, and other substances relate to the development of tumors. In the United States, there is controversy regarding the exact role that estrogen pills, given to reduce the symptoms of menopause, play in promoting cancer of the uterus. Estrogen pills are not available in the USSR. Comparing the number and types of cancer cases in American and Soviet women, therefore, might some day be one way of looking at the question of how estrogens promote uterine cancer.

As a first step toward examining this relationship, a joint study between the National Cancer Institute and the Harvard School of Public Health, of this country, and the Cancer Research Center in Moscow and the Institute of Experimental and Clinical Medicine in Tallinn, Estonia, is now underway. The study will compare the estrogen content in urine samples of 150 Soviet and American women.

Besides these initial chemical studies, however, there are many problems involved in comparing Soviet and American cancer statistics. When beginning the cancer program exchange, one of the first questions American scientists asked was how the Soviets collected data on their cancer cases.

For twelve months in 1974 and 1975, Dr. Paul East, a public health specialist and an expert in epidemiology (the study of disease occurrence in a population), was a visiting scientist in Moscow under the terms of the health exchange. It was East's goal to examine how the Soviets gather and report their cancer statistics.

At the end of his year, East wrote a sixty-page report detailing how he had failed to accomplish any part of his research. Today, an official with the Veterans Administration in Washington, D.C., East still maintains that the Soviets had no intention of providing him with the basic or raw data.

"I was expected to accept what the Soviets gave me without question," he recalls, "but no epidemiologist is prepared to pay attention to results unless he knows how they were obtained."

Dr. Nikolai N. Blokhin, director of the Soviet Academy of Medical Sciences Oncology Center, where East worked, was quoted at the time as saying that he resented an American "inspector" coming to check on Soviet research methods, and that there was never any agreement between the two countries on the examination of raw data.

Frustrated after a year of unfulfilled requests and broken promises, East believes that the Soviet reluctance to provide him access to their methods was another example of inappropriate secrecy. The Soviets, for their part, claimed that East spoke poor Russian and spent more time complaining than working.

Regardless of the exact details, the situation East encountered, and his reaction to it, are typical of many American scientists when they are first confronted with Soviet medical research techniques. Faced with incomplete data, the conclusion often reached is that Soviet scientists are still fighting the Cold War. The truth, as far as epidemiology is concerned, may be far less sinister. Since East's return in 1975, we have learned a great deal about how Soviets gather cancer statistics.

We now know that cancer is identified quite differently in the Soviet Union and the United States. Here, there is a population-based cancer registry which searches out all cases through its own analysis of medical records from doctors and hospitals. In the USSR, the reporting of cancer is up to the doctors who take care of the cancer patients. Although the actual effect of this difference is not scientifically established, most knowledgeable observers, such as Dr. Noel Weiss of the Department of Epidemiology, University of Washington School of Public Health, believe that it could probably lead to an underestimation of cancer incidence if doctors fail to report all their cases.

Supporting this supposition is the observation made recently by Dr. David Levin, a senior investigator at the National Cancer Institute and the American editor of a joint Soviet–American monograph on the epidemiology of cancer.

"In the early period of the exchange, the Soviets presented a paper at one of our joint meetings," Levin recalls. "It was a study giving the prevalence [number of cases] and mortality [number of deaths] with a particular type of cancer. In their conclusion, the Soviets had a larger number of mortality than prevalence.

"When we pointed out that it was impossible for more people to die from a disease than have it in the first place, they didn't understand. When we insisted that the results were impossible, they replied that those were the results and therefore they had to be right," Levin says. "They had no understanding of basic epidemiologic principles. They were complete neophytes."

According to Levin and other epidemiologists I spoke with, the progress of talks between them and their Soviet collegues always followed a standard sequence: "First, the Soviet doctors try to put their best foot forward. They tell us they have already completed a study," Levin explains. "Then, as we get down to asking for data, they say the study is only in its planning phase. Finally, after three or four meetings and hours of conversation, they admit that they haven't even begun planning the study."

In addition to properly reporting and analyzing cancer statistics, there is another problem in the USSR which makes their cancer statistics suspect. According to a study performed by two Soviet pathologists, N. G. Krovobokov and A. I. Volodikitin, in the Stravropol Regional Health Division, there is substantial error in cancer diagnosis.

The pathologists reached their conclusion after analyzing records of 4,000 autopsies. When they compared the autopsy findings with the person's medical history, they found that 20 percent of the cases had cancer which was not diagnosed before the patient died. In another 17 percent, the diagnosis of cancer made prior to death was wrong—there was no tumor present. With some tumors, such as cancer of the liver, there were as many errors in diagnosis as there were correct findings.[7]

Because of these findings, it now appears that the problem East encountered with cancer statistics is more one of substance than of secrecy. They simply did not have the knowledge and the background to conduct proper studies.

The situation with regard to basic research in cancer, while not as dismal as epidemiology, also reflects the difficulties of going it alone for so long.

Dr. Ariel Hollinshead, director of the Laboratory of Virus and

---

[7] David Levin, ed. *Cancer Epidemiology in the U.S. and U.S.S.R.* (Washington, D.C., Department of Health and Human Services, 1980).

Cancer Research at the George Washington University Medical Center in Washington, D.C., recalls what she and other cancer researchers found when they first made formal contact with their Soviet counterparts in 1968.

"They were behind in cancer research in many ways," the researcher, who was named American medical woman of the year in 1976, remembers. "The laboratories that I visited in 1973—and I'm sure we saw the best—were not well equipped. There was a heavy layer of political bureaucracy within the research institute, making it difficult for the individual researcher to do his job. Most of their scientists were unaware of current advances. Some were using laboratory techniques we'd abandoned years ago."

Despite difficult beginnings, Hollinshead, along with other Americans, enjoys her association with individual Soviet scientists and is now collaborating with them in various research projects. In 1975, Hollinshead and Dr. V. V. Gorodilova of the P. A. Hertzen Oncological Institute in Moscow published a paper in *Science,* detailing the immunologic similarities of patients with malignant melanoma (a particularly virulent form of skin cancer) in both the United States and the Soviet Union.

The work these two prominent researchers are doing involves the intricate relationship between our body's immune system and the development of cancer. Researchers in both countries now feel that human cancer develops from a delicate interaction of external factors, such as cigarette smoke or environmental pollution, and internal problems, involving a breakdown of immune surveillance. As a result, most cancer treatment today is directed at eliminating potential cancer-causing substances, while stimulating the body's immunity system into doing a better job of fighting back when cancer does occur.

Currently, there are three main ways immunotherapy is done. The first, and most specific, is by preparing vaccines from human tumor cells and then injecting them into cancer patients. The vaccine, it is hoped, will stimulate the body to produce small proteins, called antibodies, that will attack and destroy the tumor. This is known as active specific immunotherapy. Dr. Hollinshead is planning to test just such a newly developed vaccine for lung cancer patients in the USSR during 1981.

A second approach, passive or adoptive immunotherapy, involves taking blood or cells from a person with a certain kind of cancer, whose own immune system has already developed antibodies, and then transferring them to a patient currently fighting the same type of cancer. The third approach is general or nonspecific immune therapy. In this case, various compounds, or other materials which have no direct relationship to the tumor, are used to enhance the patient's ability to fight his own cancer.

Nonspecific immunotherapy had its origins in the observation that cancer patients who developed infections occasionally had remissions of their tumor. This association was first noticed near the turn of the century when Dr. William B. Coley, a New York surgeon, watched a large muscle tumor disappear after his patient developed a severe bacterial infection near the cancer site. The surgeon used this observation as the basis for a series of experiments in which he treated cancer victims with varying combinations of bacteria, often injecting them directly into a tumor.

Although innovative, Coley's work failed to produce reliable results. By the time of his death in the 1940s, scientific interest in bacterial toxin treatment was shrinking. In the postwar United States, medical attention was being directed toward other cancer-killing techniques, such as a recently discovered chemical, nitrogen mustard.

But while American scientists were discovering the value of chemotherapy, a pair of Soviet researchers announced their development of a bacterial preparation that not only stopped the growth of cancer, but actually dissolved malignant tumors. Miraculous cures for cancer have been announced before, and it is only in retrospect that this particular Soviet discovery becomes intriguing.

The preparation was known as KR, after its two developers, Nina Georgiavna Klyueva and her husband, Gregory Iosifovitch Roskin. KR was an extract made from a small bacterial organism, *Trypanosoma cruzi.*

Trypanosoma cruzi are the cause of Chagas' disease, an infectious disease found mainly in Central and South America. When a person is stung by an infected insect, the spindle-shaped trypanosomes roll their way through the bloodstream until they reach the heart, stomach, and other internal organs. Once lodged in the heart, the trypanosomes multiply and, if the infection persists, heart failure can develop.

What brought this infection to Roskin's attention was that live trypanosomes, injected into mice afflicted with experimental cancer, did not follow their usual pattern of spreading throughout the body. Instead, the trypanosomes headed straight for the animal's tumor, where they "suffocated and dissolved" the cancer.

Roskin reported his findings in the American journal *Cancer Research* in 1946, one of a very limited number of Soviet papers published during the brief postwar thaw in American-Soviet relations. In his article, Roskin not only recounted slowing and dissolving tumors in mice, he also reported the case of a forty-two-year-old man with inoperable oral cancer who, after being treated with an extract of trypanosomes, recovered enough to undergo radiation treatment and was free of tumor two years later.

The discovery of KR was also announced by Klyueva at a 1946 meeting of the Soviet Academy of Sciences in Moscow. The announcement captured the imagination and attention of the world. For a few weeks in the fall of 1946, the promise of KR was widely publicized. A headline in the October 11, 1946, issue of *The New York Times* proclaimed "Cancer Solvent Tested in Russia."

On October 26, 1946, Dr. V. V. Parin, then secretary-general of the Academy of Medical Sciences of the USSR, riding the wave of Soviet-American cooperation immediately after World War II, told a Washington, D.C., news conference that the USSR planned to spend 200 million rubles (at that time approximately $20·million) on KR research that year and 300 million the next. While Parin mentioned that it was still too early to know what the eventual place of KR would be in cancer treatment, he hoped American scientists would take a close look at the Soviet success.

Unfortunately, as has been the case with many of the miracle cures for cancer, KR treatment did not survive independent inquiry. Other scientists, attempting to duplicate Roskin's animal work, failed. They attributed part of the difficulty to Roskin's failure to use control, or untreated, animals in his experiments. Stalin reportedly was furious with the embarrassment caused by KR's failure. Roskin and Klyueva, once honored as heroes of the Soviet Republic, rapidly fell into disfavor.

Today we have a different perspective on the work of Klyueva and Roskin. Although their 1946 claim still appears scientifically premature, their methods now make sense. They form the basis of modern immunology.

By injecting the products of *Trypanosomes cruzi* into mice afflicted with experimental cancer, Klyueva and Roskin were unknowingly performing nonspecific immunotherapy—encouraging the animals' immune systems to mount a more aggressive antibody attack against the tumor. The scientific leap in understanding, from blindly injecting dead bacteria to selectively prodding the body's immune system into antitumor, antibody formation took place rapidly, in less than twenty-five years. It required the development of many new research techniques, sophisticated new instruments, a better understanding of molecular biology, and the isolation of many new substances, such as antibodies. The development of immunology is one of the most detailed and significant advances in the modern history of medicine.

Unfortunately, the Soviet medical research community failed to contribute to its growth. Despite the provocative beginning provided by Klyueva and Roskin, there was no follow-up, no integration of the clinical observation with more basic experimental work, no more international exchange of theories. After its brief postwar exposure, Stalin quickly withdrew Soviet research from the world's view.

There are other explanations for its dismal record: the enforced adherence to Pavlovian theory, the political domination and insufficient funding of most institutes, and the isolation of research from patient care.

But are conditions different today? "There has been some improvement," Hollinshead observes. "Even in the seven years of my involvement, I've seen differences in the way Soviets approach the exchange program in immunology and cancer research. The scientists coming to visit my lab are more aware of the world literature. For the most part, they're up to date on new techniques and aware of clinical applications. They want to do research and they are getting a little more money.

"There are still a lot of problems," she admits. "For one thing, the Soviets take forever to plan an experiment. They'll sit for days on end, arguing over minor points and debating how to do this or that. In the time we would have finished a project, they're still planning it, getting specific approval for every step. And then there's the problem of politics. Every so often a scientist, someone you met on a previous meeting or heard about through friends, will no longer be working. If you ask about them, no one seems to know what happened."

Research on Russians

The telephone rang in Jim Muller's apartment during dinner, March 26, 1975. Through the static he heard his Soviet assistant, Natasha, tell him that a patient with a myocardial infarction had just arrived at Moscow City Hospital No. 42. The man would be a perfect subject for the U.S.–USSR research study.

Jim quickly finished eating. He told his wife, Kathleen, not to wait up for him and kissed his children, Brian and Susan, goodbye as he put on his coat. Running down the three dark flights of stairs to the street, he said good evening to the *dezhurnaia* (manager of the apartment building) and climbed into the rented *Zhiguli* (a small Soviet-made Fiat).

The trip to the hospital took ten minutes. Jim had been driving in the Soviet capital for only a week, but he had quickly learned the rules: use your parking lights, not your headlights; stay to the extreme right; and keep up your speed at intersections. At first he had slowed down at crosswalks, only to have pedestrians stare at him for this unexpected courtesy.

When Jim arrived at the hospital, his heart beat quickened and his palms began to sweat. After nearly three weeks of haggling with Soviet Customs officials to release the special electrocardiographic equipment, pleading for a telephone for his apartment, and fighting with Intourist for his own car, he was about to accomplish his purpose for being in the Soviet Union. He was entering his first heart attack victim into the carefully negotiated scientific study that would help determine whether an old drug, hyaluronidase, could be used for a new purpose, reducing the severity of heart attacks.

B. A. Petrov, a sixty-five-year-old factory worker with muscular arms and a barrel-shaped chest, lay on his back, his six-and-a-half-foot frame spilling over the small iron bed. His bright-red face was covered with sweat and he moaned softly, periodically bringing his arm across his chest as if to massage his injured heart.

Valya, the physician on duty in the coronary care unit, told Jim that Petrov had been suffering from angina for a month. That very morning he had gone to his factory's polyclinic complaining of chest pain. At that time the electrocardiogram (EKG) had been normal. But at 3 P.M. he had returned with another, more severe attack. This time the EKG had distorted complexes with massive elevation—the diagnostic hallmark of a heart attack.

Even now, four hours and three injections of narcotic later, pain from the dying segment of Petrov's heart muscle was so severe that he begged for another injection.

While the nurse ran to get the drug, Jim looked around and found that Natasha, a Soviet *aspirant* (fellow) in cardiology assigned to assist him with the research, had everything ready. The tubes for collecting the blood samples were carefully laid out on the windowsill. In her hands, Ntasha held the small, square blanket fitted with thirty-five metal electrodes that would be placed over the patient's chest. When connected to a standard EKG machine, the specially designed blanket would produce a cardiogram with thirty-five different channels, compared to the usual twelve. By examining information from the thirty-five channels, Jim would be able to plot precisely how large an area of heart muscle was being deprived of blood flow and undergoing infarction.

The technique, called electrocardiographic mapping, because it plots and measures the area under each ST elevation,[8] had been developed by Drs. Peter Maroko and Eugene Braunwald of Harvard Medical School. Since the late 1960s, Braunwald, a professor of medicine and department chairman at Harvard, had been experimenting with different ways to reduce the size of infarcts. Braunwald's and Maroko's experimental work was based on the hypothesis that the amount of heart muscle damaged when a blockage develops in one of the coronary arteries is not fixed at the moment of infarction. Instead, the destruction spreads in an ever-widening circle as the waste products of the initial injury poison neighboring heart muscle cells.

Limiting the size of this circle (Braunwald refers to the center as the zone of injury, with the perimeter being the fringe, or watershed, area) could reduce the number of serious complications, such as heart failure, that follow large infarctions.

[8] ST refers to a part of the electrocardiogram tracing that is elevated when damage to the heart muscle occurs.

Since developing this theory, Maroko, a young cardiologist, and Braunwald have used various techniques aimed at keeping the circle as small as possible. Hyaluronidase, an enzyme found in the testicles of mammals, was their latest means. By increasing the blood and oxygen supply to the heart, hyaluronidase theoretically might limit the size of infarctions. In experiments on dogs with artificially produced infarcts, the drug had done just that.

After the dog experiments, Maroko and Braunwald received permission from the U.S. Food and Drug Administration to use the old drug in this new way on humans. A study of thirteen patients, published April 1975 in the *Annals of Internal Medicine,* suggested a beneficial effect. The ST elevations decreased faster in those patients receiving hyaluronidase than in a similar group of controls.

After publication of the *Annals* article, continuing evaluation of hyaluronidase in Boston was going slowly. The problem was that, to be effective, hyaluronidase must be given within a few hours of a heart attack. The experiment was based at Peter Bent Brigham, a specialized hospital which does not receive many patients with new infarctions. Most new heart attack victims are taken to smaller community hospitals near their homes. Because most of the hospitals were not research institutions, a carefully controlled scientific study was not possible. But without more evidence that the enzyme worked in humans, the National Institutes of Health was unwilling to support a larger test, which would be necessary before hyaluronidase could be approved for general use.

The idea of using Soviet patients as part of a hyaluronidase study was conceived at a 1974 international cardiology symposium in Ponte Verde, Florida. Attending were Braunwald, Jim Muller, who was a junior member of Braunwald's department, and Dr. E. I. Chazov, Deputy Minister of Health of the USSR and director of the Myasnikov Cardiology Institute in Moscow.

The Soviets, by virtue of a centralized emergency medical transport system, quickly take most heart attack victims to a few large city hospitals. Thus, finding enough patients soon after their heart attacks in Moscow should not be a problem, Chazov told Braunwald.

Moreover, Jim was ideally suited to direct the project. A cardiologist, he had worked in Braunwald's laboratory for the past two years. He spoke Russian well and had twice visited the USSR, once as a medical student from Johns Hopkins and again as a member of the official U.S. delegation that set up the 1972 Health Exchange Agreement between the United States and USSR.

Jim's thoughts briefly touched on these personal and international milestones as he stood in the coronary care unit (CCU) of Moscow City Hospital No. 42. It was a long, nearly empty room. Compared to the CCUs back home, it was barren, containing none of the specialized monitoring and safety equipment that continuously record and store every heart beat, blood pressure rise, and temperature change occurring in the critical twenty-four to seventy-two hours after an infarction.

Moscow City Hospital No. 42's CCU had eight beds, two EKG machines, a nursing station, and a small, metal drug cabinet. Jim reached through its door for a container of salt water, which he would use to improve conduction between Petrov's skin and the thirty-five metal electrodes of the EKG blanket.

As he did, Natasha plugged in a German-made EKG machine.

When Jim attached the EKG map to the German machine, however, the recording was filled with tagged electrical interference, making it impossible to interpret the tracing. Valya recognized the problem. She placed one hand on the patient's shoulder, the other on the bed's iron-rail headboard. Acting as a human grounding mechanism, she eliminated the interference and finished the EKG.

Throughout the EKG, Petrov continued to moan softly and jerk uncomfortably from side to side. One of the nurses gruffly told him to lie still. "We're doing this for your good, not ours," she snapped. Valya told her to leave him alone, he was a sick man.

Jim took the completed tracing back to the nursing station to examine it carefully. Normal ST segments are flat. These were grossly distorted, raised four millimeters from their baseline. As Jim began to measure the total area enclosed by the ST elevations, he heard Natasha call desperately for help. Valya and the two nurses ran to Petrov's bed. The four of them tried to turn the heavy factory worker onto his back. (Natasha had rolled him over on his side so that she could listen to his heart.)

When Jim arrived at the bedside, he could see that the old man's face was blue, his teeth clenched shut from a seizure caused by a lack of oxygen to his brain. Jim put his hand on the man's groin, searching for a femoral pulse. There was none. Petrov's heart was fibrillating.

While Valya tried to attach a regular EKG, Jim called for the defibrillator. The nurse handed him a large, steel paddle covered with a wet towel. He shoved it under Petrov's back. He was handed another paddle for the chest. Jim asked Natasha if she wanted to apply the electrical charge herself. She did not. Jim held the top paddle on Petrov's chest as the 300 watt-seconds of electricity snapped between the two paddles and through Petrov's heart. His body jerked in response, but there was no return of the femoral pulse.

Jim handed the paddle back to the nurse and began cardiopulmonary resuscitation, pumping on the old man's chest, his palm over the sternum near the red circle where the defibrillator paddle had burned the skin. Valya tried to open Petrov's mouth, but his teeth was still tightly clenched. He was turning blue. There was no blood pressure.

The nurse handed the defibrillator paddle back to Jim, telling him the machine was recharged at a higher voltage. The 400 watt-second charge worked, returning a strong femoral pulse and restoring Petrov's blood pressure. Color returned to his face and he groaned softly. His EKG returned to a fast but normal rhythm.

Jim suggested that Petrov now be given lidocaine, an anesthetic drug used intravenously to numb the heart muscle and prevent a second episode of fibrillation. But Moscow City Hospital No. 42 had no lidocaine. A substitute drug, procainamide, was found, while Natasha went to the Myasnikov Heart Institute for the lidocaine.

As things settled down, Jim collected the EKG and made sure he had the blood sample. By a randomized card process, he had already decided that Petrov would not receive hyaluronidase but would serve as a control patient. When the study was complete, patients receiving hyaluronidase would be compared with the controls to see if the drug really did limit the size of infarctions.

Valya suggested that Jim might want to leave, because the coronary care unit would soon be crowded; Petrov's sister, who was the head doctor at another Moscow hospital, and a number of consultants were expected at any moment.

Jim joined Natasha, who had returned from Myasnikov with the lidocaine, and Oleg, a cardiologist. They sat in the chief resident's office, drinking tea and nibbling small pieces of red fish and black bread. Jim explained that the study protocol called for three more thirty-five-channel EKGs, one at two hours, one at six hours, and one at twenty-four hours after the first tracing. If hyaluronidase was to have an effect, it would be within this critical first day after infarction. Although Petrov was a control, it would still be necessary to have the EKGs taken at these times.

Jim slept at the hospital that night to make sure everything was done. When he awoke at seven the next morning, a nurse gave him a piece of white cheese soaked in sour milk and a container of *kifir* (yogurt) to eat.

Driving back to his two-room apartment through the cold, misty March morning, Jim felt tired but happy. Ever since his first trip to Russia, he had felt a need to do more than just be a good doctor; he saw his present work, the hyaluronidase project, as a small step in that direction.

Jim's interest in Russia began when he was a student at Notre Dame. During the early 1960s, Russian language training was still common among undergraduates; Jim took a course from a kind, patient Russian professor who provided him with a firm foundation in the language.

After entering Johns Hopkins Medical School, Jim attended a lecture by Dr. Russell Nelson, president of Johns Hopkins Hospital. Nelson described his recent visit to the Soviet Union. Impressed by the man and his experience, Jim resolved to spend part of his elective time in the USSR.

While making plans to apply to the student exchange program between the United States and USSR, Jim reacted to the pressures of medical training by becoming more and more isolated. He spent most evenings alone, studying pathology, physiology, and biochemistry and preparing for his trip to Moscow. During the day, he went to class and began making rounds in the hospital. He felt clumsy around patients. He felt out of place around residents and interns, who spent all their time talking about medicine.

Like many young people in the late 1960s, Jim began to spend more and more time thinking about the problem of world peace. The young medical student began to see disease, the kind he studied in pathology and saw on the wards of Johns Hopkins, as important individual problems, but he began to recognize another equally important threat to the human condition. He found the problem of nuclear arms proliferation elusive, far harder to comprehend than the diagnostic criteria for rheumatic fever but also more challenging. When he walked into the hospital's emergency room, he wondered what it would be like after a nuclear war. The burned bodies, the nausea and vomiting, the thousands, perhaps millions, of victims. Soon, thoughts of nuclear war dominated his thinking. Conversation about other things—classes, sports, dating—all seemed trivial by comparison.

He began reading books on the arms race. One, *The Arrogance of Power* by Senator William Fulbright, seemed to crystallize what Jim felt. There was one phrase on Soviet-American relations that seemed aimed directly at him: "The only way in which nations will eventually get along is after they have developed habits of cooperation by work in non-controversial areas of common interest." Jim saw his interest in the USSR and his commitment to medicine as an important part of the process Fulbright was writing about.

In 1968, Jim spent three months of his junior year as a student in the First Moscow Medical School as the first American medical student to participate in the official student exchange. The experience increased his interest in and knowledge of the Soviet system. When, two years later, the official U.S. health delegation to the USSR needed a translator, Jim, then a Public Health Service officer, was chosen.

It was in this capacity that, in 1970, he accompanied HEW Assistant Secretary for Health, Dr. Roger Egberg, to the Black Sea for talks with Soviet Health Minister Dr. Boris Petrovsky. A year later, Jim helped draft the first formal, five-year Health Agreement between the two superpowers. It was because of that agreement that he now was working in Moscow.

The next day, March 27, there were no phone calls. Jim returned to No. 42 in the evening to do the twenty-four-hour tracing on Petrov. The old man looked pale and exhausted, but his pain was gone. He thanked Jim for saving his life and promised he would never forget him. He also said he had no plans to return to the factory. "It's too much work, someone always wants to overfill our factory's quota."

As part of the study, Jim had to know each of the drugs given the Soviet patients. It took a long time to figure out the eighteen differ-

ent drugs Petrov had received. Unlike a typical heart attack patient
in the United States, on whom few routine drugs are used, the Soviets order a combination of traditional herbal preparations, tranquilizers, vitamins, and blood thinners for most myocardial infarct
patients.

But Jim had lots of time. The remainder of March was quiet. No
more telephone calls. No patients.

Jim used the time to get better settled. He enrolled Brian, four,
and Susan, six, in the closest *detskii sad* (nursery school). He paid a
courtesy call on the American Embassy, where he met Dr. Igon
Loebner, the scientific counselor. Loebner suggested that Jim tell
the story of his project to one of the American reporters assigned to
Moscow, maybe even grant an interview to CBS television.

Jim felt nervous about seeking publicity. He had wanted to write
a story, perhaps a book, about his experiences in the Soviet Union,
stressing his hopes for world peace. The story would be out of his
control if he gave it to a reporter. But his research did need better
financial support back home. If a story could help to generate more
funding to support more patients, then it would be worth the risk.

But foremost in Jim's mind now was finding out why there were
no telephone calls. He was concerned about the slow pace of the
study. On April 1, he drove to the Myasnikov Cardiology Institute
to see Dr. Nikoloeva, a Soviet cardiologist he had met in Ponte
Verde. Jim suggested that the *skoraya pomoshch* (emergency ambulance system) might be instructed to bring all patients with new
myocardial infarctions to the six hospitals participating in the study.

As if in response to his request, the telephone interrupted their
conversation. It was Hospital No. 42; they had another patient.
When Jim arrived at the hospital he let Olga, the doctor on duty,
pick the card that would determine whether or not the patient received hyaluronidase. The card read hyaluronidase. Jim shook
Olga's hand. Everyone was excited about using the drug for the first
time in the Soviet Union.

Before injecting the hyaluronidase intravenously, Jim did a skin
test. The introduction of a few drops of hyaluronidase immediately
under the skin would demonstrate whether the patient was allergic.
In two minutes, the site of injection on the patient's forearm had
swollen and turned an angry red—a positive test. The patient could
not receive hyaluronidase. He would have to be a control.

Since the percent of allergic reactions to hyaluronidase in the United States was less than 1 percent, Jim wondered if something was wrong with the batch he had brought to the USSR. The drug had to be stored in a cool place. While staying in London, Jim had even stored it in the hotel's wine cellar.

More frightening than a spoiled batch was the remote possibility that the entire Soviet population might be allergic to hyaluronidase. Before being permitted to bring the drug to the Soviet Union, Jim had submitted samples, along with the records of the animal and human studies submitted to the Federal Drug Administration.

Since the Soviets had never used hyaluronidase for infarcts, the drug had to clear the Soviet drug inspection process as well. In fact, waiting for Soviet approval had delayed Jim's departure from the United States for ten days. Now he wasn't sure whether he would ever be able to give hyaluronidase to a Soviet patient.

The answer came a day later. On Thursday, April 3, Jim was called to City Hospital No. 63. The patient was a seventy-five-year-old man, a Tatar. Natasha wanted to give him hyaluronidase regardless of what the card said, but Jim insisted they stick to scientific protocol.

While the Soviet physician struggled to start an intravenous (there was only one dull needle available in the CCU and the doctor had trouble piercing the skin), Jim picked the card—hyaluronidase! This time the preliminary skin test was negative, and the Soviets proceeded to draw the blood tests needed before giving the drug.

But there was another problem—the blood kept clotting before it could be properly centrifuged. Jim decided to put more anticoagulant in the collection tubes. Because later blood samples were needed, Jim gave the Soviet doctor some extra anticoagulant. The only container available for the powder was a used perfume bottle.

Further complicating the preparations was the crude hand-cranked centrifuge. Fortunately, Jim had brought an electric American model with him. Within a few hours, the preparations were completed and the first dose of hyaluronidase to be used in the USSR was given. There were no problems.

The next morning, Jim received a call from Sklifosofsky Hospital, another of the six centers assigned to the study. Built 180 years ago by Count Sheremetiev, a wealthy Moscow landowner, Sklifosofsky, named for a famous nineteenth-century Russian surgeon, is an odd mixture of the very old and the almost new. The main reception room is decorated with a huge antique crystal chandelier, ornate plastic wall moldings, and portraits of Lenin, Marx, and Brezhnev. Some floors are green marble, others vinyl tile.

Because of its age, more than half of Sklifosofsky was undergoing *remont* (renovation), as the ubiquitous Soviet signs proclaimed. To get to the CCU, Jim had to walk through hallways crowded with ladders and construction equipment. When he found the door leading directly to the unit, it was closed, and he had to walk around the hospital twice to find the right entrance.

When he finally arrived, he found that two heart attack patients had been brought in the night before. Both infarctions were now too old (over eight hours) to enter into the study. The doctor in charge said he hadn't wanted to call Jim late at night. Jim explained that he always wanted to be called, regardless of the time.

But the next call was not until Sunday, April 6, and not from Sklifosofsky, but from Hospital No. 42. The patient was a sixty-year-old, matronly looking Russian woman. It was her first infarction. The envelope specified hyaluronidase and Olga gave her the injection. Like every hyaluronidase patient, she received the drug every six hours for the first two days.

Jim had been in Moscow now for two weeks and had enrolled only four patients in the study, two hyaluronidase and two controls. Plans called for him to remain in the Soviet capital for eight more weeks. If the number of patients did not increase soon, the goal of fifty patients would not be reached.

After the weekened, the pace began to improve. One patient was added on Monday and another on Tuesday. At 3:30 Wednesday morning, a third call came. This time the doctors at Sklifosofsky had not hesitated to call at night.

The patient, an old, bearded peasant from Uzbekistan, had been in Moscow visiting his son and developed chest pains while eating dinner. It was a large infarction, extending across the entire anterior surface of his heart muscle. The old man was having trouble breathing; fluid was backing up in his lungs. His injured heart was unable to keep up its normal pumping action.

There are two major reasons people die from heart attacks. The first is an acute injury to the heart which makes the muscle irritable, as had been the case with Petrov. The area of infarction is like a fresh, raw sore and it can act as a focus for ventricular fibrillation—a life-threatening disturbance in the heart's normal rhythm. In a few days the infarct, or scar, heals and the risk of fibrillation decreases. In recent years, the routine use of lidocaine has reduced the frequency of fibrillation.

"Pump failure" is the second reason heart attacks are fatal. When the area of heart muscle destroyed by an infarction is large enough, the heart loses its ability to push blood out of the lungs to the head, kidneys, and other vital parts of the body. Unlike the risk of fibrillation, "pump failure" does not decrease with time. As more and more infarctions develop, or as the size of a single infarction spreads, a patient is more and more likely to develop irreversible cardiogenic shock or "pump failure."

Reducing the number of patients who develop pump failure is what the Soviet–American study of hyaluronidase was all about. From their experiments on animals, the Harvard group believed that hyaluronidase increased the blood flow to the injured heart muscle, thereby decreasing the size of the infarction and avoiding shock. If the drug proved successful, it could do for pump failure what lidocaine did for fibrillation.

Since the patient from Uzbekistan was already suffering from pulmonary edema, the first sign of pump failure, the Soviet doctor urged Jim to use hyaluronidase on him.

Jim objected, pointing out that the only way to scientifically test the drug was not to choose patients who might benefit (and then credit their survival to the treatment), but to randomly give the drug to two groups and then compare their overall survival.

At first, the Soviets did not seem to appreciate the need for strict controls in the research project. In fact, Jim recalled a long conversation he had had with a Soviet physician who was conducting his own experiment on reducing infarct size. In that study all patients who could not be given the drug (in this case a blood-thinner) because of other medical problems were being used as the comparison or control group. When Jim explained that the process introduced a selection basis which might prejudice the study's results, he was told that the Soviets do all their experiments in this way.

In the case of the peasant from Uzbekistan, however, Jim insisted that they stick to the rules. The envelope chosen said control and he was not given hyaluronidase.

In one of the many discussions that Jim had with the Soviets regarding the possible action of hyaluronidase and how experiments to test its action should be designed, he was criticized for acting superior. After all, he was reminded, Russian physicians had been the first to describe nonfatal heart attacks.

The claim surprised Jim. Like most U.S. medical students, he had been taught that an American, James Herrick, was the first to report a patient surviving a heart attack. Prior to Herrick's 1912 paper, it was universally taught that any severe block developing in the three pencil-sized coronary arteries that supply the heart muscle with blood would immediately kill the victim.

The Soviets claimed that in 1910 two Russian physicians, V. P. Obraztsov, a professor of pathology at the University of Kiev, and his student, N. D. Strazhesko, had described five patients who had the characteristic crushing, substernal chest pain which we now associate with a myocardial infarction. All five survived the episode.

Furthermore, in their 1910 discussion, the two Russian scientists noted that both physical and mental stress played an important role. "The infarct began in one case while climbing a steep staircase; in another, during an unpleasant conversation; and in a third, during emotional distress associated with a heated card game," read the original paper.

Confused, Jim had a copy of Herrick's original article sent to him. He found that the Soviets were right; Herrick mentioned a German translation of the Russian paper in his discussion of nonfatal heart attacks.

There were no patients during the rest of the week. On Saturday night, Jim and Kathleen went to the home of Peter Osnos, then Moscow correspondent for *The Washington Post*. Kathleen had met Susan Osnos at the embassy, and the dinner was their idea.

Jim was nervous throughout the evening. Osnos asked him questions about the project and requested that he be given an exclusive on the story. Jim was not sure how to react. He was still uncomfortable with publicity and fearful of the Soviet reaction. In the end, after Osnos suggested that a story in the *Post* would do the most good for everyone concerned, Jim agreed.

The tension of the meeting and the pressure of the study caught up with Jim that night. He was nauseated when they got home.

The next week went by slowly; only two patients were added.

On Wednesday, Dr. Maroko called from Boston, wanting to know the progress of the study. Jim explained the difficulties he had had in getting trust and cooperation from the dozens of Soviet doctors at the six hospitals, the problem of getting them to call him in time to get the EKGs and blood tests, and the fact Jim was not permitted to start an experiment unless a Soviet member of the research team was also present. Considering the problems with everyone from Customs agents to nurses, and the inherent suspicion most Soviets have toward foreigners, the fact that the study was underway at all was a major accomplishment. But now Maroko and Jim were interested now in the bottom line—the number of patients. At the present rate, the study might not reach its desired goal.

Toward the end of April, the weather in Moscow began to change, with warmer air replacing the strong, cold, north wind. It rained almost continually and the long gray days futher depressed Jim. Three or four days would go by between patients. He had little to do.

On Monday, April 28, Jim attended a medical conference at the Myasnikov Cardiology Institute. The Soviets were preparing for two of their biggest celebrations—the thirtieth anniversary of the end of World War II (May 9) and International Worker's Day (May 1).

At the conference, speakers described the medical organization and first aid preparation accomplished in Moscow during the war. Jim noticed that most of the audience were reading books, talking, or involved in completing charts so they could get an early start on the holiday. The speeches were largely ignored. As May Day approached, normal hospital routine also slowed and there were even fewer calls.

Then, on April 30, Jim got a call from Intourist asking for return of his car. There was a standard requirement, it seemed, that all cars rented to tourists had to be returned for the holidays. Jim would have his car back on May 10. He was furious. It had taken delicate negotiations to arrange for the car in the first place, and without it, successful completion of the study was impossible. As he was thinking how to convince Intourist that his case was special, there was a knock on the door.

Two men, the *dezhurnaia* (manager) of the apartment building told him, were in the parking lot to pick up his car. When Jim arrived, the two men, dressed in dark brown raincoats, told him to empty the equipment from the car. Jim protested, with help from the *dezhurnaia*. She explained how Jim had to work at night, when it was impossible to get a taxi. The two men said they were under orders, however, and they left with Jim's only form of transportation.

During the remainder of the day, Jim fought a frustrating verbal battle with the Intourist bureaucracy. Beginning at the lowest level, Jim quickly found it impossible to find anyone willing to discuss his problem. He turned for help to the Myasnikov Institute and Dr. Chazov. Chazov transferred the request to a cabinet-level official, Dimitri Venediktov, First Deputy minister of the USSR Ministry of Health. With Chazov's and Venediktov's help, Jim was called back to the Intourist office at the Hotel Ukraina at 5 P.M. There, the same men who had taken the car that morning handed him, with their apologies, the keys to a new Zhiguli.

On May Day, Jim got a call from Hospital No. 42. He drove his new car there, being careful to avoid the center of town and parading workers. He made a wrong turn, however, and ran directly into a line of workers carrying a fifteen-foot-high-poster of Lenin and carrying a banner proclaiming "Communism is our future."

When he finally arrived at No. 42, only a skeleton staff was on duty. He and Natasha took the EKG, performed the blood tests, and gave the patient hyaluronidase. This brought the total number of patients to nineteen.

May 5 was a busy day. At 6 A.M. a call came from the Sklifosofsky Institute about a patient. In the afternoon, Jim was to accompany the American Embassy's scientific attaché and physician on a tour of the Myasnikov Institute. Of the six hospitals at which Jim worked, the coronary care unit at the Myasnikov was by far the best equipped. All of the monitoring equipment was American made and the staff knew how to use most of it. During the tour, Dave Millet, then the embassy physician, wanted to know why Americans with heart attacks were not taken here, instead of Botkin, a hospital without a CCU. The question embarrassed Jim, for there was no way that he or the Soviet doctors he worked with could answer it.

Jim felt that many of the Americans he had met, especially those associated with the embassy, wanted Soviet medicine to be exactly like theirs. Differences never seemed to be accepted as simply that, but were always judged as deficiencies. Very few Americans, Jim thought, regarded the study as he did—a small but important step toward reducing tensions between the two countries. It was as if Americans in Moscow preferred tension to adaptation.

Jim spent the May 9 holiday at Hospital 63, enrolling two new patients. One of them, an elderly Russian told Jim he had been at the Elbe meeting of American and Soviet troops. He asked Jim why there was not free medical care in the United States, commenting "It'd be better than spending all that money in Vietnam."

That night, as part of the holiday observance, Soviet Premier Leonid Brezhnev spoke to the country on nationwide television. He stressed the need for countries with different social systems to work together to keep world peace. Brezhnev mentioned that the Saigon government had collapsed nine days ago and that this "removal of friction" could ease tension with the United States and encourage more peace.

Watching the hospital TV set, Jim noticed how tired the sixty-three-year-old premier looked, how he spoke with a lisp, and how the camera would show only the right side of his face. After his speech, a young Soviet school girl recited a poem: "We are the flowers of life—let there be peace so we can bloom." Brezhnev, along with many of the patients, cried.

After the holidays, Jim was much busier. More patients became available and cooperation seemed to improve. There was an international cardiology conference at Sochi in the Ukrainian USSR to attend. The embassy had decided to let Peter Osnos write an exclusive story and there would be a joint Soviet-American news conference at the end of June, the conclusion of Jim's stay. Jim was scheduled to present a formal talk on the study to the staff at Sklifosofsky. In addition, he and Kathleen were planning a party for all of the Soviet doctors who had worked on the project.

These events quickly took Jim out of the world of medicine and into that of international diplomacy and politics. Things did not go well. For example, many of the Soviet doctors Jim asked to be interviewed by Osnos were suspicious of an American reporter coming into their hospital, "Aren't all your reporters told to write sensational stories to sell papers?" Natasha asked. Some of the friends Jim had made turned down the invitation to visit his apartment. Chazov said he would be out of town. The conference at Sochi went badly; Dr. Nikolaeva, a Soviet cardiologist who had been especially kind to

Jim during the study, was attacked by two American scientists because a study she presented did not have proper controls.

When Jim returned to Moscow and took Osnos on a tour of the Myasnikov Institute, all the Soviet physicians were tense. Many seemed unwilling or unable to talk. The tour of Sklifosofsky went better. Jim gave his presentation, talking in Russian without notes. He ended his speech with a quote from Sklifosovsky: "Science only develops when there is cooperation from people of all countries."

The next week, as Jim began making plans to leave, he stopped to visit Petrov, his first patient. After two months, he was still in the hospital. The Soviets usually hospitalize heart attack patients for eight weeks, compared to the two or three week maximum in the United States.

As Jim walked into the room the old man smiled, shook his hand, and thanked him for his help. Petrov had one of the few semiprivate rooms in Hospital No. 42. Two vases of flowers sat on the window ledge. He wore a bright blue, terrycloth robe. Through its opening, Jim could see the angry red circles on his chest, left by the defibrillator.

They talked about that first night. Jim explained to Petrov how his heart had stopped, how he had responded to electrical shock, and the fact that the danger of more episodes of ventricular fibrillation was now past.

Petrov stood up, slowly stretching himself to his full six-and-a-half-foot height. "You've given me the dearest present possible," he said solemnly, "life." Then he grabbed Jim around the shoulder, pulled him toward him, and kissed his cheek.

Jim felt honored by such intimacy, but he was careful to explain that Soviet doctors helped to save him, too. "If I hadn't been there, I'm sure they would have done the same thing," Jim told him.

Peter Osnos's *Washington Post* article was published on Sunday, June 9. In the United States, the article attracted widespread interest, being carried by many papers outside Washington. On Monday, Jim spoke to Loebner, the science attaché. Loebner was upset, claiming that Osnos quoted him when he should not have. He told Jim it had not been a good idea to give the *Post* an exclusive.

On Wednesday, Jim met with Chazov. Just a week earlier, the high-ranking Soviet cardiologist had told Jim that all the problems with the study thus far had been minor, that he was pleased with their progress. He had even warned Jim not to appear too "pro-Soviet." "Despite being physicians, we still have our own countries," he said.

Today, Chazov was less supportive. He asked Jim whether he was sad about what his friend Osnos wrote. Chazov did not like the article's suggestion that an American physician was experimenting and trying out a new drug on Soviet patients. He did not like the idea that while private doctors in America refused to give their patients hyaluronidase, Soviets were getting the drug.

"We did start with American patients." Jim tried to explain. But Chazov was upset and the meeting ended abruptly.

When Jim got home, the problems continued. Natasha called to ask what had happened with Petrov. "You didn't tell him he was reanimated?" she demanded.

"Well, yes," Jim stammered. "I said his heart had stopped."

"You're so stupid and undiplomatic," she shot back. "Don't you know people's hearts have stopped again when they've been told that? I wouldn't be surprised if they never call us with another patient," she shouted. "You've ruined everything."

Natasha's prediction did not come true. There were other patients. But Jim's time in Moscow rapidly came to an end and the animosity caused by the *Washington Post* article put a final edge on many of the friendships he had cultivated during the project. Although uncontoversial in the United States, Osnos's precise description of the project conflicted with traditional Soviet journalism.

"The article is terrible," Alek, one of the Soviet doctors, told Jim. "Many Soviet physicians helped you, and they are not mentioned."

"It's as if you're using Soviet patients as guinea pigs," another said. "And look at this line, 'Such are the cultural differences.' Does this mean Soviets are barbarians?"

Most of the reactions were the same, a mixture of resentment and misunderstanding. Some physicians told Jim that the Soviet system, where the scientist has to sign the article before it appears, would have avoided these problems.

There was a final news conference for American and Soviet reporters. Chazov summarized the work in the hyaluronidase study and presented results of the Soviets' own research technique, which used blood thinner to reduce the severity of infarctions. Jim attended the conference, but did not speak.

He returned to Boston at the end of June, with records from twenty-four Soviet heart attack victims, twelve hyaluronidase and twelve controls. These were added to sixty-seven American patients and controls, and on April 24, 1977, the results of the hyaluronidase study were reported in the *New England Journal of Medicine*.

Jim was the third of eighteen authors, three Soviets and fifteen Americans. The results from the ninety-one patients, some of whom came from Brazil, Belgium, and Italy, suggested that the enzyme did reduce the EKG signs of heart muscle damage. The study's conclusion, which would not have been as convincing without the large number of Soviet patients, was encouraging enough for the National Heart, Lung, and Blood Institute in 1978 to begin a $7 million, five-center, three-and-one-half-year study. The study will test hyaluronidase and another drug, propanolol, in 1,500 patients. Eugene Braunwald is the principal investigator and Jim Muller is the project's main coordinator.

5

Women and Children

The Soviet doctor is a character unprecedented in the history of medicine. His undoubted superiority over the doctor in capitalist countries stands out clearly. . . . He bases his relations with the sick man on the perfectly concrete principles of humanitarian Soviet medical science, to prevent disease, to treat patients and return them to work. . . . The Soviet doctor is proudly aware that he is practicing a truly humanitarian medicine, which in a socialist state serves all without exception, not just the select few as is the case in capitalist countries.
—G. S. Pondev in *Notes of a Soviet Doctor*, 1959

We shall be fighting the evils of bureaucracy for many years to come, and whoever thinks otherwise is playing demagogue and cheating, because overcoming the evils of bureaucracy requires hundreds of measures.
—V. I. Lenin, *Draft Program of The Russian Communist Party*, 1919

Four in the morning. Tamara pushes herself from the sofa and begins another day. She folds her blanket and carefully places it in the crowded closet. Shivering in the early morning cold, she takes off her nightgown and forces her plump, swelling body into a torn, yellowed slip.

In darkness, she finds her dark-blue skirt, woolen sweater, and black plastic boots. Pushing aside the blanket that serves as a divider between her and her sleeping son, she walks quietly into the kitchen and switches on the light above a small, cracked mirror.

Blinking, she stares at her reflection. Her color is an unhealthy red. There are sleep lines crossing her cheek. Her skin is doughy. She runs a rough hand over her face, as though trying to erase all the imperfections at once. She bends over the kitchen sink and splashes cold water on her face. She runs a comb through her short, coarse, matted hair, trying to cover up the dark-brown roots that are beginning to show through the artificial red color. With great care, she puts on bright red lipstick and blue eyeshadow.

After starting the teakettle, she opens the apartment door to see if the bathroom at the end of the hall is available. Quickly finishing her toilet, she hurries back to the small kitchen and huddles near the stove, waiting for the tea water to boil. She cuts off three slices of dark bread and spreads them with plum jelly. She sits at the kitchen table chewing slowly, staring out the window at the foggy, deserted street. She finishes breakfast with a cigarette, inhaling deeply between sips of strong, dark tea.

In a few minutes she will have to leave for work. Tamara's shift at the factory begins at 6 A.M. and the bus ride takes an hour. Putting on her coat in the hallway, she looks in on Kolia, her son, sleeping fitfully in his small bed. She checks the adjacent chair where she has laid out his trousers, sweater, hat, and coat. Yesterday, Tamara's mother told her, Kolia had refused to wear his hat to the *detskii sad* (nursery school).

Being careful not to wake her sleeping parents, Tamara wraps a scarf around her head, picks up her bag, and quietly leaves the apartment.

She walks three blocks to the bus stop, her breath frosty on this cold November morning. The bus appears suddenly out of the darkness, its weak yellow lights jerking over the rough streets of Tula, a town about 125 miles from Moscow, famous for its metalworks. Tamara pulls herself aboard, drops fifteen kopecks in the fare box, and takes the seat closest to the driver. She puts her handbag on her lap, stretching her arms across her swollen abdomen, and reviews what she must do today.

After work she will go to the *zhenskii konsultatsii* (women's consultation center). It will be the first time she has seen a doctor since the visit five months ago, when the gynecologist convinced her not to have another abortion.

"Of course," Tamara thinks bitterly, "it was easy then, when Victor was still living with me, to talk about another child, to say that three was 'ideal.' " Five months ago there had even been talk about the three of them getting their own apartment.

But now Victor is gone, living someplace in Moscow, and unless he stops drinking, Tamara refuses to let her husband come back. No, she thinks, staring resolutely out the window, she would rather stay with her parents, despite their crowded apartment, than put up with the drinking, shouting, and constant fighting that marked her marriage for the past few months.

But how much easier it would be, she thinks, if only she were not seven months pregnant. If only she had gone ahead with the abortion. After all, it would only have been her fourth. Four abortions are not that many. Why, some of the women at work have had eight, even ten.

The bus comes to Tamara's stop just as the first light of the sunrise appears over the flat, snow-covered horizon. At the factory, Tamara exchanges greetings with the other women as she puts a dark-blue laboratory coat over her clothes. She begins sorting through a large pile of metal forms that, once stamped and molded, will be the factory's main product, electric irons. When Tamara first became pregnant, she asked for a transfer to another job in the factory, one where she would not have to do much lifting and bending. After all, official work policy gives Soviet women the right to such a transfer without jeopardizing their job or work record. But Tamara's factory manager told her there were no other jobs available.

"Oh well," Tamara sighs as she bends over to pick up the first form. In a week she will be on maternity leave. And this time she will take the entire 112 days to which she's entitled—two months before and two months after delivery. When Kolia was born, Tamara went back to work in two weeks "because they needed me." Maybe, she thinks, she will not go back to work for a while. She will stay home and be a mother.

Tamara works until 2 P.M., when she takes a bus to the clinic. There, she has to wait in line for an hour for an admission card, and finally, at 3:30, just before the clinic is scheduled to close, she is shown into a *kabinet*. The *vrach*, a gynecologist, begins to ask her questions. How many children? Was there any problem with your delivery? How many abortions? The questions run on. Then, "How much weight did you gain?" Tamara hesitates. She knows her weight is too high, but she doesn't want a lecture. Maybe she could hedge a bit. Finally she acknowledges the truth, fifteen kilos (thirty-two pounds).

"Why did you wait so long to come?" the *vrach* responds. "You know you're supposed to see the doctor once a month."

"I came two months ago," Tamara tries to explain, "but I was late and the clinic was closed."

The *vrach* sighs. She takes out a pink piece of paper. As she writes, she talks to Tamara; "You must not gain any more weight. Your blood pressure is already too high. You must try to eat better and get more rest. I will give you vitamins and you must come to the clinic for ultraviolet treatments, to make sure you get enough Vitamin D. And stop smoking."

Tamara shifts uncomfortably on the chair. She sits on her nicotine-stained fingers. Then, without looking up, she rises, takes the slip entitling her to maternity leave, and hurries out of the building.

The clinic is almost a mile from her parents' apartment, but she has shopping to do so she begins walking home, stopping to buy milk for Kolia. It is late in the day and when she gets to the open-air market most of the stalls are empty. Tamara finds a woman who sells her two turnips for twenty kopecks (31 cents). Her last stop is at the *gastronom*, where she waits in line for a half-kilo of frozen fish. She gets home just as the street lights come on.

In the apartment, Kolia is playing with his grandfather but when he hears Tamara open the door, he runs to meet her. She picks him up, kisses him on both cheeks, and playfully tries to throw him in the air.

In the kitchen, she puts the milk on the windowsill and pulls out a pot in which to cook the fish stew. She lights a cigarette, thinks about what the *vrach* told her today, and starts to put it out. Just then, she notices her face in the mirror. She looks old, too old. At twenty-four, she should still be having fun, the kind of fun she and her girl friends dreamed about when they were students in the gymnasium—dancing at nightclubs, trips to the seashore, concerts, rides in the country. Feeling trapped and lonely, she brings the cigarette back to her lips and inhales deeply.

Three weeks later, Tamara returns to the *zhenskii konsultatsii* for her ultraviolet treatment. She has stopped working at the factory. She has been watching her weight. The *vrach* examines her and says that her blood pressure is normal. And although Tamara has not entirely stopped smoking, the *vrach* is satisfied with her progress. She makes sure that Tamara understands that she is to call the *neotlozhnaya* (minor emergency services number) if she has any problems; there is also a number for the hospital where she is scheduled to deliver.

Tamara spends most of her days with Kolia. Each morning she carefully dresses him and takes him walking in a small park near her parents' apartment. One morning, as she and Kolia are watching a man playing an accordian in the park and three weeks before she had expected them, her labor pains begin. At home Tamara lies down; her mother rubs her swollen abdomen. When the contractions become severe, she calls the clinic, but it is closed and the woman answering the telephone tells her to go to the hospital. Tamara's mother calls the *skoraya pomoshch* (emergency ambulance system). In an hour, an ambulance with a midwife arrives. She confirms that Tamara's labor has begun and takes her to the maternity hospital.

Tamara is put into a large room with two other women also in labor. There is a midwife assigned to each. As Tamara's labor pains increase she is told to breathe slowly. She is given a small injection of a narcotic. Tamara knows she will not get more medication during delivery. Soviet doctors, drawing on a strong Pavlovian tradition, consider pain during the childbirth a reflex that can be controlled by the woman assuming a proper attitude. Therefore, unless there are complications and a Caesarean section becomes necessary, women are expected to block out the pain or, as they do their other burdens, accept it without complaining.

Tamara lies sweating on the thin mattress; the midwife wipes her forehead and checks her progress. No visitors are permitted during labor or delivery. The same idea about infection which demands that visitors to Soviet hospitals remove coats, hats, and sweaters also prohibits any contact between mother and child for the first twenty-four hours.

Six hours after entering the hospital, with only the assistance of her midwife, Tamara delivers a healthy 3.5 kilogram (7.7 pound) girl. Her baby is taken from her immediately. For another six hours she is left lying, exhausted, in the delivery room. Through its open door she can hear the nurses and *akusherki* (midwives) talking about shopping and their husbands. No one talks to her. She stares at the walls and ceilings. The room is stark white and, except for the four beds, empty.

While in the hospital for the ten days required following childbirth, Tamara becomes friends with some of the other mothers. Most of them are young. Their husbands come to the courtyard outside the hospital and wave to them as they lean out the windows. One woman, a shy, awkward young girl named Lidia, is not married. She reminds Tamara of herself at that age. Tamara also became pregnant at seventeen, before she met and married Victor. But Tamara's mother had helped her get an abortion. "A girl still in *srednaya shkola* (high school) should not have a child," she had said.

Lidia had given birth a few days before Tamara. But her baby was not doing well. "She weighed only two kilos [4.4 pounds] at birth," Lidia tells Tamara tearfully, "and she came six weeks early. Now the doctors say there's trouble with her breathing and she's too weak to eat. When I try to give her my breast, she only cries."

Once, when Tamara was breast-feeding her new daughter, the nurse pointed out Lidia's little girl. How tiny, Tamara thought. How can something that small live?

The day Tamara leaves the hospital, she sees Lidia sitting in the hallway, sobbing. "She's gone," Tamara hears her say, "my little girl died."

In 1980, there were 70 million women of childbearing age in the USSR. Today, a slim majority of them are, like Tamara, Russian women living in or near large cities. The remainder come from a mixture of more than one hundred different nationality groups. An increasing percentage live in the very un-Russian, rural Central Asian republics, where the writings of the prophet Muhammad are better known than Lenin's.

The average family size in Central Asia is 5.4 persons, compared to 3.5 in most Russian cities. According to their own national customs, each family should have no fewer than five or six children and as many as possible should be male. Very few of these rural women use any form of preventive birth control, and abortion is considered "the greatest crime." Although some rural women work on the collective and state farms, there is also a strong religious tradition that women stay home and care for their families while the husband works.

On the other hand, most Russian women have jobs. They work in service-related jobs such as health care, education, and sales. A smaller percentage are workers in light industry and construction. Faced with a declining Russian birth rate, the Soviet government, in January 1981, passed a law prohibiting women from 460 hazardous occupations. Many of these jobs, such as swinging a pickax on heavy construction, were thought to be contributing to a high rate of spontaneous abortions. Nevertheless, over 68 percent of Soviet women over age sixteen work (the U.S. figure is 51 percent). Most of them share what has become known as the "double burden" of the modern Soviet woman—working full-time while maintaining complete responsibility for raising children and running the household. As a result, Russian women are having more abortions and fewer children than their Muslim counterparts. Both are living in male-dominated societies, but the Russian woman, forced to work to support her family, sees childbirth as one of the few burdens she can still control.

The contrast between the weary Russian woman and her Muslim counterpart has important consequences for the Soviet Union. By the turn of the century, Muslim women will make up 25 percent of the female population and, because of their higher birth rate, will contribute proportionately more children to the Soviet population.

According to population specialist Murray Feshbach, chief of the USSR-East European Population, Employment, R & D branch of the Census Bureau's Foreign Demographic Analysis Division, and Soviet specialist G. A. Bondarskaya, by the year 2000 Russians will make up less than half (46 percent) of the total Soviet population. Because Russian women are having fewer sons, in a few years the majority of Soviet soldiers will be non-Russian. With a decrease in trained urban manpower, the Soviet government may also find itself with insufficient manpower to continue its slow economic and industrial growth. But of more immediate concern to leaders in Moscow is the strain on their fragile medical system from the two connecting demands—abortions in the large Soviet cities and increasing births in rural areas.

Since 1918, the Soviet medical system has placed the medical care of women at the top of its list of priorities, second only to care of military personnel and industrial workers.

To accomplish this, they have built hundreds of hospitals and trained thousands of doctors. Today, there are a quarter of a million hospital beds in the USSR reserved for childbirth. There are 25,000 consultation clinics, factory dispensaries, or maternity clinics where Soviet women can go for prenatal care, routine examinations, pap smears, or abortions. One of every twenty Soviet doctors specializes in obstetrics-gynecology. Except for elective abortions, for which there is a five ruble fee, all maternity services are free. An expectant mother is expected to visit the consultation center fourteen to seventeen times during her pregnancy.

Nevertheless, in Moscow, the jewel of the Soviet crown, existing clinic and treatment facilities are inadequate. One of the major findings of the Moscow City Committee of the Women's Deputy Council, as reported in 1977 in the journal *Biulleten*,[1] was that "the Gagarin Regional District of Moscow does not have adequate facilities and personnel to attend to the medical care of women ... the waits for examination are long and there is no policy for follow-up care or succeeding visits for women with problems peculiar to them."

One of those unique problems is obtaining periodic pap smears to detect cervical cancer in its early stages. In part, because of the widespread use of pap smears in the United States, the cure rate for cervical cancer (number of women alive five years after diagnosis) has been steadily improving. In the USSR, the technique and use of the pap smear are well known, but because of problems with laboratory supplies, clinic facilities, and public education, its use is not as efficient as it might be.

Dr. Victor Eisenberg, a prominent Kishinev gynecologic cancer surgeon, told me his biggest surprise when emigrating to the United States and studying our cancer statistics was the high percentage of cervical cancers diagnosed in their early stages. "Look at your figures," he said. "Seventy percent of cervical cancer cases are detected in Stage 1, when surgery can still cure them. Only 10 percent of U.S. patients are detected in Stage 4, too late for either surgery or other treatments. In the USSR, 60 percent of all first cases are Stage 4."[2]

Another area where, compared to her American counterpart, life is more difficult and risky for a Soviet woman is contraception. Birth

---

[1] *Biulleten ispolnitelnogo komiteta Moskovskogo gorodskogo soveta deputatov trudiashchikhsia* Moscow (April 7, 1977).

[2] The Soviets publish tables giving the prevalence (total number of cases) and incidence (total new cases) for cervical and other cancers. Both prevalence and incidence figures for cervical cancer are similar to that found in the U.S. None of these tables, however, including those contained within a recent Soviet textbook on the epidemiology, or population distribution, of cervical cancer, *Epidemiologicheskie aspekty profilaktiki i rannei diagnostiki raka matki*, by L. I. Charkviani, provides a breakdown of cervical cancer by the stage in which it was detected. I was told by Soviet health officials that such statistics are not available nationally or by region, but only for individual hospitals.

control is left entirely to the woman. Most Soviet men give little thought to the problem. Condoms are for sale in the smallest village, but they have a reputation among men of being thick, inflexible, and, from a male perspective, totally unsatisfactory. "If you feel anything through a 'galosh,' " a young Soviet husband told me, "it must be your imagination."

Withdrawal is commonly used, but some Soviet men believe if it is practiced frequently it leads to mental illness. In many cases the woman is left on her own. "She runs for the douche," one man explained.

A woman can purchase a small variety of vaginal jellies, creams, and dissolving tablets, all designed to kill sperm. But most women say they do not like the mess. Diaphragms can be purchased but, since they come in only one size, do not always work. Nationwide, the rhythm method, with all its uncertainty, remains the most common form of contraception.

A few educated Soviet women prefer intrauterine devices (IUDs) or spirals, as the domestic variety is known. To date, the supply of IUDs has not kept up with demand. Urban polyclinics have waiting lists as each year more Soviet women try to find an alternative to "an abortion a year."

Many of the Soviet women I spoke with looked to IUDs as the safest and most effective form of birth control, but felt they should be reserved for women who have had at least one child. When asked about birth control pills (which have been available on the black market from Hungary for a number of years and whose internal production in the USSR is just beginning), a frequent answer was that they are not "physiologic" and therefore are dangerous.[3]

The many newspaper articles describing the dangers of birth control pills are one of the few forms of reproductive information provided Soviet women. Formal sex education is still sporadic in most Soviet schools and families seldom discuss sex. But young girls, liberated in the sense that no religious or official stigma is attached to premarital sex, begin sexual relations early. Many feel pressured into early sex because of the desire to find a husband. There are a

---

[3] The Soviets base their skepticism toward birth control pills on their finding that after prolonged use (two years) women have "abnormal brain wave activity" as detected by an EEG, the significance of which is unknown, and on the known association between birth control pills and vascular disease, especially thrombosis.

great number of single women in the USSR, 170 single women to 100 men, according to the 1970 Census. Surveys done in the Soviet Union have shown that more than 80 percent of college-educated women have had premarital sexual relations.

Many of these initial sexual experiences are hurried, unromantic, and done more in a spirit of adventure than love. "There is no place to go to make love," a young Leningrad student lamented. "Someone is always at home and hotels, of course, are impossible. They check your passports." With the chronic housing problem in Soviet cities and the shortage of private automobiles, the only places available are park benches and, occasionally, isolated corners of museums. In the winter, a few resourceful couples take compartments on the Red Arrow Express train between Moscow and Leningrad to have a night together.

Since the majority of the young girls do not use any form of birth control, pregnancy is a common problem. Between 1959 and 1970 there was a threefold increase in the number of illegitimate births nationwide. It is estimated that one out of every ten births in the USSR today involves an unmarried woman.

The official Soviet government policy toward all pregnancies, illegitimate or not, is that they should be carried to term. There is extensive publicity provided advocating the concept of "the ideal three" family size. If a couple has a fourth child, the government will provide a small monthly payment until the child is five years old. If the woman is unmarried, the state pays support for her first child which continues until he or she is age twelve. In 1974 the government instituted a new badge, Heroine of the Soviet Union, to any woman, married or not, who had ten children.

Complementing these positive approaches is a heavy negative publicity campaign, "the fight against abortion." Its major emphasis is on the potential dangers of abortion. Infection, psychological trauma, and the possibility of permanent infertility are prominently mentioned in the brochures, posters, and newspaper articles condemning the practice.

But the demands of everyday life, the crowded apartments, the double burden of running a household while holding down a job, and the uncertainty of marriage (more than a third of marriages end in divorce) are more persuasive than the fear of surgery. The financial assistance for the child's support (from twelve to fifty rubles a month) is too small to be of much help. And, as one woman told me, "Badges do not help you raise children." What's more, public censure and criticism of unwed mothers is still strong.

As a result, in 1980, Soviet doctors performed an estimated 16 million abortions. That is 40 percent of the 40 million abortions which the Population Crisis Committee estimates occur throughout the world and ten times greater than the approximately 1.4 million legal abortions in the United States each year.

The average Soviet woman has six abortions during her reproductive lifetime. A woman in Odessa told me, without hesitation, that her mother had had twenty-four abortions.

Twice in its history the Soviet government has tried to get out of the abortion business. Immediately after the 1917 Revolution all abortions were prohibited, but on November 18, 1920, the commissariats of health and justice of the new revolutionary government reversed the ban.

The reason, as recorded in an official comment accompanying the 1920 decree, was that "up to 50 percent of women are infected in the course of the secret operation." This high infection rate was having a detrimental effect on the health of Soviet women. Moreover, in 1920 the new government believed that as soon as economic conditions improved, more women would want to have children and the need for abortions would diminish.

By 1936, economic conditions had not improved; in fact, they were worse. Nevertheless, abortions were outlawed that year under a prohibition that remained in force until 1955. Then, as it had done in 1920, the government acknowledged that making abortions illegal had only led to a vast underground system of illegal operations. In the 1940s, a Leningrad gynecologist estimated that 70 percent of patients in the female wards of hospitals were recovering from infections resulting from illegal abortions.

Today, an abortion is available on demand to every Soviet woman during the first twelve weeks of her pregnancy. There is a charge of five rubles ($7.75), unless the procedure is necessary for the health of the mother, in which case it is free. After twelve weeks, there must be some medical necessity for the operations. Most Soviet abortions are performed by scraping or aspirating the womb and the woman may be hospitalized for two or three days following. There are no medications given for anxiety before the procedure and only local anesthesia is used during the surgery.

The role of the gynecologist, who is frequently a woman, is difficult. Under official government policy, she is instructed to try to discourage her patients from going through with abortion.

"I love children," Natasha, a twenty-seven-year-old physician specializing in gynecology, told me. "And I understand how bad it is for a woman to have too many abortions, the danger of infection the risk of perforating the uterus. But when a woman comes to you in tears, telling you she has no room either in her apartment or her heart for another child, you cannot simply be a doctor, a cold, isolated scientist. You too suffer with that woman. She is working. Her husband probably drinks too much. How much can you ask her to do?

"We are directed," Natasha explained, "to send women with financial or other problems to the lawyers [they man special social service agencies set up to help pregnant women get money, a bigger apartment, or a nursery school]. I used to send many of my patients there. But most decided to have the abortion anyway. And by that time, it was later in their pregnancy when the operation is more dangerous. Now, if the woman convinces me she really wants the operation, I fill out the form right away.

"Many of my patients," she says, "especially the older ones, are suspicious and frightened of IUDs. Sometimes it's their husbands who won't let them use anything. There is one woman I saw a month ago who already had three children and six abortions and was pregnant again. I tried to tell her that she must be more careful, but it is difficult. She wanted to have the abortion quickly, while her husband was out of town, so he wouldn't find out."

Getting an abortion done in time and in privacy are two reasons why some Soviet women use unofficial methods. The number of illegal abortions performed in the USSR each year is unknown but is estimated to be small, especially when compared to the large number of legal operations.

Most illegal abortions are performed in private apartments by physicians. A commonly mentioned fee in Moscow is fifty rubles. The most frequent customers are young girls who wish to hide the abortion from their parents, wives who do not want their husbands to find out, or women who have had a government abortion within the last six months and are therefore ineligible for another.

As in other countries, self-induced abortions also occur in the Soviet Union. Increasingly common, according to Dr. A. E. Kudryavtsev of the Moscow Emergency Service, is the use of pachycarpine, a drug injected by Soviet doctors to speed labor but also prescribed in pill form for vascular insufficiency.[4] Pachycarpine pills can be obtained on the black market and, when taken in large amounts, stimulate contractions and a miscarriage. Unfortunately, the unsupervised use of pachycarpine can also lead to uncontrolled hemmorhage.

Natasha, a young gynecologist, and I became friends during the two months I lived in Odessa. I would frequently visit her and her husband, an architect, in their one-room apartment overlooking the Odessa Opera House. They had been married just two years and their only furniture was a bed, two chairs, and a table.

Natasha, despite her reservations about official abortion policies, believed that the medical care most women receive in the Soviet Union is superior to that available in the United States.

"Today, just about every birth takes place in a hospital," Natasha explained.[5] "Always, a midwife or doctor is there. And we don't use as many drugs as you do," she goes on. "I've read how you give pregnant women antibiotics and other drugs that can damage their babies. In the USSR we do not use a lot of medicines. Every mother is expected to visit her polyclinic once a month during her pregnancy. Vitamins or anything else she needs are supplied free of charge. You do not have to pay as you do in the United States. If the woman works, she's given time off from her job to come to the clinic. The Soviet Union wants to have strong, healthy children. We always have wanted healthy children."

In one way, the Soviets have led the rest of the world in trying to improve the health of the infant. Under the stimulus of Pavlov's writings (mandated by Stalin as the "science of the land"), the So-

[4] L. B. Shapiro, I. A. Ostrovskii, *Organization of Emergency Medical Care* (Baltimore: Johns Hopkins University Press, 1975); *Emergency Care in Acute Poisoning,* by A. E. Kudryautsev.

[5] Official Soviet statistics document that 98 percent of all births now occur in hospitals.

viet Union was the first nation to widely adopt the concept of "painless childbirth." But they adopted it in a particularly rigid format.

The story begins with a doctor named Velvosky, a neurologist working at the railway clinics in Dniepropetrovsk in 1920. At that time Velvosky wrote, "The teachings of Pavlov have strengthened the conviction that childbirth, insofar as it is a natural act, need not be accompanied by painful manifestations. . . . So we should try not to cure the pain of childbirth by the use of drugs . . . but to make every effort to destroy the concepts that breed this pain." Velvosky, along with other Soviet researchers, believed that if properly conditioned, a woman would not feel pain during labor and delivery.[6]

In 1923, Velvosky reported success with his early technique of "suggestive words" during delivery to the Second Pan-Russian Congress of Psychiatrists and Neurologists. He helped spread overall belief in painless childbirth throughout the scientific community. During the 1930s and '40s there were many attempts to find the best approach. Some researchers stressed hypnosis, others the suggestion, or psychoprophylactic, method, which provided the woman with "suggestive words" she could repeat through labor and delivery. Researchers reported success with both approaches, with the proportion of women completing delivery without drugs varying from 65 to 85 percent.

By 1951, during a conference on the use of analgesia during pregnancy in Leningrad, the Soviet government officially adopted the psychotherapeutic or suggestion method and mandated that it be applied in every maternity unit in the USSR. Hypnosis was rejected since it required highly trained personnel and could not be used throughout the country. But the government placed restrictions on the psychotherapeutic technique. It could be used only in normal presentations. The method used had to be precisely the same way in every hospital: slow, steady breathing throughout the period of labor and delivery. Since it was a government decree, there was no room for variation.

In 1953, 300,000 mothers were offered the benefit of the new technique, with 80 percent success. By 1955 the total reached 700,000. As

[6] Quoted in Fernand Lamaze, *Painless Childbirth*, trans. L. R. Celestin (London: Burke 1958), p. 12.

yet, however, the world knew little of what was going on in Soviet maternity wards. It was up to a French physician, Fernand Lamaze, who was present at that 1951 obstetrics conference, to popularize painless childbirth. An obstetrician-gynecologist, Lamaze was amazed at what he heard in Leningrad. Upon his return to Paris he began a trial of his own. His testing ground was the Paris hospital Maternité du Métallargiste. He decided, in his own words, to relax the "many restrictive regulations" surrounding psychotherapeutic childbirth used in the Soviet Union and to involve the mother early in her pregnancy, something the Soviets did not do.

Lamaze instituted a series of lectures for expectant mothers, instructing them about the changes that would occur in their bodies during delivery, and how to react and work with these changes. Like Velvosky before him, he wanted the woman to participate actively in childbirth.

In 1956, Lamaze published the results of his work in a book called *Painless Childbirth*. Over the years, it has become the bible of the psychotherapeutic or psychoprophylactic school of natural childbirth. Today more and more classes in the Lamaze technique are being held throughout the world, as more information becomes available regarding the side effects of many drugs on pregnant women. In the Soviet Union, the emphasis on education before delivery is less. The Soviet woman is expected to tolerate the birth with appropriate suggestion and a minimum amount of narcotic.

Infant Mortality

For twenty years, from 1951 to 1971, the overall record of the Soviet Union in regard to childbirth, and as measured by infant mortality, steadily improved. As Natasha mentioned, the high number of women seeking care before birth, and then having their children under medical supervision, has brought about significant decreases in the number of children dying during their first year of life. In 1951, at the time of the Leningrad conference, the USSR lost 84 children of every 1,000 born; by 1971, the deaths had fallen to 23 per 1,000 births. And, although the percentage was still behind that of the United States and other developed countries, in 1971 there was every indication that, as in the rest of the world, infant mortality in the Soviet Union would continue to decrease. It has not.

In fact, an upward trend began in 1971. The phenomenon was first brought to Western attention by Murray Feshbach of the U.S. Bureau of the Census. In 1974, reversing a long-established practice, the Soviets stopped publishing the nationwide infant mortality rate; that year it stood at 27.9 deaths per 1,000 births, an increase of 22 percent from 1971. In 1976, Dr. A. Boyarskiy, director of the Scientific Research Institute of the State Administration, spoke of "an alarming increase in infant mortality."

At that time, Feshbach and his co-researcher Christopher Davis, who had joined him in the analysis, estimated the 1976 infant mortality rate at 31 deaths per 1,000 births.[7]

Soviet medical leaders I spoke to acknowledged the problem of an increase in infant mortality. While admitting that there were many reasons behind the rise, many attributed at least part of the increase to improved statistics, with more accurate reports available from Soviet hospitals. This, they contend, makes the situation appear worse than it really is (an explanation Feshbach and Davis say is not supported by their analysis).

Soviet spokesmen such as Dr. Urii Lisitsin, Director of Medical Information, also told me that the rise leveled off in 1976, at approximately 28 deaths per 1,000. "In 1978 and 1979," Lisitsin said, "there has been some slight improvement, although official statistics are not available."

By recording the number of infants who die within a year of birth, a country can summarize the many medical and nonmedical factors that interact to produce that elusive concept, health. The general state of nutrition, housing conditions, cases of infectious disease, availability of basic medical services, and the amount of preventive medical care all influence a country's infant mortality rate. So do the age of most mothers and the number of children they have. Like an Impressionist painting made up of thousands of small dots, none of these factors can be interpreted by itself. But viewed together on the canvas of infant mortality, they provide an excellent picture of the health of a nation.

[7] During the same five years that Feshbach and Davis documented the increase of 34 percent in the Soviet infant mortality rate, the U.S. figures were: 1971, 19.1 per 1,000, 1976, 15.2. Rates for other countries in 1976 included Sweden, 8.7; Great Britain, 13.9; Czechoslovakia, 20.8. By 1980, infant mortality in the United States was approximately 13 per 1,000 births.

Because infant mortality rates reflect, and are in turn influenced by, so many different factors, it is important not to take the numbers simply at face value. This is especially true when it comes to the USSR. As we have learned from other contacts with the Soviets, and by their own admission, their statistics may be subject to a large degree of reporting error. Therefore, the figures obtained by Feshbach and Davis, painstakingly derived from studies of the Soviet republic for which information was available, must be viewed as close estimates, not hard facts.[8] Even with this important limitation, however, there is no disagreement that since 1971 infant mortality rates in the USSR have been increasing in direct contrast to the general U.S. and worldwide decrease.

The increase, as best as we can tell from available evidence, is taking place throughout the USSR, although some areas are clearly better off than others. Vilnius, capital of the annexed Lithuanian Republic, had an infant mortality rate in 1974 better than many American cities—14 per 1,000. Overall, however, the Lithuanian infant mortality rate has increased by 20 percent from 1971 to 1976.

Because of the increase in the number of Central Asian births, researchers originally suspected that the nationwide rise in infant mortality was coming only from these higher-risk rural births. It is well established that conditions found more commonly in rural areas— low income, poor housing, low educational levels, and inadequate medical services—can all combine to increase infant mortality. In the United States, for example, there are rural counties with infant mortality rates of 60 per 1,000 births, over four times the U.S. average.

And, as we will see later in the section on rural health, the Central Asian republics do have many serious problems, ranging from a shortage of specialists to a lack of Vitamin D, all of which seriously affect infant mortality. Tashkent, capital of the Uzbekistan Republic in Central Asia, for example, has an infant mortality rate almost

[8] For example, the Soviet statistics exclude three classes of live births who die in their first week of life: 1) premature births occurring before the twenty-eighth week of gestation; 2) babies weighing less than 1,000 grams (2.2 pounds); and 3) infants smaller than 35 centimeters (13.7 inches). These exclusions, which are not observed by other nations, underestimate the Soviet infant mortality rate by approximately 15 percent. If these births were included in the 1976 figures, the nationwide infant mortality rate would have been 36 per 1,000.

three times that of Vilnius, which is located in the European Soviet Union.

Despite these large regional differences, however, the infant mortality profile compiled by Feshbach and Davis demonstrates that the problem of the increase in infant mortality is everywhere. It is necessary, therefore, to look at some general factors that might be contributing to this important and disturbing health problem.

The first group of factors are those that affect the health of the mother before she has the baby. Like their American counterparts, more Soviet women are smoking today than ten years ago. Not only are cases of lung cancer rising among Soviet women, the increased use of tobacco has also led to a greater number of premature births and underweight babies, problems that, as we will see later, lead to pneumonia and infant deaths.

Besides smoking, we also know that the use of alcohol is increasing among Soviet women. Although the abuse of alcohol among men has been widely acknowledged by the Soviet government, there is increasing evidence, as determined by letters to the editor of national newspapers and discussion among medical professionals, that the use of alcohol is also becoming increasingly common among women.

In an oft-quoted article published in the *Literaturnaya gazeta* in 1976, alcoholism among females was given the title "The Third Disease." After heart disease and cancer, the most common reason for illness among women was the abuse of alcohol. In a reply to that 1976 article, Minister of Health Petrovsky acknowledged the problem of female alcoholism and the increased need for medical facilities to treat women drinkers.

A 1979 update in the same magazine, a liberal forum for public criticism and discussion, suggested that the problem of female drinking was getting worse. Every tenth alcoholic in the USSR is now a woman. And although the average female alcoholic begins drinking at a later age than a man, many more young women are turning to alcohol.

One link between alcohol consumption and infant mortality, like that of smoking, is low birth weight. The more alcohol consumed during pregnancy, the smaller the infant; and the smaller the infant, the more problems it will have surviving the crucial first few weeks of life. In the Soviet Union, as in the United States, about 65 percent of all infant deaths occur in babies weighing less than 5.5 pounds.

Some of the children born to alcoholic mothers in the Soviet Union in addition to being underweight are also suffering from the fetal-alcohol syndrome (FAS). First described in modern literature in 1968 by a group of researchers in Nantes, France, FAS is now recognized worldwide. Children with FAS have a higher incidence of congenital abnormalities. They do not grow as quickly as other children. They develop frequent infections. Some actually have withdrawal seizures shortly after birth since the alcohol drunk by their mother passed into their bloodstream and made them alcoholics before birth. Keeping these infants alive during the critical first days of life is a difficult and demanding challenge.

Dr. G. I. Shurygin of the Orekhovo-Zuyevo Neuropsychiatric Hospital No. 8 in Moscow reported in the journal *Pediatriya* on forty-two children born to chronic alcoholic mothers who did survive. Although some of the mothers had consumed more alcohol than others, all drank heavily. They all had a higher than normal incidence of stillbirths. Furthermore, their children had poor physical development and, in some cases, severe physical weakness. They had poor appetites, "increased emotional excitability, slept fitfully and displayed a tendency to cry often."

Those born to mothers with the heaviest drinking histories were the most severely affected and in many of them mental retardation was a common finding, an observation also seen in other countries.

Acting in combination with tobacco and alcohol on the health of the mother and her children is diet. Unlike the U.S. situation, the Soviets still are trying to provide enough animal protein in their basic diet. A quick look at the national differences between the typical diets reveals that in America 40 percent of all calories come from animal products; in the USSR only 25–30 percent. Americans also eat 30 percent more vegetables, 40 percent more eggs, and almost three times as much fruit. The Soviet diet, compared to ours, is heavy with grain products, potatoes, and fat.

Each year, throughout the USSR, there are severe food shortages. Fresh meat is infrequently available; the only reliable source is the black market, whose high prices prevent most ordinary Soviet citizens from eating meat except on holidays. Even more important, fresh vegetables and other sources of vitamins, so important for a pregnant woman, are frequently absent throughout the long Russian winter. As partial compensation, pregnant women are supposed to take vitamins. In addition, they are supposed to spend thirty minutes once a week standing nude before banks of ultraviolet lamps, wearing protective goggles which make them look like welders. But the fact that rickets, a disease caused by a deficiency of Vitamin D that was common amid the poverty of Victorian England, remains a frequent health problem in parts of the rural USSR today is a striking example of the failure of such measures to reach all mothers (see the chapter on rural medicine).

The question of prenatal care brings us to the second part of the infant mortality picture: physicians and the availability of medical care. There are two main ways that medical care can reduce infant deaths. One is to treat the woman before delivery; the other is treatment of the newborn infant.

Treating the mother means examining her in her early months of pregnancy to ensure that she follows good health practices. There is interest in good prenatal care in the Soviet Union. Dr. Benjamin Spock's handbook on child care has been translated into Russian and the government supports public education programs aimed at urging women to visit the polyclinic early in their pregnancy.

Unfortunately, the system frequently breaks down. There are so many abortions performed each year that even in the western cities of the USSR (where the number of gynecologists is six to seven times higher than in the rural republics) there are long delays in scheduling appointments.

An abortion clinic I once visited in Leningrad was one example of the process. It was a large clinic, treating 200–300 women a day. There were three waiting rooms each holding approximately 50 women who sat on benches. One woman told me she had been waiting for three hours for a nine o'clock appointment. Another admitted she was supposed to be operated on the day before but had been told to come back today.

While I was there a nurse came into the waiting room and called ten names. The women followed her to a smaller room where there were ten cots. Each woman was asked to undress and then each was given a single sheet.

After an hour, without inquiring about past medical history, important allergies or performing any laboratory tests, four women were taken into the operating room. The small room had four operating tables, two facing each other with a metal basin in the center. There was one large operating light.

The four women were treated by two physicians. Once placed in position on the table each patient received two small injections of novocaine drawn from an open bottle. Shortly after the injections the physicians began scraping the uterus. Each woman could see the results of scraping on the woman facing her. I saw one woman faint before her surgery began.

Although the entire process took only a few minutes the staff took long breaks between cases. No one seemed concerned about the women waiting.

Many women with high-risk pregnancies (very young or old mothers or those with associated medical problems such as hypertension) are first seen late in their pregnancies when the risk of premature delivery is already high. According to Dr. A. E. Serenko, writing about the polyclinic situation in Moscow, "Too many polyclinics [for women] are crowded and not fully equipped with medication. . . . There is delay and inefficient organization in the treatment and screening of women."[9] Soviet studies have also found that many women do not keep appointments because of the demands of work and family.

A look at the medical care given the woman during delivery, and then at the care given her newly born child, shows that the Soviet medical system provided a basic, no-frills service, one that performs well in normal situations but which allows no margin for error.

For example, a major cause of infant mortality in the USSR is pneumonia, an infection that can strike both newborns and infants. In the United States, the majority of the deaths occur early, in the first two weeks of life when pneumonia affects low-birth-weight, high-risk newborns. In the USSR, the timing of infant deaths is more like that found in an underdeveloped country with both newborns and older infants falling ill to infection. The reason is that many Soviet infants are undernourished and lacking in normal vitamins and nutrition. Expecting them to breathe sixty times a minute

---

[9] A. F. Serenko et al., *"Osnovy organizatsii poliklinicheskoy pomoshchi naseleniiu"* [The Bases for the Organization of Polyclinic Assistance to the Population] (Moscow 1976).

and simultaneously fight off infection is simply asking too much. Dr. V. K. Ivanov, in a paper on the role of pneumonia and infant mortality within the Soviet Union, documented that, as expected, pneumonia accounts for almost half of all infant deaths.

In the United States, infants with pneumonia or other life-threatening problems are treated in neonatal (for the newborn) intensive care units, and as a result the survival rate of high-risk, low-weight infants is improving. Such units are equipped with miniature respirators, artificial kidney machines, and sophisticated systems for feeding and monitoring infants who begin life in trouble. With the use of such technology, it is possible to save most infants born prematurely who weigh over three or four pounds. Within the last ten years, most large U.S. hospitals and many of our community hospitals have built neonatal intensive care units.

No similar technological revolution has occurred in the Soviet Union. Even Moscow, a city of 7 million people with the most sophisticated medical care available in the USSR, only one hospital, Children's Hospital No. 10, specializes in treating premature births. All others contain only simple nurseries with neither respirators nor other support technology.

One new form of technology now widely used in the United States which is generally unavailable in the USSR is electronic fetal monitoring. With it a doctor can listen to the heartbeat of an infant still in the mother's womb by means of an electrode attached to the baby's head. A U.S. study estimated that if electronic fetal monitoring were used in all high-risk deliveries, 109 babies might be saved for every 1,000 high-risk deliveries monitored. Thus the lack of neonatal intensive care units and technologies such as fetal monitoring probably form an important part of the difference between the fall in infant mortality in the United States and its rise in the Soviet Union.[10]

[10] Both neonatal intensive care units and fetal monitoring are controversial. A 1979 NIH panel concluded that fetal monitoring was being used too often in normal low-risk deliveries where it does not save lives but can lead to more Caesarean sections. With the rapid spread of neonatal intensive care units, infants weighing less than 1,000 grams (2.2 pounds) were surviving birth and the subsequent quality of their lives was questioned.

A recent study from Johns Hopkins, however, that examined birth records between 1976 and 1978 found no increase in developmental problems but a major drop in overall death rates. As a result, intensive treatment of low-birth-weight infants is now credited as a major reason behind the recent drop in U.S. infant mortality figures.

There is another explanation, according to some Soviet observers. Dr. Albert Sabin, developer of the polio vaccine, told me that during his thirty-year association with the Soviet government he had learned to distrust Soviet statistics, especially ones that were potentially embarrassing.

"There are tremendous problems interpreting numbers from the USSR," Sabin says, "Their methods for collecting and recording data are crude. I would not be surprised if all of the deterioration is because they're doing a better job of counting."

Murray Feshbach of the Foreign Demographic Analysis branch of the U.S. Census, the man primarily responsible for bringing the increase in Soviet death rates to Western attention disagrees, "The increase is too widespread, too universal to be simply due to variations in reporting techniques. No, I'm convinced it is a real increase."

Because of Soviet secrecy and current lack of scientific expertise there will not be a quick answer to the question of why the infant mortality rates of the two nations are different. Regardless of this discrepancy, however, it is clear that the USSR still faces greater challenges with medical care than the United States.

One of these challenges that directly affects infant mortality is the food the baby receives after its birth. Soviet physicians, like doctors in other countries, recognize that the best infant food is mother's milk. Breast feeding not only provides important calories and vitamins, it also transfers important disease-fighting antibodies from mother to child. Nutritionally, nothing is better. The many commercial infant formulas can, at best, only provide a close substitute.

But to breast-feed, the mother must be available throughout the day, a requirement that conflicts with the official Soviet policy of quickly returning women to their jobs and placing their children in crèches or state-supported day nurseries. A 1978 study in Dagestan, USSR, found that only a third of new mothers breast-fed their children. The rest relied upon formulas. As a Ministry of Health spokesman told me, "It looks as though we'll have to find a formula equal to mother's milk."

Because of low funding priorities, the Soviets do not make enough baby formula. Demand frequently exceeds supply. In addition, they have technical problems producing a high-protein formula that will supply essential nutrition.

Even when they improve production, there are problems. Many

of the crèches are crowded and the pay for the women who work in them is low, resulting in inadequate supervision. Occasionally infants are fed formula from the same bottle, spreading bacteria and increasing the risk of infection.

The Soviet infant formulas are similar to standard preparations in use throughout the world. But formulas for children with special needs are not available. The difference between the U.S. and the USSR approach in caring for children with unusual nutritional problems is illustrated in the case of Jessica Katz.

Jessica's case came to the attention of the world when Senator Edward Kennedy asked Soviet Premier Leonid Brezhnev to intervene and allow the year-old girl to come to the United States for treatment.

Jessica was born in Moscow in October 1977. At birth she appeared to her parents, Natalia and Boris, a healthy, normal, eight-pound baby. There had been no problems with her delivery or with Natalia's pregnancy. After a few weeks at home, however, Jessica failed to gain weight. She developed constant diarrhea, frequent rashes, and cried continuously.

In December her parents took her to Moscow Children's Hospital Number 1. They were told there was no room. Boris and Natalia were frightened. Two years ago the young couple, both Jews, had applied for exit visas to leave the Soviet Union for Israel. The visas had been refused on the ground that Mrs. Katz had had access to state secrets through her job at the Soviet Institutes of Experimental Meteorology and Geophysics. Since the refusal, both had felt discrimination in dozens of small and large ways. Now the illness of their daughter made their troubles seem overwhelming.

They sought help from Boris's mother, Mrs. Khaika Landman, who had already left the USSR and was living in Boston. With her help and that of the organization Action for Soviet Jews, a political effort was launched aimed at bringing the child to the United States for medical treatment. In the first four months of her life Jessica had gained less than half a pound.

On the board of the Jewish organization was Boston family practitioner Richard I. Feinbloom. On January 13, 1978, he contacted Jessica's parents, took a history, and came to a presumptive, long-distance diagnosis.

Dr. Feinbloom, director of the Family Health Care Program at

Harvard University, determined that a malabsorption syndrome best explained Jessica's problem. Malabsorption is a relatively unusual disorder with a number of causes, but the same end result— the child is incapable of absorbing food naturally, especially milk and milk-based foods. Jessica's persistent diarrhea and failure to gain weight were the main clues to the diagnosis.

Feinbloom recommended that the Katzes try to eliminate certain foods from Jessica's diet to see if she was more sensitive to one type of food. Just as they began the trial diet, a bed opened up at Moscow Childrens Hospital Number 1 and on February 16 Jessica was admitted. She remained there until April 4. During the forty-eight days, according to Feinbloom who maintained contact with the Katzes and later obtained Jessica's hospital records, nothing was done. "They didn't do any tests to try to find out the reason for her diarrhea. There was no biopsy of her intestine, no sweat test, no balance studies, no cultures. They didn't even try to change her diet to see if that would help," he concluded.

"From my perspective," said Feinbloom, "it was a completely inadequate diagnostic workup for a child who was obviously not doing very well. I got the impression the Soviet doctors didn't have a good understanding of the problem."

Concerned over Jessica's progress, Feinbloom began a long-distance treatment program. He still did not know the exact nature of Jessica's problem but he felt it was important for her to gain weight soon.

"We began sending cans of a special infant formula to Jessica's parents. We used tourists who were going to Moscow," Feinbloom explains. "The Soviets didn't try to stop any of these shipments and when the Katzes began giving it to Jessica, the Soviet doctors agreed. I'm sure they wanted her to get better, too."

The formula Feinbloom sent contained sugars, proteins, and amino acids—a sort of liquid protein for children. If malabsorption were Jessica's problem, her body should be able to absorb these simple calories which required no digestion.

"Jessica began getting the formula on March 30," Feinbloom recalled. "By April 4, her weight had increased almost half a pound. It worked!"

The improvement continued. By May she weighed fourteen pounds. On November 30, 1978, when, as a result of Senator Kennedy's personal intervention, Jessica and her parents arrived in Boston to live, she was almost off the formula and eating regular food.

In an interview four months after Jessica's arrival in the United States, Feinbloom told me she was a healthy, normal child. "The best I can tell is she probably had a viral infection in Moscow that caused her malabsorption. It's not unusual for such infections to last for a few months," he said.

Did the special formula save her life? "Who knows?" he concluded. "We do know that Jessica immediately began to gain weight once the formula was used and that she continued to improve with its use. Of course you could say that her improvement was because her infection was better. There's just no way to tell."

6
Polyclinics

Article 32 of the 55 Principles of Health Legislation of the USSR specifies that all Soviet citizens are entitled to free medical care whether provided through polyclinics, hospitals, the emergency ambulance system, or home visits. "Invalids of World War II," according to the law, "receive special privileges in both hospitals and outpatient treatment."

Pavel Zorin, thin, dark haired, dressed in a black suit, white shirt, but without a tie, carefully placed his special medical pass in the small wooden box designated for invalids and heroes of the Great Fatherland War. In addition to war heroes and invalids, there were slots for "Heroes of Socialist Labor," "Heroines of the USSR," "Orders of The Lenin Prize." Each cubicle had at least two dozen cards marking patients who were waiting to see the doctor. Pavel noticed that his box contained one of the smaller piles. Perhaps he would not have to wait long today.

Pavel walked slowly along the corridor of the polyclinic looking for a place to sit. Two young men smoking and talking at the end of a long bench got up and offered him a seat. Pavel accepted with a nod, his thin body barely taking up half the space. When he was younger Pavel had resented such courtesies. After all, the loss of an arm did not make a man a cripple. Besides, since the accident in 1942 when he caught his right arm in the firing mechanism of a Zenitka antiaircraft gun, he had continued to work. During the rest of the war Pavel served as a supply sergeant and for the last twenty-five years he had worked as a statistician for Gosplan, the Soviet Ministry of Finance.

But at fifty-eight, Pavel felt old and was more than happy to accept small courtesies. Positioning himself uneasily on the hard bench (his bones seemed uncomfortably close to his skin), he pulled an old copy of *The Sea Wolf* from his pocket. It was the second or third time he had read the Jack London novel but it was still a good story.

Polyclinics are the starting point for Soviet citizens when they want medical care. From age sixteen every citizen carries an internal passport book which records date of birth, nationality (Russian, Georgian, Jewish), and place of residence. On the basis of this address a polyclinic is assigned. In the past polyclinics were small neighborhood units of four to six general doctors and a half-dozen nurses, serving four to six thousand persons. Today, with the increasing trend toward specialization, the urban polyclinics are a larger part of a hospital-polyclinic complex with dozens of doctors on staff responsible for a population of 50,000 persons.

For the last six years Pavel had been coming to a small, older polyclinic in the Izmailovskoye Region of Moscow. It had ten doctors on staff but there were rumors it too would be closed with all patients reassigned to larger clinics. Pavel hoped the change would not come soon. Over the years he had grown used to the drafty examining rooms, the hard benches, and even the long waits. Over the years the inconveniences had become familiar, even strangely comforting.

When he was younger, Pavel thought, there had been little need for medicine and doctors. But a half-dozen years ago he had started getting headaches. On his first clinic visit, Pavel was afraid the doctors would find a brain tumor or some other form of *rak* (cancer). The first doctor who examined him asked a lot of questions. When did his headaches occur? How long did they last? Did he also have problems with his vision? No, Pavel said his eyes were fine. The only thing that bothered him was his head. It hurt like a bad tooth. The *vrach* told him his blood pressure was too high and that he would have to see another doctor, a specialist, before treatment could begin.

In polyclinics most Soviet patients are examined first by a general practitioner or a *terapevt* (internist) and then referred to a specialist for consultation or treatment. According to the system, Pavel had no choice in the physician who first examined him or the specialist who prescribed reserpine, an antihypertensive drug.

But Pavel, like most Soviet patients, quickly learned the polyclinic's routine. Many of the general physicians work a split day, spending three and a half hours in the clinic and three hours making house calls. The specialists, depending on their seniority and qualifications, spend more time at the polyclinic, but every physician follows a schedule.

After having trouble with his first specialist (Pavel insisted the de-

pression caused by reserpine was not worth a lower blood pressure),
Pavel varied the times of his visits. That way he was sent to different
doctors (his medical record was always kept in the polyclinic's central record room). On his fourth visit the physician, a middle-aged
Russian woman, agreed that another drug would be better.

Since then Pavel tried to schedule his arrival at the clinic during
the hours when Dr. Tamara Glotox was on duty. Over the years,
Pavel and Tamara, as she asked to be called, developed a close phy-
sician-patient relationship.

Together they discovered that Pavel's blood pressure readings
varied widely. They went up when he had to work late or when he
had fought with his *sosed* (neighbor) who was always getting drunk
and singing late into the night. Once when Tamara had gotten permission for Pavel to go to his trade union's sanatorium, or health resort, on the Black Sea, his blood pressure was normal without medication. But as soon as he got back to Moscow, away from the rest
and relaxation, he had to restart the pills.

Pavel has his blood pressure measured once a week at a small
medical station near his work manned by a *feldsher* (physician's assistant). Every three months he comes to the polyclinic and his
weekly blood pressure readings are precisely recorded on the back of
a small calender.

Occasionally, Tamara prescribes valerium in addition to Pavel's
regular pills. Extracted from the valeria root, it is widely used in the
Soviet Union as a mild tranquilizer and it helps reduce the amount
of blood pressure medication Pavel needs.

On most polyclinic visits Pavel, despite his "special consideration" as a war invalid, has a two-hour wait. "There are special consideration for many things," he told me. "Everyone has a medal.
They can't give you a raise, so they give you a medal or a special
pass. But the clinic is so crowded," he explained, "that everyone has
to wait. So I read, I try to relax." The one thing that does bother
Pavel is when, after waiting his turn, Tamara can only give him a
few minutes.

"She has too many patients," he complains. "The administration
expects the clinic to work like a factory, so many in and out each
hour. Even while she is talking to you she is writing, trying to fill out
the necessary papers."

The official Soviet norm or standard for the number of patients a polyclinic physician should see each hour is eight for general physicians, nine for surgeons. That is roughly seven minutes per consultation. Most polyclinic administrators I spoke to admitted that it was impossible to meet these goals. For one thing, the Soviets' own research demonstrates that the average polyclinic doctor needs at least five minutes to fill out the forms required for the patient's medical record, his trade union, and to excuse the patient from work. But since the norm calls for it, five to eight patients are scheduled each hour. By 10 A.M. the wait is up to an hour.

All Soviet workers are entitled to time off to visit polyclinics. Because of the long wait, however, there is at times reluctance on the part of plant managers to permit the visits. To solve the problem, many factories with more than 4,000 workers have separate physician-staffed polyclinics. Smaller factories have *feldshers* to handle small emergencies and provide routine examinations. In addition, there are first-aid stations at subway stations and other public places where any citizen can receive attention.

All of these many alternatives—neighborhood polyclinics, industrial clinics, and first-aid stations—resulted, according to Soviet health planner-economist G. A. Popov, in an incredible 4 billion contacts between Soviet citizens and their health system in 1978. This amounts to approximately fourteen contacts with the medical system a year for every man, woman, and child in the USSR (in the United States the comparable figure is six). About two-thirds of the visits are to physicians, the remainder to *feldshers* or public health nurses.

How many of these 4 billion annual visits are necessary and helpful is, of course, unknown. But as in any system where missing a few hours' work is the only reason for not going to see a doctor, there is bound to be overuse. According to a study done by Dr. E. K. Kama in the Estonian Republic of the USSR, 10 to 15 percent of clinic visits by workers from industrial establishments during working hours were "unfounded." The Soviets measure these unnecessary visits as they do other examples of inefficiency—in terms of unfulfilled industrial production. "If on each clinic visit an average of two hours is spent away from working time," the study authors conclude, "then, for the Estonian Republic as a whole, the losses total 5,000 hours each day and result in unfulfilled production of 30,000 rubles [$46,500]."

Dr. Popov's analysis supports this observation. He has found that there is less demand for polyclinic visits among retired Soviet citizens than among workers. Popov, a former practicing physician now recognized by many non-Soviet economists as the most incisive health analyst in the USSR, is also concerned that this large number of visits reflects the increasing dependence of Soviet physicians on specialists.

"It is becoming increasingly common in our country for a person to come to a polyclinic with a few vague nonspecific complaints, nothing serious, just anxiety," he says. "But because the *vrach* cannot put a name on the problem or perhaps because he doesn't want to spend time with the patient he sends her to a specialist. And that specialist sends her to another.

"The average Moscow citizen," Popov told me during a 1979 interview, "sees a doctor or *feldsher* eighteen times a year. Is that number of visits really necessary? And then there is the problem of duplication. A patient will see a *vrach* where he works, then another one at his polyclinic, and perhaps a third at the hospital. Most of them do the same thing."

But while there is concern among articulate and recognized experts like Popov over the large number of physician visits, there are no government plans to reduce them. Unlimited access to a doctor is the most popular aspect of the Soviet medical system. A Soviet citizen knows that no matter how many visits are needed, there is no problem finding a doctor. He simply goes to his polyclinic and, after waiting long enough, he will be seen. Besides, the propaganda value of the many physician visits combined with their low cost makes them attractive to Ministry of Health officials who do not share Popov's views.

Directives for the 1981–85 five-year plan call for a doubling in the number of physician visits for rural inhabitants from what Soviet leaders consider a low of four per year up to eight. A small increase is also projected for persons living in most cities. One reason for this emphasis on physician visits may be their cost, which under the Soviet system remains low.

Recent Soviet estimates, unearthed by economist Christopher Davis of the Harvard Russian Research Center, place the cost of this polyclinic care at slightly over one ruble ($1.55) a visit. This cost varies depending on which specialist the patient sees and how long he spends. But even the longer, more specialized visits seldom cost more than two or three rubles.

The reason is that the main cost (75 percent of the total budget) goes for doctors' salaries, all of which are low. Only 7 percent is spent on medicines and dressings and less than 1 percent on medical instruments. The low investment in instruments and technology is similar to that found in Soviet hospitals.

The result is a simple, "hands-on" approach to diagnosis and treatment. When Pavel first came to the polyclinic for evaluation of his hypertension, for example, no X rays, blood, or urine tests were taken. In the United States such testing would have been routine to check for any damage the high blood pressure might have caused Pavel's kidneys and heart. In some cases, depending on the patient's age and his medical history, more elaborate diagnostic tests searching for an underlying cause of the hypertension might also have been done.

With most cases the results of these tests do not change the patient's treatment since the reason behind most patients' hypertension is never discovered. Regardless of existing heart or kidney damage, the pressure must be controlled. Therefore, the Soviets take a direct approach. This means a few patients with a potentially curable form of the disease (those caused by tumor, for example) will be missed.

Large surveys estimate that 10 to 14 percent of the Soviet population have hypertension. A study of Moscow factory workers, reported by Dr. Igor K. Shkhvatsabaya at a 1978 World Health Organization (WHO) meeting on hypertension, estimated that 30 percent of people who had high blood pressure were unaware of it and that only 15 percent of identified hypertensives were being adequately treated.[1]

With this record in Moscow where the best medical services in the Soviet Union are available, it is not surprising that problems with undetected cases of hypertension occur in other parts of the USSR. A survey from the Semashko Research Institute, published in *Soviet Health Protection* in 1976, recorded that in many Soviet republics, half

[1] Comparable estimates for the United States reveal similar overall figures, with the degree of success varying widely depending on whether the population studied is urban or rural, poor or affluent.

of the newly discovered cases of hypertension were uncovered in the late, more serious stages when discovered. The same study showed that a third of patients with previously documented high blood pressure had not seen a doctor in over a year.

The problems of discovering and then treating the estimated 20 to 40 million people with hypertension in the USSR (U.S. figures are, again, roughly similar) were discussed by Shkhvatsabaya at the 1978 WHO meeting. As a director of the Myashnikov Institute of Cardiology, Shkhvatsabaya has been trying to improve public education by appearing on television and radio and by writing articles for the popular health magazine, *Zdorovya,* emphasizing the importance of detecting and treating high blood pressure.

There have even been spot announcements on *Vremya,* the main television news program which comes on at nine each night, urging people to have their blood pressure checked.

Since prevention is a basic hallmark of Soviet medical philosophy, finding large groups of untreated patients with hypertension is disturbing to its medical leadership. In the past, the concentration in both the hospital and polyclinic was on getting enough beds, clinics, and physicians. Today, with over 3 million beds and 4 billion annual clinic visits, Soviet leaders are beginning to question why these large numbers have not worked.

The problem is especially disconcerting since the Soviets now claim that approximately 100 million citizens or 40 percent of the population are examined under its *dispenserizatsiia* (follow-up center) system. *Dispenserizatsiia* refers to the practice of examining people with special medical needs, such as pregnant women, young children or hypertensives, on a regular schedule.

But getting the right persons to consult a doctor in the first place is a major problem. Although the nationwide average for medical visits per population is high, there are many parts of the USSR where people are still suspicious of medical care and many Soviet citizens, whether rural or urban, who prefer to treat themselves.

A recent article by Professor Kudrin, head of the pharmacology department at the First Moscow Medical Institute, in the nationwide daily *Izvestia,* criticized self-care:

> Self-care is one of the most widespread paradoxes of our time. In this century of amazing scientific successes and gigantic strides in enlightenment, apparently there remains in the human soul a

niche that is subject to the most absurd superstitions. I am referring to the fetishization of medicine. How else can one explain the
fact that even many highly educated people show an astonishing
thoughtlessness about repairing their bodies themselves. . . . [These
persons] have a passion for hunting out and trying everything
without consulting physicians.

Pavel explained that it is common practice among his friends to
treat many different symptoms—headaches, stomachaches, muscle
cramps—with a large variety of common herbs. Many small kiosks
around Moscow sell preparations ranging from coriander seeds to
special mountain-grown varieties of honey. Most have been used for
hundreds of years and the habits are difficult to change.

Besides established traditions, Soviet health leaders are discovering that the exact number of physician visits, especially under the
dispenserizatsiia system, may be inflated. At times forms are filled out
without actually examining the patient. The same philosophy that
ensures that polyclinic doctors always see the required number of
patients, at least on paper, leads to exaggerated estimates of preventive examinations.

Also contributing to the problem of untreated disease are the
kinds of *vrachi* the Soviet patient sees. Today, as Dr. Popov pointed
out, polyclinic patients in most Soviet cities see a specialist for most
of their problems.

Urban Soviet citizens have accepted the loss of the family physician. They acknowledge that outpatient care will be provided by
various physicians at different times. A close patient-physician relationship is increasingly rare. In fact, many citizens living in large
cities mistrust general physicians, believing their knowledge is not
sufficient to treat most problems. In large part this attitude has been
fostered by the Ministry of Health, which in the last few years has
emphasized the importance of specialists in daily medical care.

Even the treatment of hypertension, for example, which would be
routine for most U.S. physicians, involves specialists in the USSR.
Soviet recommendations include a nerve specialist to check on the
contribution of anxiety to the disease and an ophthalmologist to follow any changes in the patient's eyes. An electrocardiogram, if
needed, must also be ordered and interpreted by another specialist.

For example, Pavel's doctor, Tamara, is a general physician, a
terapevt, and she sent Pavel to an ophthalmologist for an eye exami-

nation. She does not have nor was she trained in the use of an ophthalmoscope, an instrument American general practitioners use every day. When Pavel went for an electrocardiogram a year ago, a specialist in clinical physiology performed and interpreted the EKG. A cardiorheumatologist listened to his heart, while another physician specializing in diets once told him how to cut back salt in his food to help lower his blood pressure.

With fifty-one different specialties, though, it is almost impossible for all but the largest Soviet polyclinics to have enough different kinds of doctors. Since no current Soviet medical graduates are broadly trained in all the aspects of what we would call general or family medicine, patients frequently get only part of their problem addressed at any one visit. The resulting fragmentation can lead to inadequate treatment.

Despite these problems, the Soviet leadership appears committed to increasing specialization, claiming that the amount of modern medical knowledge is now too large for any one graduate to master it all. In doing so, they seem willing to forego the benefits of the closer, if less rigorous, doctor-patient relationship that Pavel and Tamara enjoy.

Once the *apteka* (pharmacy) where Pavel bought his blood pressure medication (the prescription cost him 15 rubles or $23 a month) ran out of the pills. The pharmacy director told Pavel he did not know when they would be available. For a few weeks Pavel went back to taking reserpine, but just as before he became depressed and increasingly uninterested in his hobby, stamp collecting, and his grandchildren. Pavel tried other *apteki* in the city but the shortage was citywide. Tamara, however, had a sister who was a doctor working in Odessa. In Odessa there was plenty of guanethidine. So when her sister came to Moscow for a visit, she brought a supply of the medicine with her.

"We help each other," Pavel explained. "She once told me she would like to have a pair of blue jeans for her son. I have a friend who sometimes travels to Italy and he brought me a pair for him. She was very happy."

7
Emergency

The coronation of Nicholas II, last Tsar of Russia, took place on May 17, 1896. The following day the traditional banquet for the people of Moscow was set for Khodynka Meadow, a field normally used as a training ground for military troops. It was the only place large enough to accommodate the hundreds of thousands of Muscovites expected to honor the new Tsar. By dawn on the eighteenth, half a million people had gathered in the large open quadrangle crisscrossed by a network of shallow trenches and ditches.

As the sun rose the crowd surged forward to get close to the wagons containing beer and food. A rumor began that there wasn't enough beer for everyone. Panic raced through the crowd and people began running toward the wagons, pushing aside the small squadron of Cossacks assigned to keep the peace. Women and children were knocked down; the mob, now out of control, stepped on them, crushing them into the ground.

According to A. A. Lopakhon, then assistant procurator of the Moscow Circuit Court, the crowd rapidly became a unified mass, swaying from side to side with people so tightly packed together it was almost impossible to free one's hand and raise it. Tatiana Petrova, another observer, recalls seeing children passed from hand to hand above the crowd in a desperate attempt to save them.

In all 2,000 people, among them many women and children, lost their lives that day at Khodynka Meadow. Many were crushed to death, others suffocated.

One of the reasons for the high death toll was that in the Moscow of 1896, no organized system of emergency care existed. The few horse-drawn ambulances that existed were late in hearing of the tragedy and when finally dispatched, they could not get through the crowds. When, four hours later, the first medical aid did arrive, according to Lopakhon, they "had nothing to do except supervise the removal of the heaps of shapeless bodies."[1]

The next day Nicholas and his wife Alexandra visited the wounded at the hospitals. The Tsar personally gave each victim's family 1,000 rubles. But despite these actions, critics of the autocracy used the disaster at Khodynka to help dramatize the ineptness of the royal government.

Coronations are no longer held in Moscow. But, as in any other large city, disasters still occur. On January 8, 1977, a bomb exploded in the Moscow subway, killing seven persons and seriously injuring thirty-seven others.

Moments after the explosion a call went to the central station of the Moscow *skoraya* (the citywide emergency care system),[2] a large building on Kolkhoznaya Ploshchad adjacent to a 600-bed hospital, and to Sklifosovskii Emergency Research Institute. The physician answering the call immediately notified the center's senior physician who, by turning a switch on a central control panel, was able to hear details of the catastrophe.

He called the three *skoraya* substations closest to the subway explosion and within seconds six ambulances were on their way to the scene. Each ambulance carried a medical team consisting of a *feldsher* and a physician, both trained in emergency medicine. The first ambulance arrived five minutes after the blast. Initially there was confusion in determining the number of injured and dead. With the arrival of the second ambulance a few minutes later, however, it became obvious that there were dozens of seriously injured people. The emergency *vrach* on the second ambulance radioed back to *skoraya* headquarters requesting more ambulances and emergency supplies.

Meanwhile at *skoraya* central, the senior physician, who had already notified the Moscow Soviet (the administrative branch of city government) along with the city's police and fire departments, ordered all twenty-two of Moscow's *skoraya* substations to immediately

[1] Quoted in M. A. Messel, *Urban Emergency Medical Services of the City of Leningrad* (Washington, D.C. Department of Health, Education and Welfare, 1975), p. 5.
[2] *Skoraya* literally means quick or rapid; the full title is *Skoraya Meditsinskaya Pomoshch*, or quick medical assistance.

stop transport of nonemergency cases and divert all ambulances to the subway disaster.

Most of the ambulances sent were RAF-977-I models, white, van-type vehicles equipped with a flashing red light on the roof, an illuminated red cross above the windshield, and the inscription *Skoraya Meditsinskaya Pomoshch* along the side. Each RAF-977-I contains a stretcher, a variety of splints and fracture boards, and oxygen equipment. RAF ambulances are similar in design and equipment to commercial ambulances in the United States. Also pressed into service were the smaller and not so well equipped Volga ambulances normally used to bring less critically ill patients to hospitals from their apartments.

At the bomb scene, one of the ambulance physicians took charge of keeping the *skoraya* central office informed of the need for more supplies and of the extent and type of injuries. Treatment for the victims who were nearest the blast began at the subway station. Tourniquets were placed above broken and bloody arms and legs. One shattered arm had to be amputated at once. Persons in severe pain but not shock were given nitrous oxide (laughing gas) to breathe to relieve the pain and make their trip to the hospital easier. Morphine was administered to some. Transfusions of concentrated glucose solution were started for shock victims.

One of Moscow's specialized antishock ambulances arrived, bringing with it a portable electrocardiograph, an electric heart defibrillator, and an anesthesia machine. A man with a penetrating chest wound was treated by placing a tube into his chest to remove blood, making it easier for him to breathe.

As the injured were treated and their conditions stabilized, they were moved to Moscow hospitals. Some went to the 600-bed hospital located next to central *skoraya* headquarters, others to hospitals throughout the city. Each hospital was notified before the patient's arrival. Because of the volume of casualties and the limited number of specialized centers in Moscow capable of handling complicated trauma cases, some patients were driven long distances to find an appropriate hospital to treat them.

After the dead and injured were in hospitals, the *skoraya*'s senior physician sent his staff to canvass the hospitals and record the victims' names. Physical descriptions of the dead were recorded for the information bureaus where worried families and friends were calling.

The Moscow *skoraya*, with 22 substations and 800 emergency ambulance teams, is one of the world's largest emergency care systems. The highly organized ambulance system, along with complementary systems for less serious problems, makes finding a doctor one of the easiest things to do in most major Soviet cities.

Whether in response to the unusual occurrence of a bombing (for which three persons were later tried and executed) or for the more common, everyday demands of automobile accidents, poisonings, and heart attacks, the Soviet citizen living in or near a city has four opportunities to receive medical service. Each level is designed to bring medical care to the patient and, if possible, keep him out of the overcrowded hospitals.

Contact with the *skoraya* ambulance system is made by dialing 03 from any telephone. Pay phones are equipped so the number can be dialed without using a two-kopeck coin. This puts the caller in touch with that city's central ambulance dispatcher. The desk clerk answering the phone records the name, address, and telephone number of the caller, along with the nature of the problem. In the case of serious accident or illness, the request card is marked with an urgent red stripe before being sent by conveyor belt to the senior dispatcher. In large cities, such as Moscow with twenty-two *skoraya* substations, Leningrad with seventeen, or Kiev with eight, the dispatcher decides which substation is most convenient. By means of a large control board, he also keeps track of how many ambulances are available citywide.

Each of the first-line RAF-977-I ambulances carries a *feldsher* (physician's assistant) and an emergency physician. To qualify, the physician must take ten months of specialized training in emergency medicine. He or she is then able to perform as much diagnosis and early treatment on the spot as the patient's condition permits. If the problem is more than the regular ambulance can handle, the physician can call for help from one of the specialized ambulance teams. In Leningrad and Moscow, the *skoraya* has ambulance teams to treat victims of heart attack, poisonings, and strokes whose conditions are so critical that, in the opinion of the emergency physician, moving them without treatment would be dangerous. The ambulance specialized for poisonings is equipped with a supply of antidotes for commonly taken substances.

If the call is not about an accident but from someone ill at home, one of two courses is taken. The desk clerk, who is usually a trained nurse, may give instructions for simple remedies over the phone. Or she may transfer the call to a physician who listens to the complaint and determines whether an ambulance should be dispatched. If the physician decides the problem is not serious enough to warrant an ambulance run, he can dispatch an emergency-care physician for a home visit or refer the patient to his local polyclinic for *neotlozhnaya* (house-call service).

These two services, the emergency aid and *neotlozhnaya*, function at levels below the *skoraya*. The emergency aid service, which is available only in a few large Soviet cities, provides specially trained physicians on call at central locations to travel to homes and apartments for emergency visits. The emergency aid service does not use ambulances.

The house-call service is part of the polyclinic system. Physicians on staff at the polyclinics or outpatient departments take turns on the *neotlozhnaya*, providing home visits to patients within the polyclinic's service area. The *neotlozhnaya* is normally much slower than either the *skoraya* or emergency aid systems and is used mainly for patients with chronic problems.

But regardless of whether the caller is answered by an ambulance doctor, an emergency aid physician, or the *neotlozhnaya*, there is emphasis on immediate evaluation and treatment by a physician. Emergency systems in most other countries concentrate on transportation. The major reason a physician-run emergency system is possible is the Soviet Union's 1 million doctors. No other country, with the exception of Israel, enjoys such a high doctor-to-patient ratio—1 per 220 people.

As a result, Soviet hospitals do not have emergency rooms. Instead, a miniature emergency room comes to the patient. Whether the emergency *vrach* arrives as part of a first-line RAF-977-I ambulance, or comes from the emergency aid center, or performs a home visit through the *neotlozhnaya* program, he or she comes prepared to diagnose and, if possible, treat.

In his book describing the *skoraya* system in Leningrad, Dr. M. A. Messel tells of a seventy-five-year-old woman (Mrs. A.) who called the ambulance service because of "aching pains in the area of her heart."[3]

Because of the seriousness of her complaint the dispatcher sent a first-line RAF ambulance. The emergency physician examined her and with a portable machine took an electrocardiogram. On the basis of the EKG and his examination, the physician concluded that she was not, as first feared, having a heart attack. He diagnosed preinfarction angina, a condition one step before a complete heart attack.

The physician also decided to treat her at home, first giving injections of morphine to relieve the pain. Because the Soviets believe in the ability of blood thinners to reduce the severity of heart attacks, the patient was started on Heparin, a blood thinner prepared from beef liver. Her daughter was to give the injections every six hours. The emergency physician left instructions for Mrs. A's doctor to check on her frequently for the next two days. According to Messel, the patient went on to recover and was never hospitalized.

Although there was substantial investment of physician time (the emergency *vrach* remained at Mrs. A's apartment for three hours), his on-the-spot evaluation and treatment kept Mrs. A. out of the hospital.

Using the *skoraya*, the Soviets are also able to start treatment earlier for other diseases. Treatment for various forms of thrombophlebitis (inflammation of veins) and infectious diseases begins in the patient's apartment and, if possible, continues in the home.

The wisdom of this early treatment approach is open to debate. In the United States, most emergency treatment is provided in a hospital. In addition, many diseases, especially problems related to the heart, that were formally treated at home are now being cared for in a hospital. The growth in the last fifteen years of coronary care units and their availability in most U.S. hospitals have led to an aggressive, hospital-oriented approach to heart attack victims.

But studies in England, where the availability of coronary care units is severely limited by finances, suggest that some heart attack patients do not need the elaborate monitoring and sophisticated machines available in most U.S. hospitals. Many heart attack patients do well with simple rest and quiet. So for patients without

[3] Messel, *Urban Emergency Services*, p. 144.

clearcut evidence of a heart attack or without evidence of complications after an attack, the Soviets will frequently leave the patient at home to be treated by the family.

The results of this policy are unknown. Exact statistics comparing hospital versus home treatment for heart attack patients in the USSR are not available. In recent years some changes have occurred that make Soviet practice more like our own. A few years ago, for example, it was common for Soviet physicians to treat patients with pulmonary edema (fluid in the lungs) at home, under the belief that patients were too critically ill to move. Today, *skoraya* physicians, like doctors in most other countries, quickly move pulmonary edema patients to hospitals for treatment. But the practice of home treatment for some heart attack victims still continues.

Besides heart attack victims, the Soviet emergency system approaches injured patients somewhat differently than most other countries, providing early, on-the-spot pain relief. Dr. Messel, in his book on the Leningrad *skoraya*, describes the treatment of a twenty-eight-year-old man who fell beneath a streetcar:

> By the time the ambulance arrived he was still lying under the streetcar held down by the wheel. He was extricated by firemen. His condition was severe. Skin pale. He was anxious, trying to get up. Confused. Did not answer questions. Pulse was 60 per minute and weak. Blood pressure low at 70/50. His right shoulder was severed, hanging on only by a small piece of skin.

> Diagnosis: Traumatic severing of right shoulder and arm. On the spot 1 cc of morphine was given intravenously; nitrous oxide anesthesia was then given and patient fell asleep after four minutes. Then the hanging shoulder was amputated and a sterile bandage applied. . . . Patient delivered in a state of sleep to the Emergency Aid Institute.

Patients suffering pain from kidney stones or gallbladder attacks also get nitrous oxide on the way to the hospital. But this early approach to pain relief is potentially dangerous; patients in shock can be further compromised by it. The use of nitrous oxide at the scene is only possible because of the early evaluation by a physician who can determine when pain relief is dangerous and when it will allow for a more comfortable trip to the hospital.

The Soviets are quite proud of the *skoraya* and are expanding it, with eighty new first aid hospitals planned for major Soviet cities.

Today the *skoraya* is best developed in Moscow, Leningrad, and Kiev.

The Ministry of Health spends much time analyzing the system's functions and seeking improvements. The time taken to respond to calls is carefully monitored. In Leningrad, the average time for an ambulance and physician to arrive is eleven minutes; in Moscow, eight. (In sixteen major U.S. cities, response times for ambulances vary from 2.5 to 8.5 minutes.)

The accuracy of the emergency physician's on-the-spot diagnosis is also subject to scrutiny. In analyzing the Leningrad system, Dr. Messel discovered that when examining patients with abdominal pain, the emergency doctors frequently (as high as 25 percent of cases in one study) diagnosed appendicitis when the problem was really food poisoning, gastritis, or another nonsurgical problem.

The organization of the *skoraya* and its heavy reliance on physicians permit the Soviet Union to allocate patients only to those hospitals that are most appropriate to their problem. Patients needing specific treatment for kidney stones or a gallbladder attack, for example, are taken to hospitals having the specific facilities to treat these problems. This means that all Soviet hospitals do not have to be equipped to handle a wide range of problems. It means economy since the expensive duplication of emergency services so common in every American city is avoided in the Soviet Union.

Furthermore, many smaller Soviet hospitals have limits on the number and type of emergency patients they will accept, thus allowing them to estimate precisely their need for staff and supplies.

The attention paid to careful planning is demonstrated not only by the triaging of hospital admissions but also by the supplies each *skoraya* physician carries. Until 1965 the emergency physician's case contained, among other things, a packet of sterile gauze. A study of the usage of gauze demonstrated that many times more was used than actually needed. Smaller, individual packets were designed to replace the larger one. Instuctions were given to all physicians to put a bandage on using the minimum amount of gauze required.

The *skoraya* is often referred to by the Soviet government as an example of how strong central planning and a government-sponsored medical system is more humane than the United States' private, for-profit medical system. In the Soviet book *Emergency Medical Care*, Dr. I. A. Ostrovskii describes our uncoordinated mixture of private and public emergency medical services, with its heavy emphasis on money, as "backward."

Indeed, compared to the U.S. citizen, the average Soviet citizen is closer to medical care. There is a clinic where he works. If he has a small injury on the street, there are first aid stations at subway stations and busy intersections. Emergencies developing on the street or at home will be handled by the *skoraya* or *neotlozhnaya*. In all of these situations, with the exception of the *feldsher*-staffed first aid stations, the Soviet citizen will have early and uninhibited access to a physician. By both official and unofficial accounts, the system is popular and widely used. An average *skoraya* substation in Leningrad staffed with ten ambulances receives 7,000 calls a year. Of every 1,000 Soviet citizens living in major cities, 124 use one aspect of the emergency-care system each year. Nationwide, the 4,000 emergency stations and 70 specifically designed hospitals handled 75 million calls in 1978.

Appendectomy—The Skoraya in Action

Thursday, December 22. I go to John's room to examine him. For the last two days I have been concerned about his abdominal pain. Initially, I thought it was another case of mild gastritis, common among the staff of the exhibit. But this morning his symptoms, fever, continued nausea, vomiting, and my examination findings (pain and tenderness in his lower abdomen) all point toward another diagnosis—appendicitis.

I wait a few hours and then repeat my examination. Although there is some danger in delay—an inflamed appendix could rupture—I want to be absolutely sure of my diagnosis.

We are living in Yerevan, Armenia, a city that nudges the Soviet Union's border with Turkey and Iran. For most of the past month the valley in the southern Caucausus where Yerevan is located has been covered by a thick, dense fog. Visibility has been so restricted that on many mornings it has been impossible to mark sunrise. Aeroflot, the Soviet airline, has been canceling or delaying most flights. Evacuation is impossible. If John needs his appendix removed, it will have to be done in Yerevan.

By noon on the same day, after probing and poking John's abdomen, I am convinced. Acute appendicitis.

I place a call to the local *skoraya* emergency service, explaining the problem. A first-line ambulance team (physician and *feldsher*) arrived within fifteen minutes. The *vrach* takes a few minutes to examine John and ask him some questions. He immediately—almost too immediately, I think—agrees with my diagnosis. He tells John to dress and the two of us follow him to the street.

The white-paneled ambulance with *Skoraya Meditsinskaya Pomoshch* written on the side contains a stretcher and a long bench. Carrying an emergency bag of drugs, the *feldsher* gets into the front seat with the driver. John, the *vrach,* and I ride in back, seated on the bench.

Within three minutes, traveling without siren or flashing lights, we arrive at the entrance to a gray, four-story building, the emergency hospital of Yerevan. The ambulance physician leads us along a corridor lined with wooden benches, filled with waiting visitors. We are shown into a room divided into small cubicles. John is examined again while the ambulance doctor fills out a form giving the patient's name, age, and his presumptive diagnosis. The hospital admitting physician, after finishing his brief examination, takes the form and countersigns it, agreeing with its conclusion—*appenditsit.*

John now is asked a few questions and it is quickly agreed that he is the first American ever treated here. The admitting doctor smiles and jokes, "Are American appendixes bigger than Russian ones?" I laugh and even John manages a weak smile.

After exchanging his clothes for a set of corduroy pajamas, John is carried on a stretcher to his room. It is long and narrow with four beds, but only one other patient. The window at the far end is filled with jars of canned food and a vase of wilted flowers. A technician comes in to take a blood sample.

As I am helping John get settled, two orderlies arrive to take him to the operating room. Surprised by the rapid decision to operate, I follow behind, expecting to accompany John into surgery. But I am stopped at the operating room door by a nurse and informed that, unlike the situation I have encountered in other Soviet cities, hospital rules in Yerevan forbid any visitors in surgery.

"But I'm a doctor," I explain, "I must be with him. If anything should happen, I'm responsible."

"*Nyet nelzia,*" she shakes her head, "the rules forbid it."

I appeal to some of the doctors sitting in their nearby lounge. A small crowd gathers around. Some of them agree, saying I should be permitted into the operating room. Others argue, "It's only an appendectomy, *eto nichego* [it's nothing at all]." Besides, they say, Dr. Yolian, candidate of medical science and the deputy chief doctor of the Emergency Hospital, is doing the surgery. There is nothing to worry about.

But the memory of the young American guide who, a year ago and on a similar exhibit, died following just such an appendectomy, haunts my memory. He was twenty-two, the same age as John. I telephone the local Ministry of Health, but the line is busy. As I am trying to decide what to do next and as the Soviet doctors argue around me, a nurse motions me into the hallway and silently hands me a small white towel. Inside is John's appendix. It is inflamed.

Obviously, I think angrily, no one bothered to listen to me. The Soviets just went right ahead and operated. As I hand his appendix back to the nurse, I begin pacing the corridor, waiting for John to return.

This would not have happened in America, I think. Patients have to give written permission for surgery. I hope John is all right, that there were no complications.

"They didn't put me to sleep," is the first thing he says as they wheel him out of the operating room. "They shaved me and then injected local anesthetic into my skin.

"I could see everything they did," John tells me. He talks rapidly, in short, excited bursts. "Sometimes it really hurt, especially when they pulled on my intestines. I could feel the pain all over my body. Once the pain got so bad, they gave me some gas to breathe and I fell asleep for a few minutes. The doctor showed me my appendix at the end."

I follow John back to his room and help the orderlies put him in bed. His surgical incision is five inches long, but it is closed with only two stitches. Still, his color is good, his pulse and blood pressure are stable. With the help of the nitrous oxide, he sleeps quietly.

I look at my watch. It is 3 P.M. We arrived at the emergency hospital only two hours ago. In that time, without the help of X rays and general anesthesia, using only the results from an examination and a single blood test, the operation is over.

In the afternoon Professor S. Avdalbekian, chairman of the surgery department, and Dr. Yolian, who performed the operation, examine John's incision, probing it cautiously with two fingers. A few hours later a nurse brings in an injection of morphine. John sleeps again.

The next morning he is able to take small sips of water. Unlike the U.S. practice of keeping patients hydrated after surgery with intravenous infusions, the Soviets, in cases like John's, wait until the patient can drink.

The next day I help John to the bathroom at the end of the hall. It is his first time out of bed and he is weak. The hallway is filled with patients, most, like John, holding their right side. They look like a small, battered army, each man marching carefully in his brown corduroy pajamas, trying not to disturb his two stitches.

The 200-bed Yerevan Emergency Hospital, I learn, is designed to treat the most common kinds of surgical emergencies: appendectomies, intestinal obstructions, acute gallbladder attacks, and injuries resulting from automobile accidents. As with most Soviet hospitals, there is a large staff on duty. Eight surgeons cover the evening shift even though the hospital averages only two or three operations a night.

In their free time, the surgeons congregate in a small on-call room containing an old sofa, a large conference table, and a small stand supporting a chessboard that seems to be constantly in use. Despite the confusion of my first hours, I have made friends with several of the staff physicians, and by the second day no one looks up when I come in.

These emergency physicians take a great deal of pride in how well and how quickly they do their job. The conversation in the small room often turns to how fast an appendectomy can be completed from the first incision to the suturing, referred to as "skin to skin." The surgeon's speed is important not only for reducing blood loss, but since most appendectomies in the Soviet Union are done without general anesthesia, also for reducing pain.

Professor Kaserzhian, I am told, holds the record for the emergency hospital. Thirty minutes "skin to skin."

Some of the surgeons on call at night are still in training, completing their *ordinatura* (residency) in surgery. For them much of medical practice is still new, endlessly exciting, and dramatic. One night as I prepare to leave for the hotel, the ambulance crew carries in a middle-aged woman who is moaning softly.

Samuel, in his second year of surgical training, follows her to the ward and then runs back to the on-call room, face flushed, talking rapidly in Armenian. One of the other *aspirants* translates his description into Russian as he speaks:

"We were called to an apartment on Karl Marx Street. When we got there she was lying on the floor. Her sister told us she'd been having abdominal pain for three or four days but she didn't want to call anyone," Samuel explains, shaking his head and pausing just long enough to light a cigarette.

"She was in shock, blood pressure 70/20, and I could hardly feel her pulse. I started an infusion and told Victor [the *feldsher*] to call for the specialized antishock ambulance. She was barely breathing but when I touched her *zhivot* [belly], she would cry out," Samuel says. "It was *peritonit*." (The patient's appendix had ruptured, spilling intestinal contents and bacteria, producing a serious infection, peritonitis.)

"When the antishock team arrived we opened her belly, right there in the bedroom," Samuel said proudly. "There was infection everywhere but we took her appendix out and her blood pressure improved. We're going to take her to surgery now to finish, but Dr. Garibdzhavian says she will be all right."

John also is improving rapidly. Christmas day is quiet. Some of the other American guides stop in to sing Christmas carols and bring food. By now John's appetite has returned, but getting warm meals is a problem. Each morning one of the nurse's aides brings in a bowl of hot *kasha* (wheat grain), but the hospital's kitchen is small and, with the exception of breakfast for some patients, meals are not provided.

Most patients, like John's roommate, an engineer, rely on their families to bring them food prepared at home. At the nursing station there is a small refrigerator to store jars of pickled eggs or borsch. Patients and families can also use a small hotplate on each floor. Tea is available and milk is kept on the windowsill. For patients from the country or those without a family, the nurses or nurse's aides bring food in.

Because it is an emergency hospital for acute problems, most of the patients recover quickly from their operations. Two days after Christmas, John is walking easily and is, as far as I am concerned, ready for discharge. But on rounds today, Dr. Garibdzhavian, a staff *khirurg* (surgeon) to whom the responsibility for John's day-to-day care has fallen, emphasizes that the minimum stay for an appendectomy is ten days. But there is no need for John to stay the full ten days, I explain. I can watch him back at the hotel. There are no exceptions, he responds.

The next day I stop Professor Avdalbekian in the hallway and ask whether John can be discharged. "It's very irregular," he says, "I will have to think about it."

Two days later, December 30, eight days after his operation, John is released to my care. His stitches are still in; I will take them out in a few days. As we walk out the door, Samuel, the young doctor who operated on the woman with a perforated appendix in her bedroom, is coming in with a middle-aged patient. *"Appenditsit,"* he smiles. "This one less than thirty minutes."

8

Sanatoriums–
The Worker's Reward

In late summer the American exhibit to which I was assigned as physician went to Ufa, a city of nearly 1 million people, more than 600 miles southeast of Moscow. Ufa is typical of other workers' towns throughout the Soviet Union—austere and single-minded.

Although the city dates back to 1574, it gives the impression of being recently established. Most of its buildings—eight- to twelve-story, gray-white apartment houses crowded in the center of town—suggest a concentrated building effort using a single box design for each structure. Radiating from the center of town are smaller four- to six-story rectangular apartment buildings, all bearing the marks of recent construction. Connecting the boxes with the rectangles like spokes of a wagon wheel are heavily traveled but unpaved roads. They lead to the Ufa and the Belaya rivers, which form a semicircle around the town. On their banks stand the reason for the apartment buildings, the roads, and Ufa's durability—a series of oil refineries.

Seven out of every ten people in Ufa work in the oil refineries or related industries. Most of the city's effort and a majority of its resources are aimed not at creature comforts but at strengthening this industrial base. To Ufa come French and Italian industrial experts along with expensive German drilling equipment. In contrast to the muddy roads around the apartment buldings, roads within the oil refineries are paved.

Each morning, from my hotel window, I watched the workers leave their crowded apartments and ride on overloaded buses or in the backs of open-air trucks to the riverbank, where miles of tubing, condensers, and collecting tanks sprawl unrestrained.

On many days, fewer workers arrive at the refinery than scheduled. Ufa, like most Soviet industrial cities, wrestles daily with the problem of sick and absent workers. The problem is large. The number of days lost per worker because of illness is substantially higher in Ufa than the Soviet Union's published national average of fourteen days per worker per year. Moreover, the illness rate in Ufa is almost twice that recorded at the giant Kama River truck factory, only 185 miles to the northwest. The reason behind this difference is not well understood. The Bashkirian Minister of Health attributed much of the difference to variations in the population of the two industrial centers.

The Kama River factory, the largest truck factory in the world, is a major, widely publicized Soviet effort. It attracts workers, most of them young, from many parts of the country. The illness rate among this group should be lower than Ufa's, where the population is older and the incidence of chronic disease higher.

The loss of valuable production time, for whatever reason, is a major concern for Soviet medicine. Articles describing methods of reducing the illness rate pervade their magazines and journals. Every illness, Soviet doctors are told, is a direct threat to the completion of the five-year plan. Screening programs designed to detect and treat workers with chronic health problems are in place. The oil refinery has a special polyclinic, with doctors available at the factory to counsel workers on proper diet, eating, and exercise habits.

Extensive health records are kept, not only on the plant but on each individual worker. The number and times he or she misses work, the reasons, and the dates are carefully noted. Excessive absenteeism is investigated. Workers are part of the investigative team.

To obtain a release from work, every oil refinery worker must see a physician. If he thinks it is indicated, the *vrach* can provide an excuse for six days. After that, the worker must be examined by a special panel. Each physician is monitored on the number and duration of the work excuses he writes. Every diagnosis has a designated number of sick days assigned. The diagnosis must be supported by objective evidence of illness.

But illness is only part of the struggle. Daily life in Ufa is suffocating, with little internal and almost no outside stimulation. You will not find Ufa on the official Intourist list of approved vacation spots. It is a closed city, with no foreign guests allowed.

As a result, the arrival of our American exhibit created a sensation. It was impossible to walk along the street without attracting long and curious stares. Most of the people had never seen an American before. From the day we opened to the closing six weeks later, more than half the people in Ufa visited the exhibit. The line for admission began forming long before sunrise and stretched for a mile by noon. The average wait to get in was six hours. For a few weeks that summer, the citizens of Ufa finally had something to do.

Besides traveling exhibits, the Soviet government sponsors other programs aimed at reducing the impact of overloaded buses, crowded apartments, and endless lines that lead to worker dissatisfaction and increased absenteeism. There are trips to the opera, to the ballet, to the museum. The local labor union even sponsors group trips out of the city, bringing Soviet-style organization and mass efficiency to a day in the country or a long-awaited vacation. Even in their free time, Soviets find themselves in groups.

"How could you take a trip by yourself?" Tamara, a factory worker, asked me incredulously. "How would you know where to go or what to do? In Ufa all my activities are done together with the workers from my factory."

Tamara is a broad-shouldered, husky woman. Her face, weathered by years of working outdoors, makes her look older than thirty-eight. All her life she has lived in Ufa, working at the refineries between the births of her four children. The children, her husband, Victor, a machinist, his father, and Tamara's mother share a sixth-floor, three-bedroom apartment in one of the boxlike buildings in the center of Ufa. The apartment and the family revolve around Tamara. She does the shopping, gets the children off to school, and prepares all the meals. She worries about what would happen if she were not there to take care of everyone.

But even Tamara admitted that sometimes she has to get away. "It's my back," she explained slowly, almost apologetically, embarrassed to admit a weakness. "For the last eight years I've had a lot of pain here." She pointed to the small of her back. The problem is aggravated by her job at the refinery, which involves checking and cleaning thirty-gallon oil drums after they are unloaded from a ship.

"It's especially bad at night," she continued, talking rapidly again while she hurried to prepare dinner in the apartment's pantry-size kitchen. "The only thing that helps is the sanatorium. I go there and everything, even my back, feels better."

Sanatoriums are a privilege officially available to every Soviet factory worker. In 1978, the Soviets had 2,277 sanatoriums with 175,-

ooo beds offering medical services. There are another 1,170 rest homes and boarding houses which are closely linked to the polyclinics and medical care. Each year these institutions provide a respite for 8 million workers. The sanatoriums are one part of the Soviet Union's many efforts to reduce industrial absenteeism.

The Soviets come to the sanatoriums to have their back pain reduced, their arthritic joints massaged, their diabetes controlled, their high blood pressure treated. Others, those with no specific medical problems, come simply to get away, to relax.

Sanatoriums are not a recent invention. Health resorts in the Caucasus, the Crimea, and along the Baltic coast catered to the wealthy long before the Soviets took power. But, as all the guidebooks and Soviet textbooks emphasize, before the Revolution the resorts were only for the wealthy and it was the 1919 Decree on Therapeutic Areas of Nationwide Importance that made them the property of the workers and peasants.

In 1960, the Council of Ministers of the USSR extended the act by turning over direct control of 80 percent of the sanatoriums to the labor unions. The move was part of a general liberalization of that time, initiated by Khrushchev, to improve the position of workers in Soviet society and provide them with more benefits. The change provided the sanatorium system with more rubles from the social insurance budget and from the individual industry's own excess funds. As the labor unions took over control of the sanatoriums, they began to use them as rewards for workers who met their quotas and as privileged vacation spots for party members.

"You must remember," a labor union official told me, "that in the USSR there is only so much you can do for a worker. You can't raise his salary or give him a better apartment. What you can do is give him a medal or recommend him for a stay in the sanatorium. Of the two, sanatoriums are far more popular."

The Soviet trade union (*profsouz*) differs from the American kind because it is organized around a particular enterprise, not a certain type of work. A trade union for a scientific research institute, for example, would include senior directors, academic researchers, as well as maintenance workers and laborers. Each trade union has a limited number of *putevki*, or sanatorium/resort tickets.

Obtaining a *putevka* requires a formal medical examination with twenty-five items in all, including a chest X ray, urinalysis, blood count, and physical examination. Because of polyclinic inefficiency, the entire evaluation can often take four to five visits to complete.

With a *putevka* in hand, the worker must negotiate for one of the limited number of slots. Many Soviet sanatoriums are designed to treat a specific group of illnesses, such as heart disease, and a worker with this problem may have to wait for an opening in that institution. Location of the sanatorium is another important factor. There is strong competition for southern ones, especially in the winter months.

At the same time, a trade union may have a large number of *putevki* for a Baltic sanatorium in February. But only a few ill persons want to go to the cold climate. Rather than lose these places, the trade union persuades its workers to buy a *goriachaia putevka* ("bought pass") if his regular vacation (*otpusk*) occurs in February.

On balance, however, the *putevki* go to workers with specific health problems, and lower-paid workers in the union are given preference for places. Workers with smaller salaries do not have to pay for sanatorium services; higher-placed officials do.

The very well-placed directors and high-ranking members of the Communist Party go to special sanatoriums. These are free of charge, with private rooms and more luxuries than state facilities. At famous resort cities like Sochi, Kislovodsk, and Essentuki there are special sanatoriums for the Council of Ministers and important officials of the Central Committee and various government ministries. Similar institutions exist for the police.

In these special places the food, by Soviet standards, is elegant, with uniformed waiters; varied menus, and formal dining rooms. The mineral baths are connected to the rooms by elevators.

Because of this emphasis on politics, party privileges, and location, all Soviet sanatoriums are frequently pictured by Western observers as a "luxury hotel." Since the mud baths, mineral springs, and heat treatments used in most sanatoriums do not have a firm scientific basis, they are viewed as window dressing, designed to give the appearance of medical attention without any attention to the results.

This type of criticism bewilders Soviet physicians and public health officials. Despite their recent support from labor unions, Soviet officials argue, sanatoriums have always been under the administrative control of Soviet public health authorities. Every facility has a full-time medical staff, and each patient is given an individual medical program to follow during his stay. To the Soviet health officials I spoke with, sanatorium treatment is an integral part of their medical system. Most of them could not understand how the United States has done without them for so long.

While our exhibit was in Ufa, I arranged a weekend visit to the main sanatorium for the city. Situated about 45 miles away among gently rolling hills, it is a sharp contrast to the urban dreariness of Ufa. The air is clear and the buildings are surrounded by parks. But the purpose of the sanatorium is ever present. Along the fence, on the approach to the main gate, a series of posters reminds workers of the latest five-year production goals and figures—"Wheat harvest, 167 million tons in 1966–70, 195 in 1971–75"—and that "the triumph of Communism is certain."

The sanatorium's medical director, a middle-aged man studying for an advanced Candidate of Science degree, met me at the entrance to the main treatment and recreation building. The sanatorium, he explained, has twenty-five physicians. It can handle 600 patients but usually has about 450. He said he hoped I would enjoy my brief stay and introduced me to his assistant, Valentina Betsianov, who would serve as my guide.

Valentina, forty-seven, had graduated from the medical institute in Ufa in 1950. She has been employed as a *vrach* at the sanatorium for the last eight years. A tall, heavyset woman with dark hair pulled severely back from her face, she had a warm and constant smile.

"All patients," Valentina explained, "stay at the sanatorium for the same time, twenty-four days." According to her, the emphasis is on teaching the patient better living habits and "it takes at least three weeks for people to realize how much better they feel."

The charge for the twenty-four days is 120 rubles ($186). The labor union pays 90 rubles; the patient is responsible for the rest.

The patients at Ufa share small, brightly painted rooms with two single beds. My roommate was Boris, a construction worker from Birsk, a town north of Ufa. His large, muscular, hairy body seemed to fill the small room. When he got up at six in the morning to do push-ups on our small balcony, I could feel the floor shake. Despite the small sleeping quarters, Boris seemed to luxuriate in the space the sanatorium provided.

Dressed in a blue cotton jump suit (the only model commonly available throughout the USSR), he would walk through the adjoining park, swinging his arms and occasionally jogging in place. Every so often he would stop and breathe deeply, obviously grateful for the clean air.

Boris had hypertension. As with all patients, he had been examined upon arrival at the sanatorium, his medical history reviewed, and a treatment program outlined. Besides medication, his daily schedule called for mineral baths, heat treatments, and three "well-balanced" meals. When I arrived, Boris had been following the program for two weeks and was pleased with his progress. "One forty," he announced proudly about his blood pressure one morning. "At home it was never lower than one sixty."

The routine at the sanitorium began at 8 A.M. For a half hour each morning, everyone participated in a short series of calisthenics led by a slightly overweight but enthusiastic physical therapist. Breakfast was held in a large, airy dining hall. Along the wall a series of colorful announcements listed the eight essential vitamins and described foods where each could be found. The meals at all three sittings were attractively prepared, and served in large portions.

Because so many of the people in the dining hall looked as if they could benefit from a diet, I asked Valentina whether she had many patients on reduced calories. "Of course," she said. "Only it's a little difficult. You see, we still have so many people who remember what it was like not to have enough to eat during the war. So the people that work in the dining room always put more on people's plates than they're supposed to. I'm afraid," she said, smiling and putting her hands on her own ample waist, "that we're not very successful when it comes to losing weight."

There were special diets designated for different conditions. Most patients with digestive problems got no fatty or fried foods. Persons with diseases of the large intestine, such as colitis, were not fed potatoes; ulcer patients ate soft foods with white bread. Cardiac patients received low-salt diets and were prohibited from eating sharp or spicy foods. All these various types of foods were not always available, but Valentina assured me everyone got enough to eat.

Besides large quantities of food, the other pride of the sanatorium's cafeteria is *kumiss*—mare's milk fermented with yeast and then quickly bottled. The sanatorium's stables supply the milk; workers bottle it on the grounds. Valentina explained that the extremely sour-tasting beverage is used to treat a number of diseases, but has been found especially useful for ulcer patients. In the past, *kumiss* was used for treatment of tuberculosis.

I asked her what she thought of its use in light of the recent evidence discovered in the United States that a milk diet might actually make ulcer disease worse by stimulating production of stomach acid. She said she had not heard of the problem and regardless of what the scientists said, she had seen *kumiss* help patients. "I have all my patients drink it three times a day," she explained. "For ulcer patients I use it more often."

My first morning, Valentina took me on a tour of the sanatorium. We began in the central treatment facility, a large room divided into small cubicles by hanging curtains and movable cloth screens. Within each cubicle was a small examining table. On many of them a patient lay being treated with low-frequency sound waves or a heat lamp or being massaged with a pine-scented oil.

"Every patient," Valentina explained, "is thoroughly examined by a physician when he enters the sanatorium. On the basis of the exam, we decide what treatment and exercise he should receive. Patients recovering from heart attacks, for example, are never given hot-bath treatments. Persons with arthritis are cautioned against too strenuous exercise for the first few days."

Soviet sanatoriums are based on specific medical categories. The one in Ufa concentrated on digestive problems: ulcers, gastritis, and gallbladders. Othes specialize in hypertension and heart disease. The Truskovetz Sanatorium in the Western Ukraine is well known for treatment of kidney stones, using special spring waters. Children's sanatoriums concentrate on rheumatic fever and respiratory infections. There are also special pregnancy sanatoriums that provide rest and relief of family responsibilities for women. They are small in number and a *putevka* to one is extremely hard to get.

The treatment program varies on its location, the availability of mineral water, and the diseases treated. A general routine involves mud baths every other day with mineral baths on alternate days. For cardiac patients, there is special attention aimed at preventing streptococcal infections because of the subsequent risk of rheumatic fever. Eucalyptus and menthol mists are inhaled.

For many diseases, the use of megavitamin injections is popular along with drinking of alkaline soda water. Visits with the doctor are held every fourth day.

I asked about the program given my roommate Boris. "He's being treated with reserpine [an antihypertensive drug]," Valentina said, "and to relax the nerves leading to his arteries, we massage him once a day after he's taken his daily bath. He's responded quite well. I'm very pleased."

"What would you do for someone with back pain?" I asked, thinking of Tamara's annual visit. "It would depend," Valentina explained slowly, patiently. "If it was *artrit* [arthritis], I would begin with heat and hot-water baths to loosen the muscles. Then a series of mineral baths. The bones in arthritis are, you know, weak and in need of minerals."

Just as I was about to ask how the minerals in the bath were treatments absorbed into the bones, a patient interrupted our conversation. "Dr. Betsianov, I want to thank you for sending me to the baths this week," a small, wrinkled woman said. "For five years the pain in my neck has kept me from looking up at the stars. But last night I was able to look and turn. It was wonderful."

"I'm glad," Valentina answered, putting her arm around the woman's waist and walking with her to the door.

"The baths are very important," Valentina continued, leading me up the stairway to a central dressing area where a dozen patients, men and women, sat in light-blue terrycloth robes. "Each sanatorium has its own special mixture, depending on the content of the local mineral springs. We're fortunate in Ufa that we have to add very little to the bath. It's very therapeutic just as it comes from the ground."

After checking with the matron in charge, Valentina led me through a long, tile-lined corridor to the central bath area. There were a dozen porcelain tubs, each at different levels and all slightly larger than the standard American model. All were connected by a gravity-fed series of pipes, with the overflow from one tub spilling into the one beneath it. After they had all been filled, an attendant went around to each one and dropped a cup of purple powder into its center.

Then the patients, dressed in bath suits, were brought in to soak for thirty minutes in the purple water. Afterwards they all walked along a short hall into a central shower area, where a series of shower heads located at various levels of the three-sided compartments sprayed them with clear water. Then they were instructed to rest for an hour.

In addition to the mineral baths, the sanatorium offered mud treatments. Exactly how the treatments work was not known, Valentina told me, but somehow "it encourages healing, it stimulates the body to correct itself." The mud is put only on the affected neck, arm, or back, heated to 108 degrees, and left in place for fifteen minutes.

These routines are taken quite seriously. The Ministry of Health sponsors special research institutes that investigate balneology (bath treatment) and other sanatorium regimes. The use of herbal cures is also an officially sponsored undertaking. In 1977 the Soviet government adopted a resolution aimed at increasing the number of medicinal plants used in sanatoriums as well as those sold in Soviet pharmacies. The All-Union Medicinal Herbs Research Institute has over two hundred varieties classified, many of which grow wild while others are cultivated on special state farms.

Valentina told me how she frequently prescribed compresses of hot olive oil for the small of the back as a treatment for migraine headaches. The leaves of nettle or burdock are wrapped around arthritic fingers and tied across sprained backs. As we walked through the dormitory, the smell of mustard plaster was everywhere.

After lunch (three small smoked fish, a large helping of potatoes, bread, and a bottle of *kumiss*), we walked into a small courtyard, dominated by a two-story silver metallic statue of Lenin.

The neatly kept park was planted with rows of flowers and large shrubs. Every few feet there was a hand-painted sign emphasing the value of a balanced diet, the need for proper exercise, or the importance of periodic health examination.

Many of the sanatorium patients were walking there. One elderly gentlemen asked if he might talk to Valentina the next day. "It's my heart," he said sadly. "I'm afraid it's not any better. It still hurts when I walk up the stairs."

"Of course," she said, "be in my *kabinet* [office] at ten."

Because of the afternoon heat, Valentina suggested we walk to the river, where the sanatorium kept another small park. To get there, we had to walk through a field filled with rows of cabbage standing full and opened to the late summer sun.

As we walked, Valentina's white coat brushed against the plants and her shoes were quickly covered with dust. Her tightly knotted hair began to loosen and drop to her shoulders and she seemed to relax. She told me her son was a medical student in Tashkent and that she had had a letter from him that morning.

"He wants to be a surgeon," she told me with a smile. "He says surgery is much more challenging than other specialties. I know he thinks the work I do is too simple for him," she continued. "But I'm satisfied. I think I'm helping people with their lives and that's important."

We walked around several large puddles and came to a small beach where there were two rowboats, a few tables, and a cabin for changing clothes. Valentina took off her coat and stretched out on the ground beneath a large tree. One of the patients came over and offered her a glass of mineral water, but she refused.

"You realize," she began, "that a person's emotional reaction to disease is very important. Some of the patients come here from the city taking six pills a day to control their high blood pressure. After a week, we have them controlled with fewer pills. They feel better and go back to work happier."

"But doesn't the blood pressure problem return when they leave?" I asked.

"Sometimes," she admitted, "but many times a change in diet and the proper exercise are all that are needed."

She asked me if I'd seen any of their hospitals.

"Then you know how hard it is to get well while you're a patient. In the hospital you must stay in bed, there is no room to exercise, to stretch the muscles, to relax the nerves. We try to have all heart attack patients come to the sanatorium a few months after they've left the hospital. We explain how important exercise is to their recovery and how they must be careful to treat their injured heart with respect.

"A lot of the problems we treat we can't cure," she admitted. "But often we can make the person feel better, make it possible for them to go back to work.

"When I first came here," she said, shielding her face against the setting sun, "I planned to stay only a few years, but I've grown to like the work. There is only so much that medicine can do—doctors are not that powerful—and I think making people feel better is one of the most important ones."

That evening at dinner, I talked with some of the patients. A few said they were here simply for a vacation, a rest, and admitted that although the medical care was nice, they did not need it. Others told me the treatments did not always work. "Sometimes I feel worse right after I exercise," a woman with a severe kind of deforming arthritis told me. Holding up her two clawlike hands, she said, "But I'm thankful for what the doctors do. They try to help."

The dining room contained a mixture of people. A metalworker from Bratsk, an instructor in seventeenth-century French literature, and a government bureaucrat sat together at one table. The metalworker boasted about sneaking into town the day before for a night of drinking. The professor shook his head in disapproval.

The major source of conflict within the sanatorium, according to Valentina, was among the patients who drank and stayed up late at night.

"I have no time for the hooligans," she said. "If they want to drink, I send them home."

Except for these occasional tensions, sanatorium treatment is one of the most desired services the Soviet medical care system provides. For twenty-four days each person receives individual attention, in itself a rare Soviet privilege. The special diets, mineral waters, and baths are valued for their rejuvenating qualities regardless of whether a person is sick or not.

An old Russian woman who always went to a sanatorium instead of going on vacation explained her reasoning by reminding me that "after all, you are always sick with something."

9

Rural Medicine

Deep within the white birch forest that makes up most of eastern Siberia, about 150 miles north of Irkutsk, the area's largest city, lies a tiny logging settlement. Wooden sidewalks and dirt roads connect the village's thirty small log cabins, one restaurant, a *gastronom* (food store), and small hospital. Even in this remote spot the government is there; telephone poles are stamped with small metal circles displaying the Communist hammer and sickle. A delegation of the town's leading citizens is directing a tour of the local logging operation for members of our exhibit, "Outdoor Recreation in the U.S.A.," which is now running in Irkutsk.

When one of the townspeople, the hospital's chief doctor, Aleksandr, hears I am a physician, he pulls me away from the group. The next thing I know I am riding in the sidecar of his motorcycle, an old leather riding cap on my head. He careens down the bumpy road, dodging cows grazing along the side.

The hospital suddenly appears before us, emerging from a clearing in the woods. The small wooden building and its two doctors are the only source of medical care for the 2,000 people who live in neighboring logging camps and fishing villages. In the winter they can reach the hospital only by plane. The road is blocked with snow.

Aleksandr, a small, heavyset Russian, talks rapidly and enthusiastically about his work. Only last week, he tells me, he did two emergency appendectomies. He pulls me into the hospital's single operating room where his co-physician is performing a hysterectomy. He shows me a small cubicle used for a laboratory and demonstrates a new centrifuge.

At the end of the tour my host ushers me ceremoniously into his office. On his desk is a hastily prepared plate of black bread, pickles, and cheese along with two bottles of vodka. He offers a toast: *"C priezdom v nashu bolnitsu, za mir i druzhbu!"* (Welcome to our hospital and here's to peace and friendship!)

I return the toast, thanking him for opening his hospital on such short notice and without official approval.

"Don't worry," he replies, "I've been here for twenty years—and I don't plan on leaving. There is nothing that can happen. After all, what are they going to do?" he laughs deeply, "send me to Siberia?"

Siberia has come to be synonymous with isolation, a place so desolate that people are sent there as a form of punishment. Its vastness is almost incomprehensible. The oil-, mineral-, and lumber-rich land stretches for millions of square miles east of the Ural Mountains. Yet this immense expanse of land, almost as large as the continental United States, is only part of the approximately 4 million square miles of the Soviet Union that is designated rural.

From the vast desert areas in Central Asia to the tiny villages in the Caucasus Mountains to the large collective farms in the central steppe region, life in the Soviet countryside closely resembles that of our nineteenth-century frontier. Unlike the present-day United States, where rural areas are connected by paved highways to modern shopping centers and drive-in movies, in the USSR, rural means isolated.

Among the hundred different nationalities living in the Soviet Union, there are some groups that welcome this isolation. Within the northern and southern Caucasus there are groups of villagers who have lived apart and to a large extent unaffected by Soviet government for most of this century. Many have no desire to leave.

Others, as evidenced by the recent population studies, are trying desperately to get into what is the heart of Soviet life, its cities. According to the last Soviet census, 37 percent of the country's 265 million people live in rural areas, a large decrease from the 45 percent found ten years ago.

Better food, better clothing, better housing, and variety of life are available only in Soviet cities. "They are the center," a young nursing school graduate told me. "If you want to meet a husband and find a reasonable place to live, you have to get to a city. In the country there is only work, nothing else."

Much of this rural work is crucial to the continued growth of the Soviet Union. Production by oil fields and natural gas supplies in Siberia, mineral deposits in the Urals, and wheat in the central steppe region constitute the difference between success or failure of the precarious Soviet economy. "The country must have rural work-ers," Leonid Brezhnev emphasized recently. "They provide the fuel that keeps our cities strong."

The Soviets try to keep people in the country by making it diffi-cult for them to move into the cities. The right to live in one of the crowded apartment buildings surrounding Moscow, Leningrad, Kiev, or Odessa is carefully handed down from one generation to the next. Marriage, a well-placed bribe, development of an essential skill, are the only other ways to avoid rural exile.

Most of the graduates of Soviet colleges are sent into the country-side for three years of mandatory government service. Once there, they are encouraged to stay through an elaborate system of incen-tives ranging from larger apartments and increased salaries to the right to purchase one of the half-million private automobiles offered for sale each year.

Some, like the surgeon I met in Siberia, remain. But not because of the incentives. "If you don't want to live in Siberia," he told me, "money won't change your mind.

"For the first five years I lived here," Aleksandr explained, "we had no bathrooms, only outhouses. In the winter you were very careful about what you drank so you didn't have to make many trips. Our growing season is so short we still don't have many fresh fruits or vegetables. But," he says, pouring another round of vodka, "life is not that bad. We go hunting and fishing. I run the hospital the way I want to. Nobody bothers to check whether we meet the plan. They only check to make sure we're still here!"

Aleksandr and his co-physician, also a surgeon, respond to emer-gency calls in a single-engine plane which also serves as an ambu-lance to transport patients to Irkutsk, the closest city with full hospi-tal facilities. Aleksandr sees himself as an adventurer and views his work with a sense of romanticism. "We are pioneers," he says, open-ing his arms to encompass the sprawling countryside. "We are open-ing the land to the people."

The problem with Aleksandr's services is that his twenty-bed hos-pital is not very efficient. "We usually only have three or four pa-tients here at any time," he told me. "One winter during an *epidemiia* [epidemic] of grippe [influenza] we had all twenty beds filled, but normally we're not very busy."

The Soviet government would like to close many of these small, underused hospitals and shift their responsibility to institutions in larger cities. But there is opposition from local health councils and by 1978, 40 percent of the Soviet Union's 27,000 hospitals had fewer than fifty beds. In the Soviet Union as in the rest of the world, empty hospital beds cost money. According to Soviet calculations, the cost of an empty bed is three-fourths that of an occupied one. In Soviet studies, such empty beds accounted for a third of the losses resulting from inefficient utilization of hospitals.

Also disturbing to Soviet health officials is how to get doctors like Aleksandr to stay and work under conditions which many Soviet physicians reject.

All graduates of Soviet medical institutes are required to spend three years giving "useful service" to their country. The only exceptions are those with a near-perfect record of 5s during their education, who can go directly into advanced training. Some graduates use party or other political connections to avoid assignment to any city where the only form of diversion is a restaurant that closes at 9 P.M. One survey found 30 percent of interns failed to show up for rural assignments, preferring to work on an unofficial basis while they try to negotiate another location.

As a result, in 1974 there were about 35 doctors for every 10,000 persons in Soviet cities; rural areas had half that total, 18 for every 10,000. There were isolated areas in some of the rural republics in which the ratio was even lower.

Not only does the countryside suffer from an overall shortage of physicians, some of the doctors who do serve have only specialized training. Both Aleksandr and his co-physician are examples. Under Soviet medical education, students specialize early in their training. As surgeons, neither Aleksandr nor his partner has any formal experience in obstetrics or pediatrics. Yet delivering babies and treating children's everyday problems are a necessary part of their work.

"The problem of providing adequate outpatient care in rural areas has not been completely solved," according to Dr. G. A. Popov, one of the Soviet Union's foremost medical evaluators and planners. "This is partly because some rural medical care establishments are not fully staffed and partly because the provision of medical care in these areas is hindered by such factors as the state of the roads, transportation, and communications."

There are also logistical problems involved in moving raw materials and supplies from city to village. An article in *Meditsinskaya ga-zeta* on October 16, 1974, is a typical account of the difficulties the Soviet Union encounters when the highly centralized government tries to support projects far from Moscow.

The article describes the cotton harvest in the Uzbek Republic. In 1974 there were 10,000 workers marshaled in the Central Asian republic to pick cotton before winter. There were combines, tractors, trucks—a small armada of machines. Because of the number of workers, many of them students and housewives unfamiliar with agricultural techniques and equipment, there was concern about injuries. For this reason, according to the article, "all cotton-harvester crews should have first aid kits. . . . They should have them," the article continues, "but unfortunately they do not. When a farmer's representative goes to the rural drugstore to buy a certain number of first aid kits, he suddenly finds there are none and no one knows when any will come in.

"Returning emptyhanded, the cotton grower's emissary racks his brain over the enigma of what insoluble problems could have produced this deficiency. . . . After all, only a month ago stacks of first aid kits were lying around in every drugstore."

To solve the mystery, an investigation was launched. It was discovered that the source of the Uzbekistan's problem began in Moscow. There the Vulcan Rubber Plant failed to meet its quota of small rubber tourniquets. For a nine-month period, fully 65,000 tourniquets—twelve-inch lengths of rubber tubing—failed to arrive at the Tashkent Chemical and Pharmaceutical Plant which was responsible for assembly of the first aid kits. Without the tourniquets, the Tashkent plant manager decided to stop production of the kits. The harvest that year was completed without them.

In those areas where no doctors regardless of specialty can be found, the Soviets are forced to use physician substitutes (*feldshers*). *Feldshers* have a long history in the Soviet Union. Originally a German institution, they were first introduced into Russia at the end of the seventeenth century by Peter the Great. During the 1917 Revolution the *feldshers* broke with the physicians, providing strong support for the Bolsheviks and helping them take control of the country's medical system.

Today in the Soviet Union there are a half million *feldshers*. The emphasis during their training, according to Dr. Patrick Storey of the University of Pennsylvania, who has made an extensive study of the *feldsher* system, is on assisting the Soviet physician rather than substituting for him. Like physicians, *feldshers* specialize. Some are a vital part of the Soviet emergency ambulance system. *Akusherki* (midwives) assist in the majority of births whether in the city or the countryside. Some *feldshers* who specialize in public health are assigned to factories to monitor working conditions and provide first aid. No matter what the specialty, *feldsher* instruction lasts only two and a half years, compared to the six years given Soviet physicians. The teaching concentrates on assisting the physician in minor surgical procedures, drawing blood, and administering first aid. Compared to the training currently given physician's assistants or nurse practitioners in the United States, the Soviet approach to *feldsher* education is less scientific and more practical.

In recent years the *feldshers* have come under attack from the Soviet medical profession for assuming more responsibility than they are trained to handle. This occurs most often when a *feldsher* must, because of regional shortage, work without the direct supervision of a *vrach* (doctor). Studies done in the Soviet Union have shown that the rate of improper diagnosis among *feldshers* working alone is high. In one small survey, almost half the patients examined by a *feldsher* were given a treatment later judged inappropriate by a doctor.

Furthermore, one of the chief sources of pride in the Soviet medical system is that every Soviet citizen, no matter where he lives, has access to a physician. Thus it is only with the greatest reluctance that Soviet leaders acknowledge that in some areas of the country, *feldshers* must substitute for a physician. When it occurs it is always viewed as a temporary situation, although as in other aspects of Soviet live, temporary can often mean years.

Tanya, twenty-six, has been a *feldsher* for five years. For all of that time she has worked on a small state farm (*sovkhoz*), located in western Siberia, about 75 miles from Novosibirsk, a city of a half million people and the unofficial capital of Siberia. Tanya's *sovkhoz* is not large by Soviet standards, about 500 workers and their families farming 25,000 acres. But like all Soviet agricultural projects, it is vital. The farm produces wheat, eggs, and milk, items frequently in short supply.

To encourage them to stay, the farmworkers are given certain benefits, among them a separate apartment for each married couple, the right to use one of the farm's twelve automobiles, and two doctors. For most of the five years Tanya has worked on the farm, the promises have been kept.

"We had a husband and wife who were *vrachi*," she tells me. "He was a surgeon and she a *terapevt* [internist]. They worked for three years after finishing their *internatura* [internship]. But it's been almost a year since they left to work in Novosibirsk. There's been no replacement. We did have a doctor for a few months last summer, but he left in October. There wasn't enough for him to do in the winter and he didn't like any of the girls, so he went to stay with a friend in Moscow."

While waiting for another physician, Tanya treats patients the best she can. The infirmary contains a supply of bandages, splints, and a few emergency drugs, along with two antibiotics, and *valerianka* (valerium), a mild tranquilizer. Tanya said she has used all of them but more often relies on simple folk remedies such as the coriander seeds she prescribes for indigestion. Most of her time is spent treating minor problems and offering sympathetic counseling.

While I am visiting Tanya, a patient comes to the clinic complaining of a pain in her neck.

"I slept by an open window last night," the young farmworker explains, "and today my neck is very sore." She pointed to a spot behind her right ear.

Tanya briefly examines the spot while asking her patient to move here head from side to side.

"Your body is out of tune," she explains. "You should try a hot bath and take some aspirin."

"I've already tried that," the young girl answers, "but it still hurts."

Tanya shakes her head, reaches into a drawer, and pulls out a small vial of dark liquid, "Take some of this and rub it on your neck three times a day," she says.

After the woman left I asked Tanya what was in the bottle.

"*Apizatron*," she said, "snake venom. It's made in East Germany and very good for minor muscle problems, aches and pains."

Asked what she would do if one of the workers were seriously injured, Tanya replies, "I would try to stop the bleeding and then call for help."

There is space in the infirmary to hospitalize five patients. But

Tanya hesitates to keep patients and sends all serious problems to Chik, a town twenty-five miles away which has a larger *sovkhoz* with three doctors. Tanya admits being confused by the problems many patients bring to her. At times, she says, she is uncertain which patients to send to Chik. Although only twenty-five miles, the trip, especially in the winter, takes almost two hours and the farm manager complains when workers are sent away.

Fortunately for Tanya, most of the 500 workers are young, only a small number have chronic diseases, and so far there have been no serious injuries. But from a national perspective, the large differences in the availability and quality of medical care in the Soviet countryside are creating a variety of problems.

According to Soviet surveys, the average urban citizen visits a doctor twelve times a year while his counterpart in the country sees one only four times a year. A rural resident sees a *feldsher* four times a year compared to three visits by a city resident. Home visits by a physician are eight times more frequent in cities, with their well-developed emergency ambulance systems, than in the country.

As Aleksandr's situation demonstrated, the appropriate specialists are hard to find in many rural areas. In Central Asia there are only eight pediatricians for every 10,000 citizens, compared to eighteen in the well-developed Baltic republics and thirteen per 10,000 nationwide. In Tadzhikistan, one of the five Central Asian republics, the availability of obstetricians is critically low, with only three specialists available for every 10,000 people, compared to a national average of ten.

These numbers assume even greater importance when you realize that the greatest challenge to Soviet obstetricians and pediatricians is occurring in the rural countryside, precisely where the availability of services and physicians is the lowest. Between 1970 and 1975, the total birth rate for the USSR increased by 4 percent. But it went up by 6 percent in rural areas. Of the Soviet Union's 4 million annual births, about 50 percent now take place in the countryside. Furthermore, the Central Asian republics, where traditions and living conditions combine to produce large medical challenges, have had a larger increase in birthrate than Soviet cities.

When the world thinks of the Soviet Union, cities such as Moscow and Leningrad with their rich Russian heritage immediately come to mind. But nearly a fourth of all Soviet citizens have no more in common with Russians than say, Chinese have with Americans. They are Muslims, Buddhists and other ethnic groups with an ancestry far removed from European traditions.

It is these Central Asian people who are having the babies and the problems. Since 1971 the infant mortality rate (number of children who die within the first year of life) has been increasing in the Soviet Union. In 1971, it stood at 22.9 deaths per 1,000 births; by 1976 it had climbed to 31 per 1,000 (see the chapter on women and children).

The rising infant mortality rate illustrates the complex interaction of life-style and economics that places extreme demands on rural medical care. Many Muslim women, for example, still cradle or swaddle their children. While an age-old practice and by itself not directly harmful, cradling is symbolic of an old-fashioned attitude toward child rearing that, combined with other factors, can produce serious nutritional diseases.

According to surveys conducted in Pinsk (in Belorussia) and in Dagestan, rickets is still a major health problem in many areas of the USSR. As such it is a contributing factor in the deaths of many rural Soviet children. Rickets is caused by a lack of Vitamin D. Common during the eighteenth century in England, when poor living conditions and forced child labor combined to produce the deficiency, rickets has been entirely eliminated in most countries by a number of medical and social factors, including widescale addition of Vitamin D to milk.

In addition to obtaining it in our diet, our bodies can make Vitamin D from sunlight. Thus a child must have both an inadequate diet and lack of sunlight to produce the bone-weakening disease.[1] Infants swaddled from birth and fed a diet inadequately fortified with the vitamin are defenseless. In one study reported from Perm, a city of 972,000 people, 13.9 percent of all illness within the first year of life was associated with rickets. A separate study of 181 infant deaths occurring in a rural area demonstrated that 37.1 percent, or over a third, were associated with rickets.

---

[1] Cod liver oil, liver, eggs, butter, and milk are sources of Vitamin D. Vitamin D can also be formed when the skin is exposed to the sun. Vitamin D is essential for our bodies to use calcium to build strong bones.

One Soviet survey documented that children with rickets developed pneumonia twice as often as those without.

From their studies it is obvious the Soviets recognize this problem but, to date, have had a difficult time changing old habits. Many Muslim women refuse to seek medical attention through ignorance or suspicion. Many do so only after it is too late. In a 1978 article on deaths among rural children, reported in *Public Health of the Russian Federation*, 17 percent of children had no medical treatment at all prior to death and 22 percent had treatment delayed for three days after symptoms first developed. Most remarkable, especially from an American perspective, was the finding that of 222 deaths, 170 children died at home, having never seen a doctor.

In January 1979, a spokesman for the Soviet Ministry of Health who had participated in high-level discussions concerning what to do about the increased infant mortality rate, especially in the Central Asian republics, indicated that part of the problem was a lack of planning.

"The increase in the number of rural [Central Asian] births was much greater than we anticipated," he told me. "You know conditions there are very different than they are in our big cities. We've had problems getting the women to come to the consultation centers and to follow good medical practices. You must remember the Soviet Union is a very large country with many different kinds of people. The challenges of getting care to everyone who needs it is much greater than in the United States.

"We sent doctors, planeloads of them, into the republics where mortality rates were high and of course they needed more hospitals. These took time and money. It left us with less to spend in the cities. Getting the right treatment to everyone is a problem. But we are working on it, things are getting better, soon I think you will see an improvement."

10

The Soviet Centenarians . . .
and the "Just Old"

In the largely rural Azerbaijan Republic, Medzid Agaev is a legend. He works as a shepherd in Dikaband, the small village where he grew up. Every day he walks twenty miles, following his sheep over the rolling countryside. Agaev, like many of his villagers, eats a simple diet of goat cheese, honey, fruits, and vegetables. He drinks spring water or yogurt diluted with water. Medzid Agaev does not smoke or drink. Even his thin, heavily wrinkled body does not give away his age. Agaev is 135 years old.

According to the Institute of Gerontology in Kiev, there are 20,-000 *dolgozhiteli* (long-lifers) or people 100 years of age or older in the Soviet Union—more than in any other industrialized country in the world and nearly twice as many as the 11,992 centenarians reported in the United States in 1978.

For much of the last 100 years, the Soviet Union has written, photographed, analyzed, praised, and popularized the *dolgozhiteli*. Photographs of Agaev and other *dolgozhiteli* celebrating their 140th, 150th, or even 165th birthday appear regularly in *Pravda*. Accompanying most photographs is an admonition that their great age did not come easily.

"If you want a long life," an article in the October 7, 1978, issue of *Literaturnaya gazeta* counseled, "then engage in physical labor."

"Whoever keeps company with his pillow will not live long," warns 108-year-old Sonya Aligyzy Kerimove. "I have always gotten up at 5 A.M. sharp."

Most of the long-lifers ("long-lifer" is preferred over "old person" since to the Soviets, an old person is thought of as someone who has grown old, while a long-lifer lives *without* growing old) reside in Azerbaijan, Soviet Georgia, and the Caucasus Mountains. There, indoor plumbing, central heating, and packaged foods are unknown.

Ninety-year-old Sergei Ivanovich Khokhlov from the Kuibyshev Province reports, for the benefit of a Soviet newspaper, that he shovels snow and carries firewood and water throughout the long winter.

Most of the Soviet centenarians eat as simply as they live. All of them caution against overeating, and their diet is an embarrassment to most Americans. It is low in meat but loaded with onions, garlic, tomatoes, cucumbers, eggplant, beans, walnuts, buttermilk, honey, and, of course, yogurt. Many *dolgozhiteli* are thin; none is obese.

A U.S. yogurt company recently photographed a series of commercials in the Georgian Republic of the USSR. In one of them a weathered, heavily lined, but still bright-eyed *dolgozhitel* becomes the center of attention when she happily spoons Dannon yogurt between her thin lips. It was an unusual but surprisingly comfortable combination of American commercial appeal and Soviet propaganda.[1]

In reality the secrets of the Soviet centenarians are, like American commercials, a mixture of fact, legend, and unchallenged exaggeration.

As recently as 1975, scientists such as Dr. Alexander Leaf, a professor of clinical medicine at Harvard Medical School and chief of medical services at Massachusetts General Hospital, believed the Soviet claims of longevity. In his book *Youth in Old Age,* Leaf talks about the Georgians of the USSR, the Hunzas of Pakistan, and the Vilcabamba Region in southern Ecuador as three areas of the world where people live well beyond the standard "three score and ten."

"I was gullible then," Leaf told me. "I realize now that the aging data in the Soviet Union can't be taken at face value. We now know that around the world, a small percentage, about a quarter of a billion, or one in 20,000, will live long lives [over 100]. But before we conclude that one area or region of a country contains more centenarians than any other, we need better verification."

It was during the 1930s that the Soviets first became interested in

---

[1] Recent evidence (*American Journal of Clinical Nutrition,* January 1979) from a research team at the University of California at Los Angeles suggests that yogurt contains a substance capable of lowering serum cholesterol. If true, and if a low serum cholesterol is eventually shown to provide protection against heart disease, the yogurt-loaded diet of Caucasian shepherds may prove scientifically valid. This is remarkable since it was almost a century ago that the famous Russian biologist Ilya Metchnikoff advanced his hypothesis that a fermentative agent in yogurt was responsible for the number of older persons along the Black Sea coast.

aging. Then, as now, they relied on an informal, anecdotal method to determine age. Since most of the rural villagers lack birth certificates or other written evidence, events are used to determine age. How old were you during the cholera epidemic in the summer of 1892? Were you in school during the abolition of serfdom in 1896? At the time of the 1917 Revolution, were you married?

Besides such questioning, Soviet researchers interview relatives and children and check gravestones in local cemeteries. Combining all of these sources, an age is determined, ages which, according to Leaf, are not very reliable.

"When I was in the Soviet Union," Leaf explains, "I went on one of their field trips, trying to verify ages. We met one 109-year-old woman who told us she had a baby at fifty-five [delayed menopause and the ability to have children late in life are part of the Soviet mythology of extraordinary aging]. But then, as we were leaving the village, we found out that it was not her son, but her stepson."

Also disillusioning to Leaf was his discovery that a photograph of Shirali Mislimov, reported to have died at age 168, kept reappearing each year in *Pravda* with claims that he was the oldest man in the world. "The last time he was 170," Leaf says. From a scientific viewpoint, the most substantial defect in the Soviet claims for unusual longevity come not from the Caucasus but the tropical mountains of Ecuador.

There, researchers from many countries have been carefully analyzing the ages and physical condition of villagers in Vilcabamba, rumored like the Georgians to often live beyond 100 years. By constructing family trees and comparing them with existing birth and baptismal records, they found widespread exaggeration of age beginning at age seventy. In most cases, persons claimed they were twenty to forty years older than their family histories indicated.

In fact, none of the twenty-three claimed centenarians in Ecuador had reached 100. The oldest was ninety-six at the time of his death.

Although the techniques used in Ecuador have not been applied to Soviet Georgia, most scientific researchers, including Leaf, believe that the same well-meaning but age-inflating tendency occurs in the USSR. One way to resolve the problem would be to examine the teeth of the *dolgozhiteli*. Recently a new form of protein analysis used to date prehistoric fossils has been adapted to human aging.

During life, the proteins in our teeth slowly but steadily change their molecular configuration. At birth, all of the small amino acids that are building blocks for protein are stacked on the left side of a large central molecule; as we age, they shift to the right. Since this turning, or racemization, is associated with permanent changes in the tooth, many scientists believe it is an integral part of the aging process. New protein cannot be made to replace the transformed fraction.

But whether or not racemization proves to be an important aging discovery, it is an accurate and completely objective method for determining age. The further right your amino acids are, the older your teeth. Dr. Leaf and others have been trying to get the Soviets to provide a tooth from one of their centenarians but, to date, have been unsuccessful. "I'd think that at least one must have fallen out by now," Leaf says.

For their part, the Soviets seem content to accept the ages, inflated or not, at face value. Dr. N. Sachuk of the Institute of Gerontology in Kiev, for example, uses the ages to develop an index of maximum longevity. Calculated by taking the number of persons age 110 and over and dividing this by the number over 100, she determined that areas in Caucasus have 20 percent of their centenarians living beyond 110.

Unfortunately, all this concentration on and controversy over numbers, according to Leaf, obscures the real lessons that the *dolgozhiteli* may be able to give us. Although the claims of longevity are probably exaggerated, he emphasizes that there is no disagreement with the Soviet finding that a great many older people living in these rural areas are in remarkably good health.

"On my trip to the Caucasus I found a number of older persons on sparse diets, mostly from habit since all had lived through years of severe shortages. Some of the foods were not what we could call healthy, like goat cheese and fat," he says. "But there seems to be something about the combination of hard work, a rural life-style and a close-knit family-community structure that enables seventy-year-olds to still walk twenty miles a day."

Some of the villagers do not have medical registration cards. They have never needed the services of Soviet medicine. Many refuse to take chemical prescriptions, relying on their own herbal preparations.

Another observation recorded by all visitors making the pilgrimage to the Caucasus is the closeness of the family and village structure. Elder members, regardless of their ages, are respected and looked to for advice. In some villages a council of elders (minimum age for election ninety) settled all disputes.

How important this extended family environment is in relation to other external factors such as diet and exercise is unknown. Separating individual factors and isolating them from the powerful influence of heredity is like trying to excavate ancient architectural ruins: you cannot move a stone without affecting and perhaps destroying others.

In the past the legends surrounding the *dolgozhiteli* encouraged many persons, among them some of the Soviet Union's leading scientists, to try to find a single reason for their long lives—the elusive "fountain of youth." In 1943, Professor Alexandr A. Bogomolets, the founder of the Institute of Gerontology in Kiev, thought he had come close.

Bogomolets's brief encounter with a "youth serum" began during the 1930s. Working with a preparation then known as anti-cytotoxic reticular serum (ACS)—prepared by taking cells from the spleen and bone marrow of human corpses, injecting it into horses, and then extracting it in purified form—the physiologist claimed to have a powerful weapon against ageing. During World War II, Bogomolets said ACS improved the healing of fractures caused by bullet wounds. He used ACS three times a day on soldiers and reduced disability from several months to a few weeks. For his war work he was awarded the Hero of Socialist Labor medal.

After this success, Professor Bogomolets, who was also vice president of the Academy of Sciences of the USSR, began using ACS for other diseases. He claimed it was useful in the fight against infections, could assist in preventing surgically removed tumors from reappearing, and could stop premature ageing by halting the breakdown of the body's connective tissue.

"Normally a man should live to the age of 150 years," Bogomolets told Drew Middleton of *The New York Times* in a June 1, 1946, interview, "that is, if he starts to use my serum when his connective tissues begin to deteriorate and takes reasonable care of himself otherwise."

There were rumors that Stalin was using ACS so he could dominate the Soviet Union until the year 2000. But by June 1946, Bogomolets's work was already under heavy attack from medical scientists in the United States and Great Britain. They had tested ACS and found its claims to cure cancer or enable women to have children at the age of ninety were false.

Bogomolets argued that he had never made such outrageous claims for ACS. "It was intended to stimulate the system's defenses against diseases that intrude on normal life," he explained, "not to be a magic elixir of long life for everyone.

"To be completely successful," Bogomolets maintained, "it must be injected systematically from birth to death, and even into the mother before giving birth."

Bogomolets died at age sixty-five, six weeks after his *New York Times* interview, a thin, bent man. Because he had heart disease he never felt it was safe to use ACS on himself. Experiments with the serum continued for a while after his death, but its popularity slowly faded.

Today, Soviet scientists along with their counterparts from other countries continue the search for an answer to why we grow old. The location of most activity is still the Institute of Gerontology in Kiev (an institution similar to the Institute of Ageing of our National Institutes of Health), which Bogomolets founded. The focus today is more on analyzing the changes that take place in ageing rather than in attempting to influence them.

"For a long time old age itself was viewed as an illness," explains Academician Dimitri F. Chebotarev, current director of the institute. "Now this viewpoint is obsolete. Studies on the physiology of the ageing process of healthy people have helped us determine what changes are a function of illness and what are a result of age."

A book of biological essays, *Why Death Comes,* by one of the Soviet Union's most knowledgeable scientists in this area, V. M. Dilman, provides a sharp contrast to the newspaper articles which talk of 140-year-old villagers and the exaggerated claims for ACS. Dilman believes that ageing results from an orderly and predictable breakdown in the body's nervous and hormonal control systems. External factors such as exercise, diet, and stress express their effects by either hastening or slowing this internal breakdown. Other factors such as heredity are also important. According to Dilman, any success in preventing ageing will, of necessity, operate through these hormonal and nervous pathways. Such actions, he cautions, are still experimental, for the hypothalamus, the area at the base of the brain which appears to control most ageing, is giving up its secrets slowly.

Whatever the outcome of Dilman's and other scientists' investigations, however, the legends surrounding the *dolgozhiteli* are sure to persist. The Soviet government seems to prefer preserving the mystique surrounding them. But future visitors may find the "long-lifers" harder to find. Leaf and more recent pilgrims to the famed mountain villages observe that children of the thin *dolgozhiteli* are putting on weight.

"The diet is improving—at least in quantity," Leaf observes, "some of the children are now fat. And they don't walk twenty miles every day."

The "Just Old"

For weeks Vladimir had wanted me to visit his mother. She was old, he explained, and too feeble to go out of the house. But he had told her about me and she wanted very much to meet the American with whom her son had become such friends. Sunday afternoon was the best time.

Vladimir's parents live in one of the few remaining log cabin homes in Irkutsk, USSR. Vladimir, thirty-four, is an anatomy professor at the Irkutsk Medical Institute. After completing his three-year stint in government service following his internship, he came back to Irkutsk to become an *aspirant* (doctoral candidate) in anatomy. Although he, his wife, and four-year-old son live in a newly constructed one-bedroom apartment, he spends much of his time at his parents'. The three-room house contains many memories.

Vladimir's grandfather built the house over a generation ago. He was one of the last exiles sent to Siberia by Nicholas II in 1902, only a few years before the revolution. Since then it has been the place of birth and death for three generations of Vladimir's family.

We entered through a small cubicle designed to seal off the rest of the house from the cold and hold in its precious heat during the long winter. Passing from this entrance to the kitchen meant walking bent over. High ceilings waste heat.

Once in the kitchen, the house's central room, I could stand erect. Vladimir's father, a shrunken miniature of his tall, thin son, sat eating pine nuts at the kitchen table. He acknowledged my greeting politely but without enthusiasm.

I sat and we drank vodka. The cloudy liquid was Ekstra, a cheaper form of vodka manufactured only for sale inside the Soviet Union. It made my throat burn and the small room with its wood-burning stove soon seemed uncomfortably warm. I noticed the walls were sweating, forming small pools of water in each corner. The room's only picture was a brown photograph of a young man standing in an open field holding a large scythe.

Vladimir's father asked me what America was like. When I began to answer, he took down a copy of the large Soviet Encyclopedia from the shelf above the sink. He showed me the two pages marked "Amerika." There was one photograph of a white mob hanging a black slave. I started to explain about the history of slavery in the United States, but Vladimir's father interrupted, saying the fire needed more wood. He went out through the small entrance to get it.

Vladimir, embarrassed but anxious that I should not feel unwelcome, motioned me into the back bedroom. The room was dark. The only window was covered with a dark cloth. There was a small candle burning on a bedside table. As my eyes adjusted, I could see two icon images of Christ and *Bogoroditsa* (the Madonna) shimmering in the candlelight.

Vladimir's mother was partly sitting, partly lying on a low single bed. She was dressed in a black dress, a black shawl around her shoulders. At first I was not sure she was breathing.

Vladimir motioned me to sit on a small stool placed close to the head of the bed. As I sat down, she opened her eyes slowly, as if the effort tired her. She immediately closed them.

"She's been very weak lately," Vladimir explained, whispering softly in my ear. "Her heart is not strong. But take her hand so she'll know you are here."

I searched for it under the heavy woolen blanket, afraid of upsetting her precarious balance between the bed and the pillows. Finding it beneath the sheet, I gingerly placed it on top of mine. Her hand was thin, its skin so transparent it seemed I could see through it. Holding it gently, I tried to feel for a pulse. It arrived weak and at irregular intervals.

"This is the doctor I told you about," Vladimir said to his mother, speaking slightly above a whisper. "He's from America."

Her eyes opened again. This time I could see they were black and glistening. She stared at me and I thought I felt her hand move in mine.

"She's tired now," Vladimir said and we quietly left. Her eyes followed us out of the room.

"Thank you," Vladimir said later, standing outside in the crisp October air. "She will probably die soon. There is not much I can do for her. She is getting too weak to eat. The nurse used to come and visit but she stopped. Medicine is of no use. My father and I will take care of her now. She is just old."

According to the Central Statistical Administration, in 1939 only 6.8 percent of the Soviet population was over the age of sixty. By 1974, the proportion had risen to 13 percent. By the year 2000 it is expected to reach 20 percent. As in the rest of the world, the Soviet population is graying.

Today there are 45 million people receiving pensions in the Soviet Union. Retirement age is set at fifty-five for women and sixty for men. The pensions, which average about 50 percent of the worker's last monthly pay check, begin at 45 rubles ($70) a month and go up a maximum of 120 rubles ($186). With this sum the retired worker is expected to buy food and clothing while keeping up with a modest rent payment. The offical Soviet poverty line is 51.5 rubles per month per person.

If the retired worker becomes ill, medical care is free, but there are almost no nursing homes. Fortunately, most of the elderly, like Vladimir's mother, have sons or daughters to help them. But as the population ages and the historically solid Russian family unit begins to disappear, there is concern over how the Soviet government—especially its medical system—will accommodate the increasing number of old people.

"A number of new social questions are arising," explained Dr. Chebotarev, Director of Kiev's Institute of Gerontology in a 1978 interview with visiting American reporters. "They involve not only medical care but the economy, social insurance, food needs, and the design of our cities. The elderly have chronic diseases and we need to create a new medical social service to meet these special problems."

Throughout all its development the Soviet medical system has

emphasized the health of its working population. The extensive system of polyclinic and preventive services, organized around large
and small factories, concentrated most services where they would
provide the most benefit.

The elderly, especially retirees, have not been given priority.
"When I visit my polyclinic," a retiree in Odessa told me, "I always
plan on waiting three hours. All of the young people ask to be taken
before me," she explains. "They say they're still working and are
'busy.' It's as if my time were not worth anything."

Until 1978, the government's response to this and related complaints by the elderly about inadequate medical services has been
well intentioned but not well supported. During the 1960s and early
'70s, geriatric rooms were established at a few of the country's larger
polyclinics. Within these rooms the elderly, who on any given day
constitute nearly a third of the clinic's patients, are evaluated separately. In a geriatric room the *terapevt* (internist) is permitted to
allow the patient thirty minutes for the first visit and fifteen to
twenty minutes for each follow-up visit, compared to the five minutes per patient allocated under normal conditions.

An article in the September 15, 1976, issue of *Literaturnaya gazeta*
reported on a survey of 3,000 persons who had visited geriatric
rooms in Moscow, Kiev, Lvov, and Tashkent. The majority preferred to be treated there. Unfortunately, because of overcrowding
and inadequate staffing, the number of rooms decreased from 134 in
1972 to less than 100 today.

One out of every ten pensioners needing medical attention is
treated by the *neotlozhnaya* (home-visit service). Unlike the situation
in the United States where a growing proportion of the elderly are
living in nursing homes, elder Soviet citizens remain at home. Further, Soviet hospitals have death quotas, so they usually will not
admit patients dying from a chronic disease.

Because of this record the medical system has frequently come
under attack not only from retirees but from its own professionals.
Professor V. S. Lukyanov, a noted academician, complained in 1976
that the Soviet medical schools did not offer courses in gerontology
and that, as a result, the clinical needs of the elderly were frequently
ignored. Other critics made the suggestion that, considering the increasing need, some pediatricians be retrained as geriatricians.

The medical leadership has not yet adopted such radical suggestions. In fact, among the Soviet Union's fifty-one recognized subspecialties, ranging from sports medicine to radiation hygiene, geriatrics does not appear, although I was told there are plans to add it soon.

Still, things are changing. In January 1978, Minister of Health Petrovsky announced that all Soviet medical schools and nurses' training facilities would begin teaching mandatory courses in geriatrics. To replace the rapidly disappearing geriatric rooms, community health centers emphasizing the needs of older citizens are planned. A Ministry of Health official explained to me that these new initiatives are tied to a general rethinking of the country's early retirement age and the growing labor shortage in the USSR.

In describing these changes, Petrovsky emphasized how they would help prolong the population's ability to work beyond the retirement age, something that is "of great importance" to the Soviet government.

Of course, many Soviet retirees have continued to work after receiving their pensions. In some cases the fifty or sixty rubles a month was simply not enough to sustain life. "I pay only three rubles for rent," a *babushka* (old woman) living in one room in Kiev explained, "and I never eat meat, but by the end of the month there's nothing left. I'm eating only bread and tea."

To supplement her sixty-ruble pension, Marina, who had been an accountant, sells newspapers at a small kiosk near the Dnieper River park. Other retirees take jobs as elevator operators, museum guards, hospital orderlies, or street cleaners. In Odessa, I watched an old woman take a small handbroom and each morning sweep between the tracks of the train station. There are other *babushki* like her throughout the Soviet Union, performing menial tasks in exchange for a few extra rubles.

According to N. N. Sachuk, a Soviet gerontologist, a third of the male pensioners surveyed and a fifth of the women would like to return to work. Many are lonely, their lives without purpose. And recently the Soviet government has decided to rethink its practice of removing retirees from regular jobs because of age alone. "We are convinced that a person can work after sixty," explains Gerontology Director Chebotarev. "Work is good, it can invigorate. It is structure."

A return to work might not only benefit them, but also would help support the Soviet Union's precarious economy and relieve the growing labor shortage. According to U.S. population projections, the lack of trained manpower in the USSR will become prominent during the 1980s and continue well into the next century. If the government can maintain a portion of its workforce on the job beyond the usual retirement ages today, the problem could be reduced. This appears to be the major reason behind the recent stress on geriatric medicine.

The increased emphasis on geriatrics has not extended to the construction of nursing homes or extended care facilities for the elderly. Living space traditionally is handed down from one generation to the next; the need for special care in the past was handled by relatives. But with smaller families and the diminishing belief in the importance of older citizens, many pensioners, especially those in Soviet cities, find themselves not only impoverished but also alone.

"An old person may be sick and lonely," Chebotarev explains, "and the loneliness of old age is considerable. It grows and is of great importance. The younger generation separates from the older and the old ones get lonely and die."

Soviet physicians have defined what they call "pensioner's disease"—a lack of interest in life leading rapidly to death. As a result, Soviet medical leaders have targeted the two main killers of the elderly, heart disease and cancer, for special consideration in the allocation of research funds. They are also increasing research into the ageing process. They are strengthening the study of gerontology among their medical students. They are recognizing that, in the future, the older portion of their population may make a crucial difference within the Soviet economy. They can no longer afford to leave people who are "just old" out of the mainstream of society.

While shopping in Kishinev, the capitol of the Moldavian Republic, I watched a frail, bent woman gathering scraps of bread and sausage from the ground beneath an open-air restaurant. She carefully placed the crumbs and fragments into her *setka* (shopping bag), which was lined with a heavily soiled plastic bag. After filling it half full, she would sit on a nearby bench and brush off each piece before placing it into her mouth.

Since she and I came to the restaurant the same time each day, I eventually got up the courage to introduce myself. At first she was embarrassed and refused to speak. But after a minute she came up to me and demanded to know why I kept watching her. I started to stammer a reply but before I found the right words, she had pushed back a small lock of her wispy gray hair and stood directly in front of me, her *setka* forgotten on the bench.

"*Molodoi chelovek* [young man]," she lectured, "it is not your place to watch me. I am an old woman—just old—my husband is dead, my children have left, and there is nothing for me to live for. I will die soon but until then, let me have peace. . . . You do not understand why, but we all do what we must."

11

Alcoholism—
The Green Snake of Russia

For all of this century the Soviet Union has had a shortage of young men. In the early 1900s it was war, revolution, and famine, one rapidly leading into the other, that produced the scarcity.

Through the early 1930s, adequate food remained a luxury and, as has always been the case throughout history, more men than women died. Then came World War II. The five years of fighting during the forties cost the USSR 13 million men.

The numbers took time to replenish. At first there were not enough men to become fathers. Those who had survived were sick, injured, or both. But by the middle 1960s, half of the precious babies born during the postwar recovery years became young men and the Soviet Union finally seemed close to achieving a normal male-to-female ratio. Then it seemed as if an irresistible predestined cycle renewed itself. Young men again began dying.[1]

The large number of men who die in their thirties through fifties is the major reason the overall life expectancy for Soviet men has declined to 63 years. For Soviet women, it is 74. (Life expectancy in the United States is now 69.3 years for men and 77.1 for women.)

All countries have male-female differences in life expectancy. For many reasons, among them a greater resistance to disease and famine, women live longer than men. What makes the Soviet Union's statistics different from that of other countries is not that their over-

[1] Crude death rates in the Soviet Union have increased from 6.9 per 1,000 in 1964 to 9.3 in 1975. This trend begins at age thirty and continues through the rest of the normal life-span. A deterioration in age-specific death rates has also been noticed for both men and women, but is much larger for males. Moreover, results of the 1979 Soviet census confirmed the continuation of this trend, with a decrease in the growth of men as a percent of the total population and a continued fall in life expectancy. In 1979, the age-adjusted death rate for the Soviet population was estimated at 9.5 per 1,000; for the U.S. it was 6.1 per 1,000 population.

all life expectancy is lower but that, in the absence of war, so many young males (thirty to fifty-nine) are dying.

The Soviet government acknowledges the problem and, perhaps out of tradition, refers to it as the result of "trauma." Only this time it is not the trauma of war, when men kill other men. Today young men are killing themselves. They are doing it with alcohol.

As in a war, there is a unique vocabulary that accompanies the killing. Vodka, the most common form of alcohol consumed, accounting for 70 percent of commercial sales, is known as "the green snake." Illegal, home-brewed *samogon* goes by various code names, including *kerosinka* (kerosene). Delirium tremens, or hallucinations and convulsions caused by withdrawal from a steady diet of alcohol, is "the white fever." When three men stagger down the street arm-in-arm, having just split the cost of a bottle of vodka, they are *na troikh,* (slang for splitting a bottle among three persons). Finally, alcoholism is known as "the third disease," trailing only heart disease and cancer as a cause of death.

Like the more traditional wars that have dominated so much of Russia's history, alcoholism is an old problem. An oft-repeated quote traces the tradition to the tenth century when Saint Vladimir of Kiev is reported to have said, "It is Russia's joy to drink—we cannot do without it."

In more recent times (1958), Soviet Premier Nikita Khrushchev tried reducing alcohol consumption by raising prices 21 percent. He failed. "The only result [of the price increase] was that family budgets were hit harder than before and people had even less money to spend on necessary goods," Khrushchev lamented in his memoirs. "We seem driven to drink."

Although publication of national figures detailing the exact amount of alcohol consumed per person was stopped by the government in the 1960s, Soviet newspapers and medical, legal, and sociological journals frequently contain articles on alcoholism. From these studies and a review of the scientific literature come the following conclusions:

· The Soviet Union is the world leader in consumption of strong varieties of alcohol (notably vodka) per capita, with slightly more than eight liters per person per year (the U.S. estimate is 4.1).

- During the last forty years, the USSR has experienced the highest rate of increase in the amount of alcohol consumed per person among developed countries. Consumption increased by 600 percent while the population grew by only 25 percent.
- The average Soviet family spends from a quarter to a half of their monthly food budget on alcohol.
- Nationwide it is estimated that 13 to 29 billion rubles ($20 to $45 billion) is spent annually on alcohol. This is equal to and probably in excess of the Soviet Union's total budget for health. (In the United States the retail cost of alcohol consumption is estimated at $38 billion, compared to our total health budget of $200 billion.)
- The taxes imposed on alcohol bring in about 12 percent of the Soviet government's total revenues and account for more than a third of the taxes citizens pay to the government.
- Of the 2 billion liters of alcohol consumed in various forms in the USSR each year, at least a fourth or 500 million are *samogon*, illegally distilled brandy and vodka for which no taxes are collected and over which little control is possible.

The human results of these statistics are everywhere in Soviet homes, restaurants, train stations, hospitals, and polyclinics. The practice of drinking *na troikh* can be found on the most fashionable streets in Moscow as well as in the sparsely populated countryside. Vodka is used to conduct business, pass time, celebrate anniversaries, forget troubles, establish new friendships, and break old ones. *Sto gram* (100 grams) of vodka is as common an order in Soviet restaurants as the pre-dinner cocktail is in the United States.

The Soviets have no bars or taverns as we know them. Persons out for an evening can buy vodka at a restaurant along with their meal, but even in large cities, like Moscow, the few bars are small, unattractive, and only permitted to sell beer.

Vodka and cognac, the two most popular hard liquors sold in the USSR, are mostly sold by the bottle in Soviet *gastronomy* (food stores). The standard 500-gram bottle of "the green snake" costs 3 rubles, 62 kopecks ($5.60). It cannot be recapped and is usually finished quickly with friends while walking down the street or in an open park.

"Vodka is not like wine," a Russian friend explained. "It is something you drink fast and hard. The pleasure is not in the drinking but in its effect."

For most persons found drunk on the street there is an established acceptance, almost a sympathy, a tenderness toward the historical Russian penchant for self-destruction in the face of overwhelming odds. Some Soviet citizens, however, especially in the Baltic States, think nothing of openly berating the alcoholic. On a train I took from Tallin to Riga, an old man who had too much to drink became sick to his stomach. A fellow passenger, an elderly woman, chastised the man for his drunkenness and sloppy dress. When he tried to escape by moving to another car, she pushed him back into his seat with her cane. "Look at yourself," she demanded. "You're a disgrace. You should be afraid for people to see you." Other passengers joined in the public lecture.

Most drinking in the Soviet Union is done at home. Drinking is a major reason behind the high divorce rate, and the example provided by an alcoholic husband, according to recent articles, is spreading to other family members. An analysis in the January 15, 1979, issue of *Pravda* said that the average age for *chronic* alcoholism among Soviet youth had been falling over the last few years: "It is now in the fifteen- to seventeen-year-old bracket."

Teenage drinking is especially worrisome to Soviet authorities since it frequently leads to addiction. Soviet studies indicate that 90 percent of the country's alcoholics began drinking before the legal age of sixteen and 33 percent of them before the age of ten. In one survey, between 70 and 90 percent of schoolchildren under age sixteen admitted they drank alcohol. The Komosomol, the youth branch of the Communist Party, had passed major resolutions declaring the fight against teenage alcoholism as one of its most important goals. But laws restricting the sale of alcoholic beverages to minors are violated. The government's economic plans provide sales quotas for all goods, including alcohol. "We do have a conscience," one Moscow food store manager told *Pravda* in October 1978, "and we also have children. We do not want them to become drunkards. But we have our plan, and we want to receive a bonus."

Although the problem is still mainly with Soviet men, women are increasingly turning to alcohol. Unlike men, female alcoholics in the Soviet Union begin drinking at an older age (thirty to forty) in the throes of juggling a job and a family and often after the loss of their husbands through divorce or death.

In a survey of female alcoholics published in the *Literaturnaya gazeta* in March 1979, more than half the women replied they had begun drinking to keep their husbands company. Others drank for a sense of well-being or because there was nothing better to do and everyone else was drinking. Loneliness was another major cause; half the women who had been patients at the *vytrezviteli* (sobering-up stations) were widowed, divorced, or single. They said that loneliness and the burden of being without a husband had precipitated their drinking.

Most of the women questioned drank at home or at a friend's apartment. Only 3 percent admitted to drinking *na troikh* or in the parks. Despite their drinking problems, almost all the women (80 percent) considered vodka, cognac, or champagne essential for entertaining guests. The 1979 survey concluded that, unlike the situation that had existed before the Revolution, when female alcoholics were found mainly among prostitutes and women of lower economic classes, alcoholism now affects women of all backgrounds and professions.

Some Soviet scientists advance the theory that women are more susceptible than men to the physiological and addicting properties of alcohol. "Cells of the female organism go mad from alcohol at a much faster rate, more terribly, and more conclusively than male cells," a scientist wrote in a newspaper article based on his preliminary studies of the internal metabolism of cells. Although there is not enough data available to judge the validity of these early cellular studies, there is evidence that the Soviets do have a double standard for female alcoholics.

Public drunkenness is poorly tolerated and more severely criticized in women than in men. "Despite the genetically inherent sweetness of the delicate sex, drunkenness and alcoholism take on a peculiarly vulgar form in the female. In a drunken state, they easily become unbalanced, lose self-control, and become aggressive. In this condition they not only scandalize but also initiate arguments and brawls," according to the Dr. B. Levin writing in *Literaturaya Gazeta*. Because of public prejudice against female alcoholics, they frequently receive medical attention later than men.

"Women usually wait until they have reached the final extreme stages of alcoholism," says Dr. A. D. Vasilivskaya, director of the alcoholic rehabilitation ward in Moscow's Hospital Psychiatric Number 13. "To cure a woman at this stage is almost impossible. Her disintegrated personality has to be reassembled by blueprints and then only in scraps."

The Soviet approach to treatment and prevention of alcoholism is a very practical one. For besides its medical consequences, alcoholism causes economic loss. The Soviets estimate that alcoholism accounts for a 10 percent loss of production through increased worker absenteeism and alcohol-related illness.

The director of the Pyatigorsk Meat Processing Combine, in an article in *Literaturnaya gazeta,* said labor productivity would be 15 percent higher if it were not for heavy drinkers among his employees. Soviet researchers who compared workers' productivity on normal days and those immediately following paydays when drinking binges most often occur found differences of 25 to 30 percent.

Because of this, the Soviet government has concentrated on modifying the alcoholic's behavior and on reducing his impact on the nation's economy. Drawing on their strong Pavlovian tradition, Soviet physicians use drugs such as nicotinic acid and antabuse that when taken in combination with alcohol produce a violent stomach upset meant to discourage the person from taking another drink.

They also rely heavily on manipulating the alcoholic's environment. A new hospital especially for the treatment of alcoholics recently opened in Moscow. As part of its program, patients work at their regular jobs during the day and return to the hospital each night. During the treatment period, which usually lasts from five to six weeks, all patients are required to give up 40 percent of their wages to the hospital.

Most alcoholics are not hospitalized but treated as outpatients. Some 25 percent of the patient load at psychiatric polyclinics are alcoholics. In most cases the polyclinic psychiatrists, along with public health nurses, attempt to isolate factors in the patient's life-style that encourage him to drink. Since the medical and economic consequences of alcoholism are assumed to outweigh the right to privacy, the patient's family and close friends are questioned regarding his drinking habits, as are his employer and fellow workers. With this information, an aggressive program is outlined for the patient, designed to get him to stop drinking and return to work. Both family members and co-workers are involved. Fellow workers frequently are charged with joint responsibility for the person's drinking problem and told that his success or failure will also be theirs.

This approach does not always meet with cooperation, however. In writing about the problems of alcoholism in the Soviet armed forces, Colonel V. Arkhipov complained that "Those from whom active assistance should be expected" failed to help commanders prevent drunkenness. "What's more," he says, "loving mothers, fathers, aunts, and uncles even smuggled liquor into camp during their visits, directly against the orders of military physicians."[2]

Another Pavlovian tradition frequently used as a counterbalance to a patient's drinking is work, especially muscular work. Tied in with this tradition is an older belief, common in Russian history, that alcoholism was not a sickness but a crime. Even though the Soviet government today disavows that notion, current treatment today reflects this heritage.

In March 1974 the Supreme Soviet of the USSR's largest republic, the Russian, reissued a 1967 decree, never enforced, which called for putting chronic drinkers into labor camps (*trudovoe perevospitanie*). There, treatment and rehabilitation could take as long as two years. According to people who have gone through the mandatory labor camp programs, medical treatment is minimal. The emphasis is on simple living conditions, a regular work routine, and the absence of alcohol.

"We had one doctor in our camp," a man from Moscow told me. "We called him the tractorist because we didn't believe he could really be a doctor, he acted more like a tractor driver. Once I remember going to him with a terrible stomachache. He told me a good day's work would cure my pain."

Indeed, little official sympathy is given to the alcoholic by the Soviet government. A 1972 decree directed that medical problems related to or caused by heavy drinking should not be treated free of charge and that alcoholic patients should be denied sick leave if their medical problem came from drinking. In some Soviet cities, men found repeatedly drunk in public are frequently taken from the *vytrezvitel* (sobering-up station) to have their heads shaved as a public

[2] V. Arkhipov, *Krasnaya Zvezda* (Moscow), 13 March 1977, p. 2.

symbol of their drunkenness. Drivers who are involved in an accident while drunk have their licenses suspended for two years. Consistent violation can result in a heavy prison sentence, transfer to a lower-paid job, or loss of bonuses and travel privileges.

When a drunk is arrested in a major Soviet city he is usually taken to a police station and placed in a holding room, staffed by a *vrach* or *feldsher*. If the person develops any medical problems such as seizures or bleeding he will be transferred to a hospital. If he is only drunk, he or his family will be made to pay for the cost of his overnight stay.

The medical problems and complications of alcoholism do present the Soviet medical system and its physicians with difficult challenges. Studies in the United States, where the mortality and morbidity from alcoholism and related disorders have been rising as well (although not at the same level as in the USSR) indicate that many diseases, such as pneumonia and heart disease, are more difficult to treat when combined with alcoholism.

Another problem encountered by physicians in all countries but especially by Soviet doctors is deciding where alcoholism stops and sickness begins. In his description of the emergency medical system of Leningrad, Dr. M. A. Messel discusses the problem of evaluating an inebriated patient and warns Soviet physicians that sending a drunk person to the police or a *vytrezvitel* can end in disaster. Dr. Messel presents the case of Patient N, who when drunk was struck by a car on the Nevsky Prospekt, one of the main streets in Leningrad. The ambulance doctor found no sign of external injury, so Patient N was sent to the sobering-up station. In the morning the *feldsher* on duty tried to wake him but failed. The ambulance doctor was called back, examined the patient, and found that he was rapidly bleeding from a ruptured liver. The patient was taken to the hospital where he died the same day.[3]

While similar incidents occur in the United States, it is the frequency with which such problems occur in the USSR that makes them an unusual challenge. A study by Dr. V. A. Shaak in Leningrad, for example, found that of all patients with skull fractures, more than a fourth were directly related to drunkenness.

The long and extremely cold winters in the northern Soviet cities

[3] M. A. Messel, *Urban Emergency Medical Service of the City of Leningrad* (Washington: Department of Health, Education and Welfare, 1975), p. 135.

pose yet another problem for alcoholics. In Moscow, winter begins with frozen fog in December; by January there are only seven hours of weak sunlight each day and temperatures frequently drop twenty and thirty degrees below zero. To many Muscovites, this "dog cold" (so named because even pets refuse to go out) actually brings relief from some medical problems such as colds and intestinal infections. Viruses and bacteria, it seems, are as immobilized by the cold as other forms of life. But to the person who has too much to drink, the street can become a premature graveyard.

Alcohol not only blunts the body's responsiveness to cold, but by dilating the blood vessels near the skin, it increases the amount of heat lost. Soviet physicians report a large increase in the number of cases of accidental hypothermia, or extreme lowering of the body temperature, during the winter months. The emergency ambulance system keeps a special watch around the Russian New Year, when celebrations and drinking increase.

The hospital treatment of accidental hypothermia, along with that of other alcohol-related diseases such as liver cirrhosis, gastrointestinal bleeding, and "white fever" (delirium tremens) is similar to U.S. practice. Cirrhotics are prescribed a low salt diet to prevent the accumulation of fluid in the abdomen. Persons with gastrointestinal bleeding are given blood transfusions, although technical problems with needles and tubing limit the amount of blood given to severely bleeding patients.

The Soviet approach to the treatment of delirium tremens also closely follows standard practice. The patient, who is often agitated and combative, is heavily sedated and restrained. Although "white fever" is dangerous and occasionally fatal, most patients survive. A doctor who ran an alcoholic treatment ward in a large Moscow hospital expressed the universal frustration of treating alcoholics. "We can cure the white fever and the pneumonia," he told me, "but the real problem remains. Many of these patients have been here three or four times. Most of them, especially the young ones, I know I'll see again."

Considering the magnitude of the alcoholism problem and its high cost both in economic and human measures, the question frequently is asked why the Soviet government, with its unchallenged authority, does not limit the supply or availability of alcohol. The answer is that the government has tried and failed. Besides raising prices, it has limited vodka sales to certain hours (11 A.M.–8 P.M.). In a few critical industrial locations such as the showcase Kama River Plant, vodka cannot be purchased within a fifteen-mile radius of the city. But a total ban is impossible to enforce. People will simply make their own liquor.

Between 1914 and 1925, the sale of alcoholic beverages was officially prohibited throughout Russia. The response was an enormous increase in the amount of illegal liquor (*samogon*) produced by Russian peasants. It was estimated that 80 percent of peasant households were distilling *samogon* and that 9 quarts of *samogon* were produced annually for every man, woman, and child then alive.

Today there is a one- to three-year prison term for anyone caught producing and selling *samogon,* as well as a fifty-ruble fine for anyone caught buying the *kerosinka.* All authorities I spoke to, however, acknowledged that these laws have made little difference; home brew is a way of life. In many apartments I visited, *samogon* was frequently offered. When hiking in the Siberian mountains around Irkutsk, my Soviet companions carried two canteens, one for water, the other for *kerosinka.*

Most *samogon* is not made in small home stills but is produced illegally by wineries that are only licensed to produce champagne and low-alcohol-content wines.

"The recipe is simple enough," according to an article in *Pravda.* "Water from the well, yeast from the bazaar, and sugar from the grocery store. Next come the time-proven techniques of brewing and distilling. For coloring and sales appeal, some add beet juice, others an infusion of oat straw.

"And no one will blow the whistle. So long as there is even a single grapevine in their personal garden plot, they are considered to be within the law. Although nobody could mistake this stuff for wine, its aroma will knock you off your feet."[4]

Unlike the top brand of vodka, Stolichnaya, which now is made exclusively for export, *samogon* can be distilled from just about anything. Moreover, the one essential ingredient—sugar—is in good supply. Not only does Soviet domestic sugar beet production come close to fulfilling the annual goals, but the USSR's close friendship with Cuba mandates that they purchase tons of that island's only export.

---

[4] "A Glass of Nylonite," *Pravda* (Moscow), 14 November 1975, p. 6.

"B. Gorvat of the village of Beregi," the *Pravda* article continues, "has more than a ton of sugar in reserve. Other vintners have 850, 500, and 403 kilograms. Could it be that these people are heavy tea drinkers?"

While the Soviets occasionally do make light of the illegal alcohol problem, most observers think they are especially disturbed by its production since it not only increases alcohol consumption, but its sale provides no revenue to the state.

The high tax (about 80 percent) on most alcoholic beverages is a major source of income for the Soviet government. It supplies a third of the total taxes obtained from Soviet citizens and accounts for roughly 12 percent of the government's total revenues. Some foreign observers claim the Soviet government really does not want to restrict the sales of alcohol because it would so radically reduce its income.

"Nonsense," a Ministry of Health Official told me. "We lose far more from alcohol abuse than we gain in taxes." He gave me an article by a noted Soviet economist, Dr. Arlanis, who demonstrated that overall economic losses from alcohol exceeded all state revenues from its sale.[5]

Since 1970, the Soviet government has carried on a wide-scale publicity campaign aimed at bringing public and professional attention to alcoholism. Posters and slogans are displayed in all Soviet factories; television programs pointing out the dangers of alcohol abuse frequently appear.

Precise statistics on alcohol consumption are not published, so the results of the fight against alcoholism are difficult to measure. Since the launching of the campaign, there has been a nationwide decrease in the amount of vodka, brandy, and cognac sold but an increase in wine and champagne sales. From a medical viewpoint, the type of alcohol consumed is of only minor importance. Cirrhosis is just as devastating and difficult to treat whether it results from too much wine or too much vodka.

Many of the reasons behind the rise of alcoholism in the Soviet

---

[5] In terms of relative magnitude, an analysis by U.S. Economist Vladimir G. Treml estimated that the economic losses caused by alcohol abuse as a share of national income are from two to two and a half times greater in the USSR than in the United States; see e.g. "Alcohol in the USSR: A Fiscal Dilemma." In the United States it is estimated that the total medical and social costs of alcoholism exceed $15 billion.

Union—crowded living conditions, lack of entertainment outlets, borderline poverty, combined with a long tradition of drinking—are beyond the control of Soviet psychiatrists or medications. Until these fundamental driving forces are changed, many Soviet physicians I spoke with felt the struggle against alcoholism is futile.

"You do everything you can to help your patient," a middle-aged Soviet psychiatrist told me, "show them how they are hurting themselves and their families. But what do you do about the things that are producing the problem in the first place? I am a doctor but I cannot change the person's life, and sometimes life is the problem." Her private frustration was publicly acknowledged in the Soviet newspaper *Sovetskaya Rossiya* in December 1978, where it was suggested that an improvement in the standard of living, better housing, and "more nightclubs with snappier entertainment" would help to lower the high rate of alcohol abuse.

This is an unusual pronouncement for a Soviet newspaper since it ties the problem of alcoholism directly to the failure of Soviet society to provide alternatives to heavy drinking. Its publication along with similar articles is symbolic, according to the Soviet physicians I spoke with, of the seriousness with which the government now views the problem of alcoholism.

"Fifty years ago," one of them told me, "Lenin said that either socialism will defeat the louse or the louse will defeat socialism. The threat is the same today, only the problem is not lice—it's vodka."

12

Psychiatry

In the summer of 1978, a young man wielding an ax attacked a group of Swedish tourists outside Moscow's Intourist Hotel. More than three hundred people witnessed the assault. The tall, muscular, 220-pound man, later identified as Alexander Nazhinsky, a twenty-four-year-old night watchman, brutally murdered two elderly tourists and severely injured a third. Militia officials who quickly subdued Nazhinsky in the hotel's lobby described him as a "schizophrenic" who had "felt like killing someone."

The violent and bloody incident shocked Moscow. Not only are such attacks rare in the Soviet Union, but violence, when it occurs, is seldom so visible, so public. Compared to the United States, few Soviet citizens own guns and while assaults with deadly weapons such as knives or axes do occur, most are in connection with clandestine robberies. The random daytime slaughter of two elderly tourists (Nazhinsky's victims were age eighty-three and sixty-seven) was the main topic of conversation in the capital city for weeks.

The ax-wielding night watchman now is heavily sedated and under tight security in a "special" Moscow psychiatric hospital. There is no talk of rehabilitating him. He is diagnosed as a severely deranged schizophrenic, a condition he is presumed to have inherited; his schizophrenic genes will be with him for life. Under the Soviet system, for his own good and for the protection of society, he will never be released.

Nazhinsky's treatment is typical of the Soviet approach to psychiatry—society is considered before individual needs. Unfortunately, such a system sets up the conditions for abuse, particularly political abuse.

Among the many books devoted to the subject, two recent ones, Peter Reddaway's *Psychiatric Terror: How Soviet Psychiatry Is Used to Suppress Dissent* and Vladimir Bukovsky's *To Build a Castle, My Life as a Dissenter* provide, respectively, a comprehensive and personal description of the extent to which good medical practices have been subverted to political ideals. I will not repeat or attempt to elaborate on these excellent descriptions except to acknowledge that mental institutions and psychiatric treatment are used as a form of political punishment in the USSR. This is both tragic and unfortunate since these abuses, by insinuation, discredit many Soviet psychiatrists and psychiatric workers who neither participate in nor approve of such practices.

The "special" psychiatric hospitals or the psychiatric-prison hospitals where the schizophrenics, the violent prisoners, and the dissenters are kept are separate from the regular psychiatric hospitals. Instead of the Ministry of Health, they are under control of the Ministry of Internal Affairs (MVD). According to Amnesty International, which claims that approximately 100 political dissenters have been illegally imprisoned in these "special" hospitals, some of the "psychiatrists" are really MVD officers and have no training in psychiatry. The orderlies are convicted criminals who at times abuse the patients. Alexander Nazhinsky will be kept for life in just such a high-security, minimal-treatment hospital.

Throughout the Soviet Union and especially in Moscow, Nazhinsky's diagnosis, schizophrenia, is considered a genetic or inherited disease. The reason, to a large degree, is Dr. Andrei V. Snezhnevsky. Over the past fifteen years, by careful maneuvering, much political skill, and some luck, Snezhnevsky has assumed a position of dominance in Soviet psychiatry. His influence extends well beyond Moscow, where he is the unchallenged leader of the Moscow School of Psychiatry. Snezhnevsky's classification system for schizophrenia is used throughout the Soviet Union. He controls the country's two major psychiatric journals and influences most of the research. He is director of the Kremlin's psychiatric clinic. He is the author of major Soviet psychiatric textbooks.

A knowledge of Snezhnevsky's teaching is important not only because of the pervasive influence he has over Soviet psychiatry but also because it provides a key to understanding how both abuses and everyday treatment take place. According to Dr. Walter Reich, a Washington, D.C., psychiatrist, lecturer in psychiatry at Yale University, and student of Soviet psychiatric methods, Snezhnevsky divides schizophrenia into three categories.

The first category is "continuous," in which the patient will always be mentally ill, with the severity of the illness increasing as he grows older. The second category is "periodic," in which the attacks of schizophrenic behavior come and go; between attacks the person appears entirely well. The final Snezhnevsky category is "shiftlike," where the patient can switch back and forth between "periodic" and "continuous" forms.

The major reason the Snezhnevsky approach is so dangerous, says Reich, is not the three categories, but that his approach permits a wide range of symptoms to be called schizophrenia. Violent attacks such as the one at the Intourist Hotel are obviously the result of severe mental problems. But Snezhnevsky's classification system also permits milder symptoms to be classified as schizophrenia. Symptoms such as depression, guilt, fear, a desire for change, which most U.S. psychiatrists would consider normal responses to stressful situations or, at worst, label as neurotic behavior, can be symptoms of severe mental illness in the USSR. Furthermore, since schizophrenia is genetic, once it is diagnosed, the Soviets believe it can never be cured. Schizophrenia is a label the Soviet citizen wears for life regardless of how much treatment he receives or how his behavior may change. He may be discharged greatly improved, return to work (employment is guaranteed), and not have problems for twenty years. But at any time the diagnosis can come back to haunt him.

The firmness of Snezhnevsky's hold over Soviet psychiatry and the danger of opposing him is illustrated by the case of Dr. Etely Kazanetz. Kazanetz is a respected Soviet psychiatrist who, until recently, was on the faculty of the prestigious Serbski Institute of Forensic Psychiatry in Moscow.

In July, 1979 Dr. Kazanetz published in the American journal *Archives of General Psychiatry* the results of an intensive study of 312 psychiatric patients. The aim of his research was to discover how many of the 312, all of whom had been diagnosed as mentally ill between 1952 and 1959, could still be diagnosed as schizophrenic fifteen to twenty years later.

Although working in Moscow Kazanetz is a member of the rival nosologist or classical school. Nosologists believe that the label schizophrenia should be cautiously applied and that the influence of external factors such as physical illness should be considered when evaluating acute mental disturbances. The classical school is worried that Snezhnevsky and his Moscow school are distorting the practice of psychiatry in the USSR.

Instead of labeling all patients with psychotic reactions schizophrenic, the nosologists prefer to use the term "exogenous psychosis" to refer to patients who, because of a physical accident or an acute emotional stress, suffer a mental breakdown. The disagreement between the Moscow and classical schools has been going on for some time. Snezhnevsky was not the first Soviet psychiatrist to push the genetic and continuous nature of schizophrenia. He simply elaborated on a three-part classification system for schizophrenia originally suggested in the USSR in the 1930s. Kazanetz's 1979 study, however, was the first attempt to actually compare the diagnosis with the subsequent course of the patient.

Kazanetz began by reviewing the original records of the 312 patients and, based on the description provided at that time, reclassified each into one of two groups: schizophrenia or exogenous psychosis. When he then compared the reclassified diagnosis with the original made in the 1950s, he found that instead of 267 only 142 patients met the classical criteria for the diagnosis of schizophrenia and, instead of 45 exogenous psychotic reactions diagnosed by Soviet psychiatrists in 1950 Kazanetz found 170.

To prove that the reclassified diagnoses were correct, Kazanetz and his team interviewed all of the 312 (the fact that he was able to find all of the original patients is an indication of the non-mobility of Soviet society) and reviewed their medical and social history. In almost all cases he found that the patients he and his team had reclassified as suffering from exogenous psychoses rather than schizophrenia had returned to work and were leading normal lives. A few patients, whose original psychiatric problems had resulted from infection or trauma, had suffered relapses.

In contrast, all of the patients whose original diagnosis of schizophrenia was confirmed by Kazanetz had, during the intervening years, continued to have important psychiatric problems.

Kazanetz concluded that, since definitions had changed little since the 1950s, Moscow psychiatrists were over-diagnosing schizophrenia and that these diagnoses, once made, were almost never reviewed.

For many of the patients Kazanetz interviewed, being labeled schizophrenic had interfered with their career. Some had been refused driving permits, others the right to a higher education.

Kazanetz also confirmed an observation he had made earlier that mental patients treated with insulin shock were permanently scarred by the treatment. They had short attention spans, poor intellects and suffered frequent headaches. By rapidly injecting insulin until the patient's blood sugar fell and tremors and unconsciousness developed, researchers thought they would ameliorate mental illness. This form of treatment is no longer used in most of the world. Its use is also almost eliminated in the USSR, being reserved now only for dangerous patients.

Kazanetz hoped that his study would encourage Soviet psychiatry, and especially the Moscow school, to reexamine its practice of diagnosing schizophrenia in persons with prominent environmental stress. Aware of the political controversy his findings might create, Kazanetz was careful not to mention or even allude to the practice of diagnosing dissidents as schizophrenic in order to silence their dissent. Rather he emphasized the scientific basis of his conclusions and the need for caution in their interpretation.

But Snezhnevsky read between the lines and interpreted Kazanetz's paper as an attack on his philosophy. Kazanetz, a prominent and respected research psychiatrist and the author of many important studies, was summarily fired from his position at the Serbski Institute. Kazanetz's career was ruined by a study that in another country would have earned him accolades.

This black-and-white approach to mental illness by both patient and physicians is one reason few patients progress beyond the local polyclinic doctor. "What do you want to go to the psychiatric polyclinic for?" the local *vrach* will frequently ask his patient. "They are all crazy up there. You don't need that."

One alternative exists for those few who can afford it. There are state-sponsored private psychiatric polyclinics where, for a fee, a person can get counseling. The chief advantage of these clinics, beyond the increased time available for private treatment, is privacy. Records are kept for only a year and the clinic is not required to contact the patient's employer. In other facilities, privacy is nonexistent.

As with other behavioral problems, such as alcoholism, the Soviets draw on their Pavlovian traditions and prescribe work therapy to rehabilitate and treat the mentally ill. Most mental patients are treated intensively with drugs and team counseling during their first three to five weeks in the hospital, until acute symptoms, delusions, hallucinations, or bizarre behavior are controlled. They then are placed into work-treatment programs where they receive part of a regular salary for the work they complete. Even the severely emotionally disabled, the retarded (*nadomniki*), are given piecework to do at home.

This emphasis on work, stemming from the ubiquitous Soviet "dignity of work" ethic and the Pavlovian concept of conditioning reflexes is more than the random, nonproductive occupational therapy frequently used in many American hospitals. Soviet mental patients assist in the production of useful goods and services. They make machine parts, repair appliances, or provide community services. There is no problem obtaining employment since the work recommendations made for the patient are binding on the factory or office where the patient is assigned. While this helps the patient quickly integrate himself back into society, it also makes it impossible for him to hide his mental problem from friends and fellow employees.

Moreover, while the employer must accept the patient as a worker, he also has the right under Soviet law to initiate commitment proceedings for any of his workers. This means that an employer who thinks one of his workers is acting strangely can ask for a formal psychiatric evaluation. If the evaluation, which can also be requested by a family member or a physician, concludes that the person is in need of hospitalization, the patient has no opportunity to appeal the ruling in the courts.

As part of its emergency ambulance system (*skoraya pomoshch*), every large Soviet city maintains a separate section for acute psychiatric patients. A psychiatrist is on duty around the clock to answer all calls to the emergency "03" number for such help. Under Soviet practice, only a psychiatrist can admit a patient to a psychiatric hospital. Special ambulances transport psychiatric patients.

Every city keeps an index file on patients in the area who have a history of severe mental problems. A call concerning a patient with a past history of bizarre behavior would bring an immediate response from the *skoraya pomoshch* doctor.

But, except for those very extreme cases of violent acts such as occurred at the Intourist Hotel, the goal of Soviet psychiatry is the same for all mental patients whether retarded, situationally depressed, or delusional—encourage them to modify their symptoms so they can get back to work. Unlike the situation in the United States where therapy is directed toward the individual and "working out" his or her particular problem, the emphasis in the USSR is on the needs of society. Until recently there was little one-on-one treatment.

A pioneer in encouraging and protecting the value of an individual approach to mental illness is the Bekhterev Psychoneurologic Research Institute in Leningrad. It is named after a well known Soviet neurologist, V. M. Bekhterev, whose work coincided with and benefited from the writings of Sigmund Freud.

Like Freud, Bekhterev emphasized the role of social and environmental factors in the causation of mental illness. During Stalin's regime, followers of Bekhterev's teaching came under severe criticism for not adhering rigidly enough to Pavlovian teaching in their practice of psychiatry. During the thirties and forties and culminating in 1950 when a joint meeting of The Soviet Academy of Sciences and Academy of Medicine was officially told to use only Pavlovian theory, open discussion of psychiatric methods was dangerous. Then, and the legacy persists today, drugs were heavily relied upon to correct "physiologic deficiencies." Adversive or conditioning behavior such as insulin shock therapy was also common.

Since Stalin's death the emphasis has slowly shifted. The Bekhterev Institute has emerged as a leader in psychotherapy but individual and group psychotherapy is still uncommon. Lara was fortunate enough to be treated at Bekhterev.

Lara

The evaluation session is held in a large, high-ceilinged room in famous Leningrad Psychiatric Institute. The patient's name, Larisa (Lara). She is twenty-two years old, tall and thin, with long dark hair and brown eyes. She is wearing light-blue hospital pajamas. As she enters the room, Lara looks down at the panel seated before her. It includes a professor, three staff doctors, and four psychiatric nurses. She nods to them, then takes her seat on a straight-back chair facing the eight professionals. One of the staff physicians, a resident (*ordinatura*), presents Lara's case.

"The patient is from Tikhvin," he begins (Tikhvin is a town 125 miles from Leningrad). "Six months ago she went to see her polyclinic doctor, a *terapevt*, complaining of trouble sleeping. He prescribed valerium [a mild tranquilizer] and asked her if she was having any problems. The patient said that a month before she had broken her engagement. She'd heard her former fiancé was planning to marry another woman. She told the doctor she knew her fiancé still loved her and couldn't possibly marry someone else."

One of the psychiatric nurses nods slowly as if in silent sympathy, but doesn't speak.

"The *terapevt* told her not to worry, that such things happened frequently between men and women and that, given time, everything would be better." The *ordinatura* pauses to look at the professor. He motions for him to continue. "Over the next few weeks the patient became more withdrawn. Her family said she refused to eat. Her *sotrudniki* [fellow workers] at the bookstore told their supervisor she no longer paid attention to her work. She was frequently heard to say that her former fiancé was still in love with her and would never marry anyone else."

Lara listens to the presentation carefully, trying to catch every word. It sounds interesting, almost as if they were talking about someone else. But suddenly she hears something familiar. It makes her head ache.

"The whole time the patient was acting in this manner," the resident continues, "her former fiancé repeatedly talked to her, explaining that he was married. He even brought his new wife to meet Lara. But the patient refused to acknowledge these meetings.

"As she became more withdrawn her parents demanded that she be sent to a psychiatrist and Dr. Strakhov of Volkhov District in the Leningrad Oblast [region] saw her in consulation. He considered her depressed and suffering from paranoid delusions. She was given stelazine [a much stronger tranquilizer]. She failed to improve and a week later took an overdose of stelazine in a suicide attempt. Following this she was sent here for evaluation and treatment."

The young resident puts down his stack of papers and the professor takes over the meeting.

"Do you still believe that your fiancé is waiting to marry you?" he asks softly.

"Yes," Lara answers.

"How many men did you know before you met Sasha?"

"None."

"Why did you try to kill yourself?"

"No one understood."

"Do you want to get better?"

"I don't know."

The professor turns to the group and asks their opinion of Lara's case. One of the younger doctors, the one who had presented Lara's history, thinks her problem suggests a schizophrenic condition.

"Possibly," said the professor thoughtfully, "but I think not. What you are seeing is more of a situational problem, more of a circumscribed paranoia, an exogenous psychosis, than a frank schizophrenic condition."

There is a lively and, at times, heated discussion. Most of the staff agree with the professor that Lara's problem is the result of her immaturity and that after proper treatment she will have no residual problems. Two of the younger doctors, though, both of whom did most of their training in Moscow, maintain that Lara's problem indicates a more serious and chronic mental disorder. After a half hour of discussion the professor signals the end of the meeting.

"The young girl is obviously suffering," he says. "I suggest we start treatment immediately."

I spoke with Lara and her parents two months after the evaluation. The professor's treatment recommendations had included three weeks of what we would call group psychological counseling. Lara, along with a group of other patients, had been asked to recount details of her illness. She was encouraged to examine how she had created the problem in her mind and why it was important for her to return to real life. While in the hospital she was also treated with strong tranquilizers, a prescription she was still using when we first talked.

Lara told me she was still depressed and lonely but that she had accepted her boyfriend's marriage. She was back at work and the previous week had even gone to a dance with her girl friends. She no longer wanted to kill herself, "but I know someone must have told Sasha [her ex-fiancé] lies about me," she insisted. "Otherwise he never would have married someone else."

Lara's parents were relieved that she had improved so rapidly and that she was not a "schizophrenic." They were satisfied with her hosptial care, but Lara's father, an official of a trade union and a member of the Communist Party, recalled that getting her admitted to the Leningrad specialty hospital had not been easy.

"Dr. Levin at the district polyclinic tried to help her," he explained, "but he is so busy. There are many patients for him to see so he can spend only a little time with each one. We were lucky even to get a pass to see him. When Lara took the overdose of pills he was out of town and the *terapevt* at our local polyclinic told us there was nothing he could do. He had no authority to send a patient to a psychiatric hospital." (A Soviet patient can be committed only by a psychiatrist whose decision is reviewed "as soon as possible" by a three-member panel. Unlike the U.S. system, there is no mandatory or periodic review of the legal rights of persons involuntarily committed.)

Frightened that she might attempt suicide again, Lara's father turned to his contacts in the trade union. Through a series of friends he eventually found someone who knew the chief doctor at the psychiatric institute. If her parents could get Lara to the hospital's clinic on Monday morning, his contact would try to get her admitted.

"We borrowed my neighbor's car," her father explained, "and got there at 7 A.M. We had to wait all morning, but after they talked with Lara and saw how depressed she was they admitted her immediately."

Just as with the broader practice of medicine, there are large geographic and regional variations in the practice of Soviet psychiatry. Most of the country's 22,000 psychiatrists and 23,000 neuropathologists (who besides neurological problems also treat neurosis and other milder forms of nervous disorders) are concentrated near cities. In rural areas, first-line psychiatric treatment and counseling are provided by the internists and general practitioners within the local polyclinics. They frequently use mild tranquilizers and tell their patients "to relax and not be nervous."

As in Lara's case, referral to psychiatrists at district polyclinics is possible. But difficulty getting a pass, the long waits, and the problems with transportation discourage many potential patients from seeking treatment beyond the polyclinic.

Each district polyclinic has a staff of twenty-five to thirty psychiatrists who serve a population of about 400,000—one doctor for every

16,000 persons. Thus, even those who live in Soviet cities seldom consult a psychiatrist. Besides, the Russians do not yet have a tradition of seeking medical assistance for minor behavioral problems or occasional episodes of depression. It is the family rather than the medical system that modifies and counsels the majority of minor psychiatric problems.

In addition to having little access to a psychiatrist, the patient who gets as far as the psychiatric hospital will find conditions crowded. Despite a two-to-one overall superiority in the number of hospital beds, the USSR has fewer psychiatric beds (300,000) than the United States (375,000). This means that many Soviet patients who in the United States would probably be institutionalized remain at home with their families and are partially integrated into Soviet society. Soviet regulations state that persons with a documented psychiatric illness are entitled to additional living space, a larger apartment so the strain on family members will be less.

The families of patients with problems that cannot be treated as outpatients, such as severe depression or mental retardation, have a dilemma. They frequently have to negotiate for years and occasionally bribe hospital officials to get their brother, son, or daughter admitted to one of the "good" psychiatric hospitals. Short-term admissions such as Lara's are somewhat easier to negotiate, but even here connections are important.

"The doctors and nurses in Leningrad," Lara told me, "explained how my grief over losing Sasha interfered with my work. They said that only by realizing I was wrong and getting back into my work could I forget him. I told them what I thought had really happened—how someone had lied to Sasha—but they said I was simply deluding myself. They called it paranoid thinking and said if I kept bringing it up someone might think I was crazy."

Lara's case reflects the influence of environmental or life-style factors on mental problems, a factor only recently acknowledged by Soviet science. To most foreigners, the everyday characteristics of Soviet life—the long lines, the crowded apartments, the lack of basic consumer goods, much less luxuries—are both frustrating and anxiety-producing. For Soviet women, who carry a large percentage of the country's economic and personal burden, the frustrations are especially severe.

From the time a woman finishes the Soviet gymnasium, or high school, there is an intense competition and fierce peer pressure to find a husband. But since there are only 100 single men for every 170 single Soviet women, many young girls are disappointed and rejected. Some are used badly by Soviet men who, fully aware of their numerical superiority, take advantage of the situation.

The loss of a prospective husband, someone to share or at least assist in the problems of "making it" in the USSR, can be devastating. Many young girls write to Soviet newspapers complaining that there is no loyalty among Soviet men, that they have no respect for a woman's feelings.

"I didn't know what to do when Sasha left," Lara told me "I felt my life was over. I wanted to die. Now I see how foolish that was."

I spoke with Lara in the living room of her parents' apartment. She sat on the edge of the sofa, her hair was carefully combed, she wore a white lace blouse and a dark skirt. She spoke rapidly and her parents told me her voice was getting back the animation and spirit lost during her illness.

"I'm not crazy. I knew that after I saw some of the other patients at the hospital and talked to the nurses. Some of my friends told me not to go to the hospital, that only crazy people went there and that once admitted, I would never be allowed out. Even the doctor at the polyclinic told me not to go.

"They were all wrong. I'm better. Of course," she started to smile, "many of them still think I'm sick, that once you're crazy you can never get better. But I know better."

13

Special Care for
Special People

The clinic on Moscow's Kalinin Prospekt (Avenue) looks no different from most other buildings in the center of the busy Soviet capital except for the carefully placed guards. In Leningrad the clinic is found just off Nevsky Prospekt, not far from the Neva River and the Winter Palace, the symbolic birthplace of the Soviet Revolution. It is also heavily guarded. The location in Irkutsk is a pink and white four-story building surrounded by large shade trees and protected by a high iron fence.

The clinics are part of the Fourth Department of the Ministry of Health. They are found in every major city throughout the USSR. Special sections dot the Black Sea Coast, and others are hidden deep within the Siberian forest. The Fourth Department clinics, sanatoriums, and hospitals (the total number is unknown) are reserved for the exclusive use of members of the Communist Party. But just being one of the 9 percent of the Soviet population carrying a party card is not enough.[1]

The Fourth Department clinics are reserved specifically for the Soviet *nachalstvo* (elite)—top party officials, the heads of large bureaus, institute directors, famous actors and musicians—the privileged of Soviet Communists.

The *nachalstvo* drive down the private center lane in Moscow traf-

[1] Admission to the Communist Party is not granted to all Soviet citizens. Persons who want to join must first obtain recommendations from three members each of whom has been in the party for at least five years. Prospective members also need approval from the local party branch where they work. They then undergo a year of probation following which a vote on membership of both the local party and district communist committee is taken.

Once voted in, all Communists place their career at the party's disposal. A member must move when directed and cannot change jobs without official permission.

About 25 percent of Soviet physicians are card-carrying Communists. The majority of them are male.

299

fic in black limousines. They shop in restricted state stores for Western goods unavailable to the average Soviet citizen. They travel to France, Italy, and the Middle East. Their children wear blue jeans and listen to American rock music on German phonographs. They eat frozen food from Denmark and drink Finnish milk. They read American and British newspapers. The higher their rank, the less Russian their life-style, including medical care.

All Fourth Department clinics and hospitals have imported diagnostic and treatment equipment not available in most regular facilities. An endocrinologist who had been called into Moscow's Kremlinovka clinic as a consultant on the case of a minister suffering from diabetes found a German-made electromyelogram (a machine used to test nerve conduction) and a slit lamp for examining eyes, both of which were unavailable to him in his faculty position at the prestigious Second Moscow Medical Institute. Blood tests that were not routinely available to Soviet doctors could be ordered in the Kremlinovka. The blood samples, the endocrinologist explained, were flown to Finland where the special tests were run by a laboratory in Helsinki. Completed, the results were flown back to Moscow in time for the *nachalnik's* (minister's) next visit.

My friend the endocrinologist told me that within the Kremlin's Fourth Department clinic there were important distinctions made for rank and position.

"Deputy ministers and persons of lower rank are seen in regular private cubicles but ministers have special examining rooms," he said. "There are carpets on the floor, bookcases, a leather couch, and heavy red drapes over the windows. It is like a living room, not a clinic."

The existence of these special clinics and hospitals is widely known throughout the USSR and rumors concerning what goes on inside their carefully guarded walls are a favorite topic of conversation among the *intelligentsia* in Moscow, Leningrad, and other large Soviet cities.

"Our great leaders go there to get their syphilis treated and to dry out," a student from Leningrad told me. "The Kremlin doctors have special machines that can diagnose cancer by heat waves," an engineer told me. (A test known as thermography that uses heat to detect tumors does exist. It is not generally available in the USSR.)

"They may have better equipment," a medical student in Moscow said, "but Fourth Department doctors are picked because they're good Communists, not good doctors. Whenever the *nachalstvo* have any real medical problems their doctors call in specialists from the university. Look at Brezhnev," he said. "You think he would be alive today if he had to rely on fourth-department doctors? Never! He's too sick."

In addition to keeping the existence of the fourth-department clinics an official secret, the Soviet government also carefully avoids any public disclosure of the medical problems of its political leaders. Unlike the U.S. practice of providing detailed daily bulletins on everything from the late Hubert Humphrey's bladder cancer to former President Jimmy Carter's hemorrhoids, Soviet citizens are told of an illness only when the official dies and even then, few details are disclosed.

Most Soviet citizens, for example, know that their Secretary General Leonid Brezhnev, a man upon whose shoulders so much of the world's future rests, is sick. When he appears on television the film is carefully edited so the public will not see his staggering gait, but the Soviet public recognizes his need for constant assistance. They hear how he garbles words during long televised speeches despite the announcer's attempts at cover-up. They notice when he disappears for a month, ostensibly to the Black Sea for a vacation but in reality for treatment of frequent lung infections.

Once a heavy smoker, Brezhnev has quit, while at official receptions he drinks sparingly. During a 1979 state dinner with French President Valery Giscard d'Estaing the Soviet menu made it possible for Brezhnev to use only a spoon for eating.

Western officials meeting with the premier report his attention span is about an hour. At times he seems disoriented.

From secret intelligence analysis and the reports of persons who have met with the secretary general, Western observers have concluded that Brezhnev does have a number of significant medical problems: The left side of his body is weak and his smile crooked, the obvious result of a stroke. This has also caused most of his problems with his speech, but compounding it is a severe degenerative hearing loss. Aides frequently have to repeat questions Brezhnev did not hear the first time.

The seventy-two-year-old leader has also had two serious heart attacks, one of which left him with heart block, a disruption in the heart's normal rhythm. Most Soviet patients with heart block go without treatment. Sometimes the problem improves on its own; often there is a progressive deterioration leading to death.

Both times Brezhnev was given an electronic pacemaker. A slender wire was inserted into his heart and then connected to a portable electrical power supply implanted under the skin of his chest. This power source guarantees that if the Soviet premier's heart fails to beat, the pacemaker will take over.

There are only a few hundred pacemakers in use in the Soviet Union. All of them are imported. In Brezhnev's case, foreign experts along with the best Soviet physicians, including E. I. Chazov, a widely respected cardiologist, deputy minister of health, and director of the cardiology division of the special Fourth Department, were consulted.

The details of Brezhnev's medical problems is the subject of constant speculation and rumor, none of which has ever officially been acknowledged by the Soviet government. Rumors occasionally appear that much of Brezhnev's problems could be due to amyotrophic lateral sclerosis, a progressive muscle-wasting problem, also known as Lou Gehrig's Disease. Other persons have claimed that the Soviet premier suffers from leukemia and that the occasional puffiness of his face is caused by steroid therapy given to control the condition.

The actual explanation behind Brezhnev's medical history, however, appears less dramatic. A prominent Moscow surgeon told me he had been asked in the late 1960s to review Brezhnev's medical history concerning possible open-heart surgery. The aim of the operation was to relieve the premier's then recurrent attacks of angina.

"He had severe arteriosclerosis (hardening of the arteries) that led to his stroke," the surgeon told me. "His rich diet and lack of exercise—he's over thirty pounds overweight—may have also contributed to his atherosclerosis (narrowing of the coronary arteries that supply the heart muscle).

"When I was first consulted, in 1969, Brezhnev's doctors were considering operating to open up the block in his coronary arteries. I thought they were crazy. Even if the surgery could have been done at that time in the Soviet Union, Brezhnev was a very high-risk candidate.

"Besides the problems with his arteries he had chronic bronchitis, hypertension and occasional attacks of severe vertigo. He was a wreck. I told them, as diplomatically as possible, that our best course of action was to treat him conservatively, with drugs, not surgery.

"Brezhnev was placed on beta-blockers, a drug that in addition to controlling hypertension reduces the oxygen demands of the heart, thereby lessening the frequency of anginal attacks. At that time beta-blockers were not approved for use in the United States and were certainly not used in Moscow. A group of English cardiologists were consulted in the use of the drug.

"Since then, although I've never been asked again for my opinion, I've watched Brezhnev on television and at official receptions. He's doing remarkably well. Frankly I'm surprised he's still alive. If you'd asked me in 1970 to predict, I would have said he'd be dead in a year."

Because of the increased contact between American and Soviet physicians through the U.S.–USSR health exchange, American experts are now occasionally asked to consult on medical problems that, while attributed to ordinary citzens, obviously belong to someone special.

One American physician I spoke to, who has an ongoing association with Soviet scientists through the official exchange and therefore does not want to be personally identified, told me of receiving an unexpected late night telephone request from Moscow. The call came a few days before he was to leave on a regularly scheduled visit.

"The caller," he told me, "was a Moscow physician I knew well. He said they had a case which might be of special interest to me, and could I bring along a sample of new medication I was experimenting with?

"Although it was a strange request I told him I would. When I arrived at Moscow Airport the Customs official seemed to know who I was and motioned me right through the gate and toward two waiting limousines. I'd never been given such treatment before. In one of the cars was the Moscow physician who had called. He took the medicine and gave it to the driver of the other car, who immediately drove off.

"I then proceeded with my tour. It called for visits to a number of Soviet institutes both in Moscow and in Kiev. While I was in Kiev the director of the local institute suddenly called me out of the tour and into his office for what he called a special consultation.

"I was shown X rays, the results of extensive laboratory tests, along with a complete medical history. All of the papers came out of a locked briefcase.

"I asked if I could examine the patient. His history indicated he had cancer, disseminated cancer in what we would call a late stage. They brought in a patient and I examined him. Although it was obvious he'd been sick, he appeared much healthier than his test results indicated. He also seemed larger than his X rays.

"When I asked to talk to the surgeon who did the original cancer operation, I was told he would have to be flown in from Moscow. He arrived the next day, one of the most prominent surgeons in the entire Soviet Union, an internationally recognized expert.

"I talked with him about the case and he described the findings at surgery. The whole time I kept thinking, who was the real patient? Who did he really operate on? Was it a member of the Politburo or some other high-ranking official?

"I never found out, but to this day I feel sure it wasn't the patient I examined. He was just an ordinary factory worker and I doubt whether the Soviets would have gone to all the trouble and secrecy for him. No, I'm convinced it was someone important, someone the Soviets wanted to have the best, not only Soviet Fourth Department specialists, but also American experts."

Because their services are not available to most Soviet citizens, there is widespread criticism of physicians who work within the Fourth Department. "You can't be a good Communist and a good doctor," a popular saying goes. But while it may be true that most Fourth Department doctors have political aspirations, they also are some of the best Soviet doctors. Many have combined the personal contacts made in the Kremlinovka and their medical expertise into a successful public career.

Boris Petrovsky, the current minister of health, was formerly head surgeon of the Fourth Department. Before that, the rotund, friendly, gregarious Petrovsky was a professor at the Second Moscow Medical Institute. There he had completed research into the repair of injured blood vessels, the use of blood transfusions, and developed new techniques of heart surgery. Since being appointed to the top health position in the Soviet government in 1964, Petrovsky has continued to work part-time as a surgeon, completing two or three operations each week. When it came time for the Soviet Union to demonstrate to the medical world that they were up to date with modern techniques, it was Petrovsky who performed the Soviet Union's first kidney transplant.

American medical leaders who have worked closely with Petrovsky have been impressed with his ability to get what he wants from the bulky Soviet bureaucracy and with his political savvy. "He's built a strong series of research institutes in Moscow, emphasizing cancer and heart disease," comments Dr. Paul Ehrlich, former director of HEW's Office of International Health and U.S. representative to the World Health Organization (WHO), where he frequently met Petrovsky. "Personally, he was very warm, but obviously powerful. I think most other WHO representatives were quite attracted to him."

"Petrovsky's a remarkable man," according to another well-known surgeon, Michael DeBakey. "Over the years I've developed tremendous respect for his ability to work within the Soviet system and get things done. He is a strong, important force moving the Soviet medical system forward."

DeBakey's relationship with Petrovksy dates back two decades to the first time the world-famous Houston surgeon visited the USSR. It was in 1958 at the International Surgical Congress in Leningrad. Under Khrushchev's leadership, tensions were easing between the United States and the USSR. A few Soviet scientists, including Petrovsky, had visited the United States. But for all of the four thousand Soviet surgeons assembled in Leningrad, DeBakey's speech was the first time any of them had seen or heard an American physician.

"I stood at the microphone for twenty minutes after the talk," DeBakey recalls. "Everyone in the audience clapped and shouted. I thought they would never stop."

The Ministry of Health took DeBakey's slides, transcribed his talk, and turned them into a book in Russian on cardiovascular surgery. It sold out immediately.

Since this initial visit, DeBakey has made many trips to the USSR. In 1962, he received the Vishnevsky Medal from the USSR Academy of Medical Sciences. During these many visits, DeBakey has become a folk hero to many Soviet physicians.

"Does he really own his own hospital?" Soviet doctors would ask me. "How big is Houston? Is it true he controls the whole town? Does he do six operations at a time? Is he the most powerful doctor in America?"

Many Soviet physicians I spoke to had read about his practice of operating on poor persons from around the world without charge and how, in the 1960s, he broke ranks with organized American medicine to support Senator Edward Kennedy in his early battles for national health insurance. But even more impressive to the average Soviet physician is the image they have of DeBakey as a skilled surgeon who, by developing and perfecting new surgical techniques, has achieved international scientific recognition and personal fame—something none of them can ever hope to achieve.

Over the years, DeBakey's frequent contacts with Petrovksy have resulted in a close friendship between the two surgeons and medical leaders. Both born in 1908, each spent part of his early training in Europe—DeBakey in Germany, Petrovksy in Hungary. Both specialized in cardiovascular surgery and both have operated on some of the world's most powerful leaders.

In April 1972, Petrovsky asked DeBakey to come to Moscow to consult on the treatment of just such an individual, Mstislav Keldysh, then president of the USSR Academy of Sciences. The unusual request and the events that followed it not only illustrate the friendship between DeBakey and Petrovsky, but also provide a unique glimpse into the way the *nachalstvo* are treated and how the Fourth Department operates.

The request to have DeBakey come to Moscow was unusual because the Soviets seldom consult American physicians openly regarding medical treatment of their leaders.[2] In fact, the Soviets frequently bring foreign dignitaries from other countries, mainly Third World nations, to be treated by Soviet medical experts. In 1978, for example, ailing Algerian President Houari Boumedienne was flown to Moscow in an effort to diagnose a mysterious and ultimately fatal illness. Although the Soviets were unable to help Boumedienne (he died a few months later of a rare blood disease), they have over the years diagnosed and treated many foreign dignitaries.

But in 1972 a peculiar set of political and medical problems re-

[2] The one notable exception is former premier Khrushchev, who for years was treated by A. McGehee Harvey, professor of medicine at Johns Hopkins University.

sulted in the call from Moscow to Houston. The medical problem was aortoiliac occlusive disease—atherosclerotic plaques blocking the large arteries in Academician Keldysh's legs. In the forties and fifties, DeBakey had pioneered many of the current operations used to cut out and replace the diseased arteries with synthetic grafts. No surgeon in the world was more qualified to operate on Keldysh than DeBakey.

But of more importance was the political consideration that in 1972 no physician in the Soviet Union would accept the risk of operating on the high-ranking scientist.

Within the strict Soviet hierarchy, important persons like Keldysh can only be operated on by an equally prominent surgeon. But, unlike the United States, where there are a number of prestigious centers and surgeons from which to choose, the Soviets have only a few. According to Michael Ravitch, professor of surgery at the University of Pittsburgh and a longtime confidant of Soviet medical leaders, in 1972 there were only two Moscow surgeons to whom the Soviets would entrust Keldysh's care. "The problem was that both Petrov and Vishnevsky[3] had recently lost patients after similar operations. Both of them were reluctant to operate on someone of Keldysh's prominence and possibly fail. Neither wanted the case."

So Michael DeBakey was summoned. To determine how extensive Keldysh's problem was, DeBakey asked for an arteriogram, the injection of dye into the diseased arteries to pinpoint the location and extent of blockage.

"I cautioned them beforehand," DeBakey recalls, "to be very careful injecting the dye so it wouldn't create a false channel, a dissection, in his aorta. Unfortunately, that's exactly what happened. There was no way I could operate in April. I told Petrovsky the surgery would have to wait."

DeBakey saw Keldysh a second time six months later when the high-ranking scientist headed a delegation of Soviet space experts to NASA headquarters in Houston. There DeBakey reaffirmed that Keldysh had extensive disease cutting off blood supply to both legs, but most severe to his left foot. If the seventy-two-year-old scientist were going to continue functioning, an operation was essential.

[3] Drs. Boris Petrov and Aleksandr Vishnevsky, both prominent Soviet surgeons, are now deceased.

"I told him I would rather do the surgery in Houston," DeBakey told me. "But Keldysh gripped my hand and said pleadingly but firmly that he wanted to have the operation in Moscow."

No date was set, but shortly after New Years Day 1973, DeBakey received an urgent call from the Soviet Embassy saying that Keldysh was in trouble and asking if he could come at once. After checking with the U.S. Department of State, which immediately approved of the trip, DeBakey hurriedly rearranged his schedule and, along with his fellow surgeon Dr. George P. Noon and two surgical nurses, flew to the Soviet capital. The delegation was met at the airport by Keldysh's personal physician and cardiologist, E. I. Chazov, Deputy Minister of Health.

The next morning DeBakey examined Keldysh and found the disease indeed advanced. His famous patient was in constant pain and there were signs of gangrene in the left foot.

The operation took place the next morning and, according to De-Bakey, "Everything went well. Of course, it was just like being at home. We had brought my instruments along with our own sutures and grafts.

"We placed a graft from his abdominal aorta to both external iliac arteries. We replaced both femoral arteries and, since he had stones, we also removed his gallbladder. Keldysh did fine," DeBakey recalls. "Pulses returned to both of his feet and the signs of gangrene receded."

Following the surgery, DeBakey and his team were given a series of banquets by various medical and political organizations. At one of the final ceremonies he became the first foreigner to receive the USSR's Fiftieth Anniversary Jubilee Medal.

"It was overwhelming," the famous surgeon told me. "The Soviets were so appreciative and, of course, receiving the medal was a total surprise. But what I remember most was Mrs. Keldysh. It was after one of the banquets, I'm not sure which one, she came up to me, kissed me on the cheek, and grabbed me in a tremendous embrace. She was crying, crying, and thanking me for operating on her husband."[4]

---

[4] Mistislav Keldysh died June 24, 1979, from advanced artherosclerosis. DeBakey's operation in 1973 had enabled him to function as president of the Academy of Sciences for two more years, until 1975.

Since September 7, 1973, there has been a hot-line Telex linking the U.S. Department of Health and Human Services in Washington, D.C., with the Soviet Ministry of Health in Moscow. Most of the time it is used for communications related to the official exchange of Soviet and American scientists, the details of conferences, the arrival times of delegations. But in late February 1979 it printed out an urgent request for help.

The message came from Dr. George Falkovsky, a Soviet physician from Moscow's 31st General Hospital. Dr. Falkovsky had a young female patient dying from acute lung failure and he was calling to ask for professional consultation, the first time the Washington-Moscow Telex had been used for such a human emergency.

Peter Frommer, M.D., of the National Institutes of Health's Heart and Lung Institute took the call and assembled a four-person team. The team could, if requested, fly to Moscow with the machines and expertise to support a patient whose lungs were acutely and severely damaged. The director of the team was Warren Zapol, M.D., an anesthesiologist on the staff of the Massachusets General Hospital and an authority on acute respiratory failure.

The first call that Dr. Zapol received directly from Moscow, from Dr. Falkovsky, was in the early morning of March 2, 1979. It was encouraging. The patient, described to Dr. Zapol as a twenty-eight-year-old woman who had developed respiratory failure following removal of an infected ovarian cyst, was "doing much better."

"We appreciate your willingness to help," Dr. Falkovsky told Zapol, "but you will not be needed." Dr. Zapol called the other members of the team.

But by noon of the same day he received another call from Moscow. "She's failing again," Falkovsky said. "You must come. Be on the 5 P.M. Aeroflot flight out of New York. Come alone."

Zapol had neither ticket nor visa, but he packed his bags and caught the shuttle from Boston to New York's La Guardia Airport where he took a cab to Kennedy International. Before leaving home, he talked to the Department of State, which cautioned him about going on such short notice. "You do not have a ticket or visa," a department spokesman told him. "It is very unlikely the Soviets will go through with this. You may as well stay home."

But at the Aeroflot ticket counter "two big men came out of the shadows and walked me right through to the airplane. I flew alone in first class. They treated me very nicely."

Zapol arrived in Moscow on Saturday morning, March 3. He asked to be driven to the hospital immediately. "She was almost dead," Zapol recalls, "in a coma, a blood pressure of only 80, her pupils fixed and dilated. I put her chances [of living] at about 8 percent."

The patient was Marina Burakovsky, a pediatrician who is the oldest daughter of Dr. Vladimir Burakovsky, director of Moscow's Bakulev Institute of Cardiovascular Surgery. Dr. Burakovsky is an internationally known specialist and has frequently treated many prominent Soviet citizens.[5]

"Everyone was very concerned about Marina," a Soviet physician told me later. "At first her infection seemed only a minor problem but it spread quickly. During surgery she had a cardiac arrest, then her lungs and kidneys failed. When Falkovsky called the United States he had done everything he could."

But why had he contacted the Americans? Surely there had been other desperate cases where the Soviets had gone it alone.

"It is difficult to say," a Moscow physician who had followed the case through one of his friends who was on the staff of Hospital 31 explained. "Of course, Dr. Burakovsky is an important man, a member of the *nachalstvo*. It could be expected that his daughter would get the best. But, in my view, a lot of the initiative came from Falkovsky. He speaks excellent English and has traveled widely. He recognized that he had a young patient with a potentially curable problem but he was having trouble keeping her alive through the crises. Falkovsky knew the Americans had more experience and better machines. He [Falkovsky] is a product of the U.S.–USSR health exchange so he took a chance and asked for permission to call in help. Older Soviet physicians, without his exposure and experience, would not have considered asking an American."

At first Dr. Zapol and the Soviet physicians disagreed over the cause of her respiratory problem. "My hunch was she had septicemia [infection in her blood]," Dr. Zapol said in an interview shortly

---

[5] The identity of the patient was never officially acknowledged. My information comes from knowledgeable Soviet and American sources. The interview with Dr. Zapol was conducted by Dennis Breo and reported in *American Medical News* Apr. 13, 1979.

after returning home to Boston. "Her lungs were being clogged with excess fluid seeping in from infected blood capillaries. The lungs are meant to be light, airy organs to transfer gases. Hers were filled with fluid. I told the Soviet physicians, 'She is septic.' They replied, 'No, no, she has shock lung.'"[6]

A few days later a blood culture grew out a particularly virulent bacteria, pseudomonas. Fortunately, Zapol had brought a supply of a new antibiotic, amikacin, with him. Unavailable in the USSR, it is used in life-threatening infections from pseudomonas.

"We also used hyperimmune polyvalent pseudomonas antisera," Zapol said, "a Soviet drug we do not use in the United States, but one that is possibly very useful. So we had found the bug [pseudomonas], which is half the battle," Zapol continued, "but now we faced the tough half. Finding the source of the blood infection."

Zapol and the Soviet doctors examined Marina Burakovsky's urine, spinal fluid, and sputum for evidence of the infection's origin. All were negative. An emergency operation was performed to see if the infection was near the site of her original surgery. Again, negative.

According to Zapol, "Things looked grim. Marina's father broke into tears."

For the next few days Marina required frequent transfusions of blood plasma as well as constant attention to her lungs and kidneys.

"We used percussion [chest thumping] and position changes to clear her lungs and suction to clear the fluids from her trachea. She had developed a kidney injury and we reduced [the] amikacin dosage to prevent further renal failure."

"In the meantime," Zapol explained, "we had to feed her. We arranged for the Massachusetts General to ship via Aeroflot, three times a week, supplies of a concentrated solution of sugars and amino acids for intravenous infusion.

"As the days crawled by," Zapol said, "her blood pressure gradually rose . . . her urine output rose, she required less oxygen."

A week after Zapol's arrival in Moscow the patient was well enough to be transferred to her father's Bakalev Institute of Cardio-

---

[6] The damage caused to a lung when, for a variety of reasons, it does not receive enough blood and oxygen.

vascular Surgery. It was there, on March 16, that Marina Burakovsky woke up.

"She looked around the room and said a few things," Zapol recalls. "We were euphoric.

"We went to the Aragvi [a Soviet restaurant specializing in Georgian food] and had a feast: fresh Georgian bread, fine-grained Beluga caviar, smoked Siberian salmon, chicken with ground walnuts. And, of course, several toasts with vodka.

"Before, my toasts with the Soviets had always been general—good health, happiness, the 1972 accord between the United States and the Soviet Union that made an exchange of medical views and my visit possible. But this day, we toasted our patient."

Zapol remained in the Soviet Union for another eleven days. He wanted to make sure his patient's recovery was complete, that she could be taken off the ventilator and would no longer be dependent on intravenous feedings. During that time he was honored at a series of dinners and parties hosted by the Soviet doctors. He was taken to Moscow's best restaurants, to the Moscow Circus, the Bolshoi Ballet, the Writers' Club, the Journalists' Club.

On March 20, he and his Soviet colleagues held a joint press conference describing their efforts. It was later reported in *Izvestia* under the title, "For Health."

"This is not a story," Dr. Zapol told the Moscow press conference, "of how one Massachusetts General Intensive Care specialist and a lot of U.S. medical technology saved a patient. Machines don't cure patients; good intensive care does. This patient got superb care. A team of Soviet physicians treated her with me, and the hard work—the chest physiotherapy, the turning, the suctioning, the blood gas analysis, the lab work—was mostly done by the Soviets.

"Today, our patient has recovered beautifully. Her brain is fine, she reads and watches TV, her kidneys function normally. . . . In two weeks or so she will be strong enough to go home. Few hospitals in America can give such fine care. She is very lucky."

14
Solzhenitsyn's Cancer–
A Case History

The first Russian-language edition of *The Gulag Archipelago I* was published in Paris in December, 1973. A few months later, while I was living in Kishinev, I secretly obtained a copy through the State Department diplomatic pouch. Carefully wrapping it in a recent issue of *Pravda* and concealing it in my *setka* (shopping bag) along with a loaf of bread and some rolls, I took it to the apartment of an old physician with whom I had become close friends. I knew that of all the gifts I could bring him, this book would be the most appreciated.

As my friend removed the layers of newspaper and saw the gray cover with red-lettered title, his hands began to shake. When it was clear it really was the *Gulag*, he shut his eyes and brought it to his lips. His wife, sitting on the other side of the room, stood up as if a fourth person had entered the room.

It was March 1974. The book's author, Aleksandr Solzhenitsyn, had just been expelled from the Soviet Union.

Today the sixty-two-year-old Nobel Prize-winning writer lives in the United States in a tightly fenced country house near Cavendish, Vermont. The three volumes of his largest work, *The Gulag Archipelago,* are now complete. Much of its 1,800 pages are documentation, providing names and histories for a few of the 20 million people who died in Stalin's vast system of prison camps. Despite its length there is a raging will throughout, a defiance of fatigue in the face of overwhelming suffering. The book is Solzhenitsyn's tribute to the strength and limitless resilience of the human mind. Its completion was a major accomplishment, one which would satisfy most men. But after writing *The Gulag,* three major novels (*The First Circle, Cancer Ward,* and *August 1914*), and numerous short stories and plays, Aleksandr Isaevich Solzhenitsyn is still a man obsessed with work. He is now finishing his long awaited account of the February 1917

Revolution. He is arranging the publication of a series of scholarly books on modern Russian history.

At times he works in a barren one-room cabin isolated by thick woods from the main house. No visitors are permitted. Each day he is at his desk by seven. His thin legs are clad in an old, loose-fitting pair of trousers. He wears a flannel shirt and, on cool New England mornings, a sweater. His eyes squint as his clubbed, calloused fingers search for a pen. For at least ten and often as long as sixteen hours, he writes. The words fill all the available spaces on many small scraps of paper. He is careful not to waste anything.

Many days Aleksandr Isaevich is so involved with writing that he forgets to eat and his wife, a precise, determined woman who handles all of his daily affairs, never disturbs him. When he does stop for food it is not at the standard times the rest of the world uses to divide the day. He believes setting a time for eating is wasteful, extravagant.

His tastes in food are simple. He avoids beef and refuses to eat any smoked or dried fish. Fresh vegetables, dark bread, a bowl of soup, and fruit are enough. His favorite dish is a single, peeled, boiled potato. His stomach fills quickly and he seldom asks for seconds. If we are what we eat, then Aleksandr Isaevich Solzhenitsyn is, like his writing, pure. But what else is there about this man that enables or indeed forces him on? Why, after so much success, does he still struggle against a constantly elusive deadline?

The details of Solzhenitsyn's early life, his education and his imprisonment at age twenty-six are well documented. He was raised in Rostov. His father died in a hunting accident six months before he was born. As a child he was constantly catching cold. He never enjoyed good health and avoided physical sports. One of his favorite activities was visiting the local theatrical school. For a time he even considered becoming an actor. Repeated infections of his larynx, however, ended any thought of an acting career.

After graduating from the University of Rostov, a quiet, reserved Solzhenitsyn became a *prepodovatel* (high school instructor), teaching physics and mathematics. The position was short-lived. Within four months, on October 18, 1941, he was drafted into the Red Army.

Initially, because of his poor health, he drove trucks. Within three years, however, by drawing on his mathematical background and a year of artillery training, Private Solzhenitsyn was promoted to cap-

tain. He took command of an artillery battery and fought in the famous armored conflict at Kursk-Orgol. His unit also helped batter
down the German defenses at Konigsberg.

Throughout the fighting Artillery Captain Solzhenitsyn maintained a dream of someday becoming a writer. He outlined short
stories on the back of battle plans. He wrote long and detailed letters
to friends and former schoolmates.

According to Solzhenitsyn, it was story outlines found by members of the NKVD's (secret police) counterespionage section
SMERSH (*Smert Shpionam,* Death to Spies) in his map case that led
to his arrest in February 1945. For the crime of referring to Stalin as
"the moustached one," along with other slanders against the Soviet
state, Solzhenitsyn received eight years at forced labor plus three
years in exile.

One of his first prison assignments was a construction project in
Moscow. Then, just as it had in the army, his mathematical background improved his position and *Zek* (prisoner) Solzhenitsyn was
reassigned to a scientific institute at Marfino. He was there a year
and his experience served as the basis for his novel *The First Circle.*
From Marfino prison, Solzhenitsyn went to Ekibastuz, a large labor
camp in Eastern Kazakhstan which he described as "the lowest circle of hell." At Ekibastuz, a camp exclusively for political criminals,
prisoners wore numbers on their chest, back, and on one knee.

It was while imprisoned at Ekibasinz that Solzhenitsyn's health,
never robust, first became a major influence in his life and his writing. But unlike much of Solzhenitsyn's public life, the details of his
very private fight against death are a mixture of partial fact, rumor,
and speculation.

It is widely known, for example, that in the early 1950s Solzhenitsyn's body developed cancer. The emphasis on body is important
because, except for a few months at the end of 1953, at no time did
his mind acknowledge the malignancy. It is also known that Solzhenitsyn's novel *Cancer Ward* was largely autobiographical. In the
novel Kostoglotov, the character who most persons believe represents Solzhenitsyn, is afflicted with a large abdominal tumor and
has come to Tashkent for radiation treatment. But how closely do
the events described for Kostoglotov mirror Solzhenitsyn's medical
history? What kind of tumor did Solzhenitsyn have and how did he
manage to survive? Did Soviet doctors really have the ability to de-

stroy his cancer in 1954 or, as some persons suggest, did Solzhenitsyn cure himself?

A major reason behind this confusion is that Solzhenitsyn does not discuss the details of his illness. Today, even his wife and close friends avoid the topic. Solzhenitsyn maintains that details of his private life are not important; only his work, his writing, matters. Yet many people close to the writer acknowledge that his illness thirty-five years ago remains the major influence in his writing today.

"He came very close to death in Tashkent," one of his close Washington friends told me. "He believes he was saved by a combination of medical treatment and his own *stoikost,* or determination to survive. If he ever stops working he's convinced his cancer will come back, and to continue to live he must write. To him, living and writing are inseparable."

Solzhenitsyn's medical history begins in January 1952. It was then he noticed a small swelling in his right groin. At first he ignored it. By the end of January, however, the lump was the size of a small lemon and growing larger every day. At the end of the month Solzhenitsyn entered the Ekibastuz prison hospital for surgery.

The doctors in Ekibastuz were, like Solzhenitsyn, prisoners. The day before his operation the camp surgeon was transported to another prison. Solzhenitsyn waited for almost two weeks for another doctor to arrive.

On February 12, a German prisoner-surgeon removed Solzhenitsyn's tumor, using local anesthesia. After the operation, sandbags were placed over his incision to stop bleeding and prevent further swelling. At the time Solzhenitsyn understood little except that the removed lump was a small cancer, a malignant lymph node. The cancer, he was told, had not invaded the surrounding tissues. From his bed in the prison hospital, Solzhenitsyn wrote his first wife, Natalya Reshetovskaya, whom he had married in 1940, that "there are no grounds for further concern."

Because there was no laboratory at the small hospital, sections of Solzhenitsyn's tumor were sent to the Department of Pathology at the Omsk Medical Institute. A microscopic analysis was necessary to tell what kind of tumor it was and whether further treatment was indicated.

Meanwhile Solzhenitsyn recovered quickly. He was discharged

from the prison hospital on February 26, 1953. In a few weeks the pain of the incision disappeared. He went back to his construction work and later as a smelter in the camp's foundry. The prison doctors did not reexamine Solzhenitsyn nor did they tell him the results of the microscopic analysis. After all, he was still a prisoner with limited and frequently ignored rights.

A year later, in March 1953, following Stalin's death, Solzhenitsyn along with thousands of other political prisoners was released from Ekibastuz. As a former "political," however, Solzhenitsyn was still not free to live and travel as he wished. He was forced into exile in the Uzbek village of Kok-Terek. He lived in a mud hut and taught the village children mathematics and physics. In Kok-Terek, Solzhenitsyn began writing furiously, anxious to put his prison experiences and those of his fellow inmates on paper.

During his first summer in Kok-Terek, Solzhenitsyn did not think much about his operation. Except for an occasional fever he felt well. He had even forgotten about getting the microscopic type of his tumor back from Omsk. There did not seem any reason. He was doing fine.

By the autumn of 1953, Solzhenitsyn's optimism was gone. In September he developed stomach pains. He lost his appetite. His weight, always precariously low, began to fall. At first Solzhenitsyn thought his problem might be from gastritis or a stomach ulcer. While in prison he had complained bitterly about the diet. Watery fish stew, gruel made from boiled grass and *sto gram* (100 grams) of bread were the daily ration. What little protein there was came in the form of dried, smoked fish.

This diet, especially the fish, Solzhenitsyn believed, had poisoned his stomach. For help, he turned to Nikolai Ivanovich Zubov, an older man, a gynecologist whom Solzhenitsyn had first met after arriving in Kok-Terek.

Dr. Zubov, a character Solzhenitsyn describes as an old-fashioned private practitioner (Dr. Kadmins) in *Cancer Ward*, urged his friend to write to Ekibastuz and obtain the exact type of his tumor. Although not a specialist in cancer, Zubov was concerned that Solzhenitsyn's current problems were not gastritis but were related to the operation and his malignant lymph node.

Because there were no cancer specialists in Kok-Terek, Solzhenitsyn applied to the local NKVD authorities (to whom he reported every two weeks under the conditions of his exile) for permission to go to Dzhambul, the closest town with specialized medical facilities.

At Dzhambul, a stomach X ray found not an ulcer but a tumor mass the size of a large fist. The mass was outside Solzhenitsyn's stomach, growing up from the back of his abdominal wall, pushing his stomach up and out. It was almost certainly cancer.

Some of the doctors at Dzhambul thought the tumor was a new cancer unrelated to Solzhenitsyn's original operation. Others argued that, although the exact type of the first tumor was unknown (the officials at Ekibastuz had written Solzhenitsyn there was no hope of tracing his diagnosis), it was very likely that this new mass was the result of cells left behind after removal of the lymph node. These malignant cells could have spread from his groin through lymphatic channels to the space behind his stomach.

Solzhenitsyn returned to Kok-Terek in early December 1953. Before leaving Dzhambul he had obtained extract from a mandrake root plant (*issyk kul*), a dark, thick liquid that, according to Russian folk lore, cured cancer. His symptoms were becoming worse. Stomach pain kept him from eating. He lost more weight. The Dzhambul doctors told Solzhenitsyn he would have to go to the Tashkent Oncological (Cancer) Health Center for treatment. But travel to Tashkent required official permission, and when Solzhenitsyn first applied the local NKVD administrator refused.

During the final weeks of 1953, in constant pain, nauseated every time he tried to eat, living on tea with sugar, "poisoned with cancer," Solzhenitsyn was convinced he was dying. His belly was swollen with ascites (fluid from the rapidly growing tumor), making it painful to breathe and excruciating to cough.

"I was a sorry sight," he wrote in his short story *The Right Hand.* "My sallow face wore vestiges of the past . . . wrinkles of forced camp moroseness, deathly ashen hardness of the skin . . . my face had the hue of green. My striped, foolish-looking jacket barely reached my stomach, my pants ended above my ankles."

The doctors told Solzhenitsyn he had at most three weeks to live. It was, according to him, the most dreadful moment of his life, "to die on the threshold of freedom, to see all I had written, all that gave meaning to my life thus far, about to perish with me," he wrote in his literary biography *The Oak and the Calf.* "I hurriedly copied things out in tiny handwriting, rolled them several pages at a time, into tight cylinders and squeezed these into a champagne bottle. I buried the bottle in my garden—and set off for Tashkent to meet the new year (1954) and to die."

Prior to leaving for Tashkent, Solzhenitsyn did write a desperate letter to the Omsk Medical Institute asking for any information they had on his tumor. To his surprise, a reply arrived in a few days. It was a letter from a worker in the pathology laboratory. She wrote that she remembered the day his tissue specimen arrived from Ekibastuz. She said the tissue had been sent without a name but since there was only one specimen from Ekibastuz it must have been his. She even remembered the diagnosis which had been sent. . . .

A few days after the letter arrived, Solzhenitsyn received an exit permit for Tashkent but he hesitated before leaving. Going to Tashkent meant the possibility of more surgery, an alternative Solzhenitsyn refused to accept. Although his body was severely weakened by the tumor, the man who had survived the Gulag and had witnessed the victory of human beings over enormous odds considered doing without traditional medical care. After all, he was taking the *issyk kul* root. Perhaps his own determination to live would be enough.

Throughout his years as a prisoner Solzhenitsyn developed a strong belief in the ability of an individual to overcome tremendous odds. He believed in himself more than in the scientific estimates of physicians. Although they were convinced he was going to die Solzhenitsyn was not sure.

In early January, a weakened Solzhenitsyn struggled to the Tashkent Oncological Health Center. On January 4, 1954, he was admitted to Ward 13 for radiation treatment. Lidia Aleksandrovna Dunayeva was chief of the irradiation department. Irina Eyelyanovna Meike was in charge of his treatment. Solzhenitsyn's treatment began immediately, for Dunayeva was convinced that the mass she could feel "deep down beside his stomach" was a "secondary" or metastasis from his malignant lymph node. Before Solzhenitsyn told her of the diagnosis from Omsk, Dr. Dunayeva had already decided the tumor had not started in that node. It had to be a seminoma, she thought. His cancer started in his testicle and has now spread throughout his abdomen.

Seminomas are part of a class of tumors known as germinomas. They get their name from the fact that all members of the class arise from germ cells, the earliest, most primitive parts of our body. During the initial weeks of human development, before the embryo assumes any shape, the germinal cell center forms the beginnings of our nervous and reproductive systems. The rest of our body is built around this early framework.

Although all types of cancer are a form of revolution against normal biology, it seems ironic that the type to affect Solzhenitsyn, a man who argues for a return to older Russian origins, should be a form of germinoma, a primitive cancer recalling his body's own origin.

It is also unusual because seminoma is a rare form of cancer. Each year it accounts for less than one half of one percent of all new cases. When it does occur, it most often strikes men thirty-five to fifty years old. Solzhenitsyn was thirty-three when he first noticed his tumor.

In adult males, seminomas (from the Latin for seed or semen) start growing in the testis. In many cases the original tumor may be small, noticed only by a careful examination. Sometimes, as was the situation with Solzhenitsyn, the first evidence of a seminoma is not a lump in the testicle but an enlarged lymph node in the groin.

Because Solzhenitsyn's tumor had already spread at the time of his first operation, he should have undergone either a second operation to remove his cancer or have immediate X-ray treatment to the testicle along with radiation to the draining lymph nodes.

Dr. John G. Maier is a radiotherapist, a doctor who specializes in destruction of cancer cells by radiation. Today he is chairman of the department of radiation oncology at the Fairfax Hospital in Fairfax, Virginia, but for many years Dr. Maier directed radiation treatment at the Walter Reed General Hospital in Washington, D.C. It was while at Walter Reed that he began studying the treatment of seminomas. Over the past two decades he has analyzed more than 1,000 cases of the rare tumor.

According to Maier, the standard approach used today against seminoma is surgery, removal of the testis along with its spermatic cord. Radiation treatment is then given to all draining lymph nodes. Using this approach, the cure rate, or percentage of persons alive five years after diagnosis, is good, over 95 percent. As in other forms of cancer, the later the cancer is detected, the less chance there is for cure.

Under current practice, physicians place seminoma patients into one of three stages (I, II or III) depending on whether or not the tumor has spread to local lymph nodes or has metastasized throughout the abdomen and chest.

According to the description of Kostoglotov's tumor in *Cancer Ward* (a description Solzhenitsyn assured me mirrors his own), the seminoma cells had spread only to his abdomen. There was no evidence of tumor in his chest. "This meant Solzhenitsyn's tumor was Stage II," Maier explains. "Today we expect approximately half of Stage II patients to be cured. In the early 1950s the percentage was lower, about a third."

Dr. Dunayeva, the chief radiotherapist at Tashkent, began radiation treatment on January 5, 1954, Solzhenitsyn's first full day in Ward 13. A large purple cross was drawn across his stomach. The cross divided his abdomen into four quadrants each of which would, in a rotating schedule, be bombarded with radiation. During his treatments three heavy rubber mats filled with lead wire were placed over the other quadrants to protect them from receiving too much radiation. Sometimes a thin copper shield was also used to protect Solzhenitsyn's skin from the effects of the radiation beam.

"His treatment program sounds very close to what he would have received in this country at that time," Maier says. "In the early fifties only a few large centers in the United States had the capability to give high voltage or cobalt radiotherapy. Most hospitals were still using the 200,000 volt X-ray machines Solzhenitsyn describes in *Cancer Ward*. These older machines were less efficient than our current models. Because their X-ray beam could not be precisely focused, they scattered or wasted a lot of radiation. They gave more exposure to the skin, required longer exposure times, and produced more side effects.

"In his novel, Solzhenitsyn records that he received between 12,-000 and 18,000 ER (rads) during the first course of radiation," Maier continues. "Those are what we call 'air doses' or the amount of radiation emitted directly from the X-ray tube. Today we use the term *rad* to refer only to the amount of radiation actually absorbed by the tumor. This difference is important because a dose of 18,000 rads would have caused serious damage to Solzhenitsyn's stomach and intestines. Intestinal cells can take only 4,000, perhaps 4,500 rads before they die.

"To determine exactly the number of rads Solzhenitsyn's tumor received, I would have to know how efficient the machine used was, its field size, and how thick his abdomen was," Maier explains. "But estimating on the basis of the equipment available at that time and knowing that he was very sick, emaciated, I'd guess that he got from 2,000 to 3,000 rads to his abdomen along with a smaller dose directed at his testis to treat the primary tumor. That dose is just about what we use today for Stage II seminoma patients."

Solzhenitsyn remained in the Tashkent Oncological Center from January 4, 1954, until the middle of February. During this month and a half he had about fifty X-ray treatments, each lasting thirty minutes. They had a remarkable effect.

Within two weeks of entering the hospital, Solzhenitsyn's pain decreased and he gained his first small but important victory. His arms, previously too weak to hold a book, now permitted him hours of uninterrupted reading. He still could not lie flat because his tumor mass pressed up against his diaphragm, making it difficult for him to breathe.

"Not unusual," Maier says. "If radiation is going to work in seminoma the response is usually quite rapid. But it takes longer for the tumor mass to shrink."

Along with radiation, Solzhenitsyn swallowed tablets of sinestrol, a form of estrogen, the major female hormone. Since seminoma is a male tumor, the Soviet doctors at that time thought that large doses of a female hormone might help prevent its growth. Later, when evidence demonstrated it did not help, use of sinestrol was discontinued.

"We never used estrogens for seminoma in the United States," Maier comments. "To my knowledge there was never any evidence that the tumor was hormone-related, so I really can't explain the use of the drug. Perhaps they knew something we didn't."[1]

Between his other hospitalizations in 1974, staggered to permit his body time to recover from the side effects of the X-rays, Solzhenitsyn returned to Kok-Terek for a fresh supply of *issyk kul*. The mandrake root, from which *issyk kul* is prepared, is a well-known Russian folk remedy. Used mainly in the form of home-brewed tea, it contains

---

[1] In *Cancer Ward*, Solzhenitsyn mentions other unconventional treatment given hospital patients, such as milk injections. It should be remembered that, in the early fifties, physicians in many countries were just beginning to discover how cancer cells behaved and what compounds might stop their growth.

the chemical scopolamine, which is used in some commercial sleeping preparations. Besides making a person sleepy, scopolamine can also cause a dry mouth. It cannot cure cancer.

"Solzhenitsyn is a fortunate man," Maier concludes. "His radiation treatment was delayed and any number of things could have gone wrong. He could have developed peritonitis, intestinal perforation, or his tumor could have spread so widely that radiation wouldn't have been effective. And then there was the type of cancer. In 1954 there were only two types of cancer that could be cured by radiation. One was a particular form of lymphoma, the other seminoma. Both are quite rare."

Solzhenitsyn's medical history is also an example of how the Soviet medical system, inefficient and frequently primitive, manages to get by. Although the 1950 American approach to metastatic seminoma would have involved more precise measurement and delivery of radiation, more attention to diagnostic tests prior to treatment, and more follow-up exams after treatment, the final results could not have been better.

In *Cancer Ward*, Dr. Dontsova, who represents Dr. Dunayeva, Solzhenitsyn's radiotherapist, tells Kostoglotov (Solzhenitsyn) that his case is special because of the exceptionally rapid revival initiated by the X rays. "Twelve sessions have turned you from a corpse into a living human being!" she exclaims. She points out the case of Azovkin, a young patient with a seminoma who today would be classified as Stage III. The tumor nodules in Azovkin's lungs, unlike Kostoglotov's abdominal masses, were not responding to radiation.

But Kostoglotov is not so sure of the reason for his improvement. In the novel he tells his fellow patients about a medical book he is reading. "It says here that the link between the development of tumors and the central nervous system has been very little studied. . . . It happens rarely, but there are cases of self-induced healing. Not recovery through treatment, but actual healing."

Throughout *Cancer Ward*, Kostoglotov has a running argument with Dr. Dontsova over his treatment, much as Solzhenitsyn must have argued with the actual Dunayeva. He wants to stop the treatment before Dontsova is ready.

"As far as I'm concerned, " Kostoglotov says, "it's enough that you've driven back the tumor and stopped it. It's on the defensive. I'm on the defensive, too. Fine. A soldier has a much better life in defense. And whatever happens you'll never be able to cure me completely. There's no such thing as a complete cure in cancer."

But Dontsova, who is writing the dissertation for her candidate of science degree on seminoma, prevails on her patient to finish the prescribed course of radiation treatments, take the injections of sinestrol, and even accept a dreaded blood transfusion. Through it all, however, Kostoglotov continues secretly to take extracts of the mandrake root and to believe in the importance of "the natural defenses of [his] organism." He knows that doctors do not have absolute knowledge about the bodies they treat and he wants to maintain control of his own destiny. He also knows that mental attitudes frequently determine physical conditions.

In Solzhenitsyn's writing there are frequent references to the inseparable relationship of mind and body. In his 1978 Harvard University Commencement speech he reiterated the theme that hardship was essential to well being and that, without a strong purpose, all living things become susceptible to disease and destruction.

In Solzhenitsyn's view, his own case history is a striking example of this interdependence. In December 1953 he was dying of cancer. He then began writing feverishly, trying to record as much as possible before it became too late. By February the cancer was receding and suddenly there was the possibility of more time. Of course there was also the radiation therapy and sinestrol treatments. There was even the *issyk kul*. But above all there was his dedication to writing. That, Solzhenitsyn maintains, is the reason he is alive today.

In his literary autobiography *The Oak and the Calf*, Solzhenitsyn refers to his victory over cancer as a "divine miracle; I could see no other explanation. Since then all the life that has been given back to me has not been mine in the full sense: it is built around a purpose."

Solzhenitsyn's victory over cancer also provides him with an analogy he frequently uses in his writing. "Russia is to the Soviet Union as a man is to the disease afflicting him," he once wrote. At the same time he was conquering his tumor Solzhenitsyn believes his country was ridding itself of its malignant dictator, Stalin. Since then, however, Russia and its people have not been dedicated enough in their fight against the "disease of Communism" which Solzhenitsyn believes will spread cancer-like "to destroy mankind, or else mankind will have to rid itself of Communism (and even then face lengthy treatment for secondary tumors)."

Solzhenitsyn has not been to a doctor since leaving the Soviet Union in 1974. Having personally overcome cancer there seems little reason for the examinations or other preventive medical services typically given to a man Solzhenitsyn's age.

In the writing center he has established in the Vermont countryside Solzhenitsyn, surrounded by friends, family, and the latest in word processing devices, considers himself self-sufficient. It is the perfect spot from which to wage his campaign against Soviet Communism and to, as he told *New York Times* art critic Hilton Kramer in a 1980 interview, "race against time."

To those critics who view Solzhenitsyn's dream of returning Russia to its former glory as a futile, unrealistic dream Solzhenitsyn scoffs.

To a man who has conquered cancer, anything is possible.

15

Free of Charge—Medicine and Money in the USSR

There is a belief [in the United States] that all the vast regions of our planet should develop and mature to the level of contemporary Western systems . . . but in fact such a conception is a fruit of Western incomprehension of the essence of other worlds, a result of mistakenly measuring them all with a Western yardstick. . . .

Every ancient and deeply rooted self-contained culture, especially if it is spread over a wide part of the earth's surface, constitutes a self-contained world, full of riddles and surprises to Western thinking. —ALEKSANDR SOLZHENITSYN IN HIS 1978 HARVARD COMMENCEMENT ADDRESS.

An American tourist hospitalized recently in Leningrad attempted, upon his discharge, to pay for his treatment. No office in the hospital would accept his money. He was told that all hospital care is *besplatno* (free of charge) in the Soviet Union.

A news program on an Odessa radio station begins, "Today in America only the rich can afford to get sick. The total cost for an appendectomy is now over $2,000—almost 1,300 rubles—and according to our American correspondent, the average worker in the United States can be financially ruined by a simple illness like appendicitis. Furthermore," the radio announcer continues, "American ambulances now refuse to pick up sick persons from the streets unless they can prove they have money or credit cards. Many workers are turned away from hospitals because they cannot pay. How much better," the announcer concludes, "the USSR system is where every worker, regardless of salary, is guaranteed high-quality medical care, where all medical treatment is *besplatno*."

"If you're a doctor in America then you must be very wealthy," a Soviet friend once told me. "American doctors are always overcharging their patients for their services. In this country it's different. The government hires the doctors, the *vrachi* have to worry only about practicing medicine, not being businessmen. I think it's better when a doctor's care is *besplatno.*"

The Soviet patient, like his counterpart in Britain or Sweden, where government-sponsored medical systems also exist, does not have to pay directly for most of his medical care. The Soviet Union, however, is the only nation to declare its medical system *besplatno*, free to all its citizens.

The noted Stanford University economist Victor Fuchs, however, in his book on health economics, *Who Shall Live,* emphasizes that no matter what financial system a country uses, it is the public who must finally pay for medical care. According to Fuchs, "There is no magic wand of finance that can divert labor, capital, and other resources to medical care without resulting in a reduction in resources . . . for other goods and services. Nor is there any secret formula that can transfer the cost of health care to 'government' or 'business' without the burden eventually being borne by the public through more taxes, higher prices, or lower wages."

In the United States, with our fee-for-service system paid for by a mixture of public and private funds, the rising cost of medical care over the last two decades is a major national problem. From 1960 to 1979 the total amount spent on all medical care in the United States increased almost ten times. Today a tenth of all the goods and services the United States produces goes directly to provide some form of medical service.

The factors behind this enormous price rise are inflation, new high-technology medical services, and government action. In the mid-1960s the U.S. Congress passed two landmark bills, Medicare and Medicaid, aimed at improving the availability of medical services. The bills provided, respectively, government-financed health insurance to the aged and the poor. As a result, the majority of the U.S. population now has some form of health insurance and the demand for medical care services is at an all-time high.

No such increase in demand, services, or cost has occurred in the Soviet Union. The USSR, like most Eastern European countries, has a "command economy." The central government and the government alone determines what services will be provided and at what price. Because the government assumes responsibility for most medical costs, Soviet spokesmen emphasize that a typical patient is better off in the USSR than the United States. Only 4 percent of the average Soviet citizen's medical expenses are paid for out of his monthly paycheck. In the United States, out-of-pocket expenditures are larger, about 25 percent of total medical costs. Another important distinction, frequently made by Soviet analysts, is that a citizen of the USSR cannot suffer a financial loss because of a prolonged illness. All hospital care is provided by the government. While a person is hospitalized his salary continues and his job is held open. But does this mean medical care is really free?

"Konechno nyet [of course not]" a young engineer in Kishinev told me. "The government wants us to think that all medicine is free, but it's not true. We may not pay for it directly, but it isn't free. We pay for it by taxes. No one officially talks about taxes, but we pay them. Look at me," he goes on. "I'm an engineer. I graduated from the institute four years ago. I make 210 rubles a month, how much is that in dollars, $300, $200? Now how much would I make if I lived in America—$2,000, $3,000 a month. There, that difference, that's what I'm paying for my 'free' medical care."

Not all Soviet citizens know or acknowledge this distinction as readily as my friend in Kishinev. Relying, as most of them must, on information from official government newspapers and radio stations, they hear only of the United States' continuing inability to control medical costs. The charges for individual services, such as an appendectomy, and the fees paid to U.S. physicians appear astronomical to the Soviet worker living on a few hundred rubles a month. The use of medical insurance is unknown to the Soviet citizen and the concept difficult to explain. One can hardly expect the Soviets to understand our complicated, overlapping, and frequently redundant methods of paying for medical care when few Americans fully grasp the system.

Similarly, when comparing the U.S. and USSR systems of financing medical care it is important not to simply compare the total budgets. As my friend emphasized, there are so many parts of the Soviet economy that are hidden from direct analysis and accounting; so much that is not written down.

In 1979, for example, the cost of all government-sponsored medical care in the USSR totaled about 18 billion rubles. This amounts to 68 rubles or $105 for every man, woman, and child. In the United States, 1979 expenditures totaled $212 billion, or $956 per person.

But while the Soviet total takes into account rubles spent for non-medical services such as physical culture and some sports medicine, it excludes the rubles Soviet citizens must pay for elective abortions, sanatorium treatment, and for most prescription drugs. (Only vitamins for expectant mothers and infants and drugs for chronic diseases like tuberculosis, schizophrenia, and epilepsy are prescribed free of charge.)

In the United States, drugs and related supplies make up approximately 8 percent of our national medical bill. In the Soviet Union, many prescription and over-the-counter medications are also expensive and are increasing in cost. A two-week's supply of antibiotics now costs ten rubles; pills for high blood pressure, as much as 150 rubles a year. Michael Kaser, in his analysis of the USSR's finances, estimates that Soviet citizens spent about 600 million rubles on drugs in 1975, an amount double that spent in 1968.[1]

Other items that do not get counted into the official Soviet total are the rubles exchanged through the elaborate gray and black markets. Within the gray market are included payments to hospital aides, the five- or ten-ruble note given under the table (*na levo*) to the *neotlozhnaya* physician visiting a patient at home, or the money required to attend one of the *platnye polikliniki* (paying polyclinics) which operate in major Soviet towns. Additional payments are common in most areas of the Soviet economy. They are an essential step in getting meat reserved at the *gastronom* (food store) or stopping a cab after midnight.

The story about a resident of Odessa, published in a national Soviet newspaper, *Izvestia,* describes how the medical gray market functions. The man, referred to as Citizen K by the newspaper, developed acute appendicitis. Before being taken to the hospital he filled his pockets with one-ruble notes. With these, he bargained with the hospital attendants to give him prompt service and to carry him to the operating room. After his surgery, everything went well—until his money ran out. Then most of his care—injections,

---

[1] Kaser's estimate increases total Soviet medical care costs by about 3 percent. Michael C. Kaser, *Health Care in the Soviet Union and Eastern Europe* (London: Groom Helm, 1976), 64. A 1981 Joint Economic Committee publication, "Consumption in the USSR: An International Comparison," estimated expenditures for drugs in 1976 at 978 million rubles.

thermometers, and even bedpans—arrived late or not at all. It was only after his wife brought more money that his care improved.

Less extensive but also increasing the national bill for medical care is the private or black-market practice. All private medical practice in the Soviet Union is secret. The heavy taxation (up to 90 percent) and other harsh administrative penalties imposed on private physicians make it impossible to practice openly.

The black-market charges for medical care vary, depending on the type of illness and the status of the physician. Private treatment for venereal disease is one of the most expensive, up to 500 rubles.[2] A visit after hours to the office-home of a high-ranking professor averages 150 rubles.

Most charges are much less. The standard rate in 1979 for an abortion performed secretly at a physician's home was 50 rubles. For an X ray taken after hours to avoid the long wait in the clinic, 40 rubles.

A woman living in Odessa told me why she preferred going to a neighboring vrach's apartment for a 40 ruble abortion, rather than the local free polyclinic: "There are no forms to fill in. There are no babushki [older women] standing around wagging their finger at you, criticizing you for not having more children. Furthermore," she explained, "at her home, the doctor takes more time with the novocaine. It's less painful."

"But what if something happened," I asked. "Suppose you started bleeding?"

"Then I would go to the hospital," she shrugged, "There would be no problem, many people have abortions na levo [on the side]."

There is also widespread use of the black-market system in dentistry. Traditional Soviet dentistry is crude and universally feared by all Soviet citizens. Pain-killers are seldom used and teeth are frequently pulled out rather than repaired. A private dentist can get 150 rubles for extensive repairing and filling done with local anesthestics. If the customer wants gold fillings, he must supply his own gold, bringing in old jewelry or other items to be melted down.

---

[2] In 1979 the Soviet government established fines equivalent to $75 for persons concealing venereal infections and made examinations and treatment in a polyclinic compulsory.

How common the system of personal private medical care is and how much it subsidizes the official government contribution is unknown. In large cities, such as Moscow and Leningrad, and in the Republic of Georgia, where all forms of the black market flourish, the system appears active and growing. In rural areas, where there are few physicians available in the first place, private payment for medical services appears less important.

Along with the black market, a Soviet citizen living in a large city can, if he wants medical care outside the regular system, visit one of the legally established fee-for-service polyclinics. An article in *Literaturnaya gazeta* described the people who visited the *platnaya poliklinika* (paying polyclinic) at 15 Kirov Street in Moscow. It is one of an estimated 130 such clinics in the USSR administered by the Board of Non-Financed Medical Establishments. At the Kirov Street clinic, unlike the situation at the standard free polyclinics, patients can choose their own physician and, by making a payment direct to the polyclinic, avoid a long wait.

According to the article, of 1,616 persons who visited the clinic in one day, 410 said they liked the paying clinic because they were treated by older and more experienced doctors; 230 had come because the polyclinics near their homes did not have the required specialists; 443 said that they not only received medical attention at the clinic, but were treated as human beings as well. Since the publication of this article in October 1965, however, the Moscow City Health Department has cut back the services offered by the paying clinics. It has also reduced the space provided for examining patients.

Vera Karbobskaya, the author of the *Literaturnaya gazeta* article, is upset about these changes. She wrote, "If thousands of people ask for the right to paid medical care, over and above free state medical care, it should be done."

Given the record of the Soviet government, however, such radical change is unlikely. Providing "free" medical care for all its citizens is viewed as a cornerstone of Soviet domestic policy. Admitting there is an unfulfilled demand for a different type of medical care by allowing the number of paying polyclinics to increase would be embarrassing. It would challenge the government claim of medical superiority.

As in other areas of the Soviet economy, there is no direct admission of problems with medical care. Officially, the health protection system of the USSR is well and growing. There are over 1 million doctors and 3 million hospital beds, a polyclinic in every neighborhood and at most factories. But, as evidenced by citizen complaints to a special Ministry of Health office, articles in Soviet newspapers and magazines, carefully worded statements by medical officials, and most importantly by the recent deterioration in life expectancy and infant mortality, there are problems. It appears that the resources devoted to medical care have been inadequate not only to fulfill consumer demands but also to meet basic needs.

Soviet hospitals and polyclinics are a good example. Despite numerous articles describing new building projects and a 1978 allotment of 5 percent of the total health budget to capital investment or improvement, many Soviet hospitals and polyclinics are housed in prerevolutionary Russian buildings. Their elaborate nineteenth-century spires and graceful arches contrast with the stark simplicity of the medical care given within. Even the new buildings appear poorly finished and old before their time.

One of the recurrent themes in the Soviet medical literature is criticism of the inadequate funding given hospital construction. Professor Burenkov, writing in 1976 in *Sovetskaya Meditsina,* said: "In Chita . . . a 1,000-bed hospital with a total cost of 12 million rubles was begun in 1974. But by the end of 1975, two years later, only 1.3 million rubles had been allocated. With such financing, a delay in hospital construction is inevitable . . . and further increases in the volume and quality of medical aid for the public are impeded. . . ."

The consequences of this relatively low priority for medical care are evident in all aspects of daily medical care. Soviet hospitals are continually running out of basic supplies such as antibiotics, sutures, and even rubber gloves. A surgeon who worked in a small town near Khabarovsk, on the Sea of Japan, complained to me that "for three months I operated with my bare hands. There was some sort of delay in getting the gloves manufactured. Furthermore," the doctor went on, eager to tell someone about his frustration, "we once ran out of vascular sutures [the kind used to sew blood vessels together]. One night a young boy came in after he'd fallen off a tractor. His popliteal artery [one of the main vessels supplying blood to the leg below the knee] was ripped open. If I'd had some vascular suture I'd been able to save his leg. As it was," he concluded, slamming his fist on the table, "I had to cut off his leg! Nine years old and with only one leg."

Some possible reasons for the shortages, according to Dr. A. Melnichenko, Minister of Medical Industries of the USSR, writing in 1977 in *Trud,* the worker's newspaper, are that "the medical industry is not provided with some types of intermediate goods produced by other industries, [and] the procurement organizations also do not make full use of the possibilities for obtaining raw materials. In the future, we hope for more understanding and financial support in the production of medicines and articles of medical technology for public health needs," Melnichenko said.

Another example of the relatively low standing accorded medicine versus other parts of the Soviet economy is the salary provided doctors. One of the most striking differences between the Soviet and American approach and attitude toward medical care is what each country pays its doctors. In a country with a government-controlled economy, most economists agree, the price paid for professional services, compared to other occupations, is a sensitive reflection of its priorities.

In the United States, the average doctor in 1980 earned $76,000, an income higher than that of 99 percent of the population. Moreover, the difference between the amount paid an American physician and the person he treats has been growing. Forty years ago, doctors made roughly three times more than the average wage earner; today, it is four times more.

Not so in the Soviet Union. There, physicians' salaries in the 1930s (when the government first estalished salary scales) were below those of skilled workers. Furthermore, from 1930 through 1970, the ratio of the salary paid physicians compared to the average wage paid all other workers actually declined, meaning that, proportionately, doctors were paid less in 1970 than in 1930. Since 1964, when the first large pay raise was announced, the Ministry of Health has tried to keep the physicians' pay level with that of other workers. Another pay raise was issued in 1972 and, according to a ministry spokesman, during 1977 and 1978 salaries were increased an additional 30 percent.[3]

[3] This low earning scale for physicians in the USSR compared to that of the United States is one factor making a comparison of exact budgets between countries extremely difficult. Referred to as the index number problem, it recognizes that countries like the

Many ministry officials I spoke to echoed the words of Professor Nikolai Gavrilov of the Semashko Institute, who in 1979 told me that "physician's salaries should be increased. But we have a budget, only so much money. Soon, however, they will go up."

Today the average Soviet physician makes about 180 rubles a month, the average skilled industrial worker 200. As in the rest of the Soviet economy, part of the reason for the low wage is the high percentage of female workers in medicine. Slightly over 70 percent of Soviet doctors and 85 percent of middle medical workers (*feldshers* and nurses) are women. In the past this policy did not attract the most qualified students to medical school. The low monthly wages provide little incentive for efficient and conscientious work.

Officially, the Soviets vigorously deny this criticism. In a recent book describing the organization of their medical system, *Soviet Public Health and the Organization of Primary Health Care for the Population of the USSR,* there is a strong defense of free-of-charge medical treatment combined with an attack on the U.S.'s fee-for-service arrangement:

> The moral and ethical consequences of free and accessible medical care are very great. The advocates of "commercial medicine" are still trying to hammer the notion in that free-of-charge medical treatment depreciates the quality of medical care, since the physician allegedly "loses material interest" in working with a patient. That it deprives the patient of a "free choice of a doctor." Such assertions are groundless. In the first place, the quality of medical care depends to a greater degree on the skill of the physician, rather than his material interest. In the second place, the doctor's material interest in a system of free medical care is not lost, because he is paid in money and rewarded morally for his work, by the state. The possibility of profiteering is eliminated, the arbitrary setting of a price on medical services and a marketable basis for medical practice are prevented. . . . In the USSR the interests of the state and the physician in protecting the health of the people fully coincide. Relations between physician and patient are free of material interest, there are no antagonistic contradictions dividing them, and their relations are based on mutual trust and respect.[4]

Soviet Union tend to use more of those resources that are relatively cheap—in this case physician services—rather than those that are expensive, like drugs and medical technology.

[4] I. P. Lidov, A. M. Stochik, G. F. Tserkovny, *Soviet Public Health and the Organization of Primary Health Care for the Population of the USSR.* (Moscow: MIR Publishers 1978). P. 38.

The typical female *vrach* in the Soviet Union is naturally close to her patients; for the most part they are facing the same struggles. But given the responsibilities of caring for her own family and knowing that no matter how hard she works, there will always be more to do, she has often adopted a nine-to-five attitude. As a result the typical *vrach* is viewed by Soviet society on a professional level equivalent to that of an elementary school teacher: kindly, well-meaning, simply trained.

Few wish to work in rural areas where doctors are in short supply. Some marry men who live in cities to avoid assignment to a rural area. Others, such as a young *vrach* I met in Irkutsk, use political connections (her father was secretary of the district Communist Committee) to get back into specialty training so they can cut short their rural service and move to a larger city where consumer goods and cultural events are readily available and life itself is fuller. As a result, there are twice as many physicians in Soviet cities per population as in the countryside. In many isolated areas there is, and probably always will be, the need to depend on physician assistants or *feldshers.*

Within the last decade the makeup of Soviet medical schools has changed. Entering classes now contain more men than women. Since Soviet society is overwhelmingly male-dominated, the increased number of males becoming doctors will probably change the nature of medical practice in the USSR as well as affecting the doctor-patient relationship.

Most male physicians are unwilling to accept the traditionally low wages and professional positions occupied by female *vrachi.* Recent Soviet medical graduates are, with the government's encouragement, going on to become specialists. They are more and more frequently looking at their jobs as careers and, through programs such as the U.S.–USSR Health Exchange, are acquiring some Western medical knowledge and skills. This change will eventually increase the professional status of the physician in the Soviet Union. Already there is evidence of this trend with more interest in professional development, a code of behavior for physicians, and emphasis on the study of deontology, or medical ethics.

This increased number of specialists is an outgrowth of the Soviet Union's exposure to Western medicine and their acceptance of the philosophy that modern medicine is too complicated for any one person to master. And to most medical leaders I spoke with, the trend toward specialization was viewed as positive, an indication that the USSR was "keeping up" with the West.

But within a few academic circles, I found the beginnings of concern, the belief that perhaps increased specialization was not the way for the country to go.

"We have so many specialists already," G. A. Popov, the prominent Moscow health economist and former physician, told me, "that no one is taking charge of the entire patient. We are duplicating services and many persons are just being shuttled from one specialist to another. Why, we found one woman in Moscow who had been to see twenty different doctors a total of seventy-three separate times in one year. She must have spent most of her time in polyclinics!

"All of these many contacts with medical care, even for the typical Moscow citizen, who averages eighteen visits per year," Popov says, "make our system very inefficient and unnecessarily expensive."

Among Ministry of Health officials, however, those who set policy and establish future priorities, there are few persons who share Dr. Popov's concern. Most high-ranking ministry officials are physicians, trained as specialists themselves and believing there is no better way to practice medicine. The problem other countries are now experiencing with an oversupply of medical specialists and a shortage of family physicians do not concern them.

"The women," one of them told me. "There are certain jobs women are better suited for and there will always be plenty of women *vrachi* to watch over the patient, to comfort him."

The masculinization of Soviet medicine may also influence research and funding priorities. If exposure to Western medical practices continues, future Soviet graduates will seek improved working conditions with modern technology. Although some changes may take place, however, it is unlikely that even a large increase in the number of male doctors will make much of a difference in the overall financing or delivery of Soviet medical care. Despite problems with supplies, hospital construction, and drugs, the Soviet government has made clear its medical care priorities.

At the top of the list, according to Professor Michael Ryan, Uni-

versity College of Swansea in England, is the protection of workers.[5]
The extensive system of factory medical units where people can go
for medical attention without leaving work; the separate system of
hospitals, polyclinics, and first aid stations reserved and designed exclusively for railway workers and other essential industries; the large
number of sanatoriums; the elaborate system of sick leave certifica-
tion to ensure that absences are limited; all point toward one conclusion: In the USSR the worker is the most important person. And
the physician is important because he protects the health of the
worker.

Professor Vincente Navarro of Johns Hopkins University agrees
that the financing and structure of the health system in the USSR
represents the Communist Party's commitment to developing a
strong, worker-based economy. While the Soviets, according to Navarro, did not change the nature of scientific medicine, they did
subvert it to their own goals, emphasizing the workers' health while
putting less effort and money into research and high-technology hospital care.[6]

Fortunately, young workers are, on average, the least expensive
portion of the population to keep healthy. In the United States we
spend only $286 each year on medical care for each person under
age nineteen and $764 for a person between the ages of nineteen and
sixty-four, compared to $2,026 for each person over sixty-five.[7]

These tight financial reins on medical technology and medical
care for the elderly have permitted the fragile Soviet economy to
spend rubles for other purposes. Many are spent for defense; others
to strengthen a weak industrial base or to open new oil fields. And,
with the arms escalation race as evidence, when the Soviets decide to
compete, they can. Although no information has ever been provided
on the financing of Soviet military medicine, intelligence analysis in

[5] Michael Ryan, *The Organization of Soviet Medical Care* (London: Martin Robertson,
    1978), p. 125.
[6] Vincente Navarro, *Social Security and Medicine in the USSR: A Marxist Critique* (Lexington,
    Mass.: Lexington Books, 1977), p. 71.
[7] The fact that the United States has made the commitment to provide full services to
the elderly is a major reason our medical costs have increased. In just two years, 1976
to 1978, Medicare's total costs went from $16 to $22 billion. Much of that increase (70
percent) went for hospital treatment where open-heart surgery, kidney dialysis, and
other high-cost technologies were provided, services unavailable to most Soviet patients.

this country supports Soviet public opinion that the medical needs of the army receive top priority for supplies and support.

"Of course if I worked for the army," a young Leningrad surgeon told me, "I wouldn't have any trouble getting the instruments I need. There would be no problem with my requisition—the army always gets what it needs." In Moscow, for example, seriously burned patients are often taken to a special military hospital on the outskirts of town. It is the only hospital in the city of eight million people equipped to handle the complex fluid, infection, and chemical problems a critically burned patient presents.

While living in Kishinev I became friends with a doctor who had decided on a military career. A soft-spoken, fleshy man in his mid-forties, he was eager, despite the risk, to make friends with an American physician. Each Thursday during the two months I lived in the Moldavian capital we met for dinner at a small isolated restaurant, a complicated two-bus and one-taxi ride out of town. On most nights Vladimir wore his uniform, a light gray wool with two royal purple epaulets decorated with a gold wine goblet and encircling snake, the symbol of medicine in the USSR. An army *terapevt* (internist), he had once spent three years of duty in the northeastern corner of Siberia. "On clear days we could see Alaska," he told me.

Vladimir confirmed that medical supplies were easier to get for the army. "My wife works with tuberculosis patients at the medical institute," he said. "Sometimes when she needs a particular medicine I'll bring some home from our pharmacy. We get first priority on all our orders." But the medical problems Vladimir said he faced most frequently with the *chast* (regiment) to which he was attached seldom needed sophisticated drugs.

"Skin problems," Vladimir complained, "I see at least six cases a day. Mostly the rashes occur when the soldiers don't wash frequently enough. It isn't enough to simply give toilet soap to a *podrazdelenie* [small troop unit]. Many of our recruits are from rural areas and have never lived so close to other men. You've got to make sure they bathe at least once a week and that they change their underwear. Cleanliness, that is my main medical problem."

Besides providing the military with enough medicine, the Soviets can, when the fancy strikes them, support a medical research institute in a style almost equal to the West. The current drive for the USSR to produce the world's first artificially powered heart is an example of the desire for *pokazukha* (show-off) appeal. But an artificial heart, although dramatic, will not solve some of the fundamental challenges still facing Soviet medicine.

When the revolutionary government took over medical responsibilities following the 1917 coup d-'état, the Russian nation was, medically speaking, in severe trouble. Epidemics were widespread and basic sanitary measures, much less medical care, were unknown in most of the country. During its first sixty years the Soviet government emphasized fundamental public health principles. They vaccinated the population, especially the children. They cleaned the water supplies. They isolated the persons with infections. They distributed more food.

The challenge was enormous. Pockets of disease were scattered throughout most of the new nation's 8.5 million square miles. Epidemics destroyed entire villages before the local health officials even heard of the problem. Starvation remained a major cause of death well into the 1930s.

Today the typical Soviet citizen no longer dies of typhus, malaria, or cholera but of the modern killers, heart disease and cancer. Changing the leading causes of death was a major, indisputable accomplishment of Soviet medicine. Starting with virtually nothing, they built a system oriented toward prevention that would attack the origins of disease. To a remarkable extent the effort was successful. But because of the size of the challenge, the enormous distances involved, and the differences in culture among the 100 nationalities living in the USSR, the victory is a fragile one.

As my friend the army captain pointed out, poor hygiene still poses significant health problems to the Soviet army. More disturbing than skin rashes among military troops, however, is the USSR's recent but continuing increase in infant mortality.

Like medical care for its workers, the protection of women and children is an area of high priority. The Soviet Union needs workers. The extensive system of state-supported nurseries, the financial incentives for having four or more children, and the emphasis given prenatal care are all aimed at encouraging more children and protecting their health.

But since 1971 more and more of these infants have died before reaching their first birthday. Although influenced by many factors, a country's infant mortality rate provides an excellent measurement of how well it is meeting medical and social needs. A national increase from 22.9 deaths per 1,000 births to 31.1, and perhaps even higher, is a cause of major concern.

Whether, as some Ministry of Health officials suggest, the rise is explained by a greater than anticipated increase in Central Asian births, improved record keeping, the demands of 16 million abortions, or the uncontrolled spread of influenza through nurseries, the conclusion remains that the challenge has not been met. The persistence of rickets as a major health problem in many parts of the Soviet Union is, by itself, a strong signal that the system is still overwhelmed by the immensity of space in the USSR.

The same conclusion comes from an examination of the recent increase in Soviet death rates and the decrease in life expectancy. Most marked among males thirty to fifty-five years old, the deterioration is presumed to be related to the ever-increasing use of vodka, cigarettes, and other "bad habits," as the Soviets call them.

This may or may not be the right answer. There are other possibilities. As in the United States, heart disease is the number-one killer in the USSR. It claims the majority of its victims in their third through fifth decades. And unlike the United States, where the death rate from heart disease is falling rapidly, there has not been a substantial decrease in Soviet figures. In fact, the life expectancy for Soviet males has actually fallen over the last decade, from sixty-five to sixty-three years. If the trend continues it could, by the end of the century, produce a severe and crippling manpower shortage in the USSR. To a Western observer, the official Soviet response to these challenges is low-keyed and somewhat confused.

All medical care in the USSR is carefully programmed, with everything decided in Five Year Plans. The plan for health originates in the Ministry of Health, one of fifteen union-republic ministries in the Soviet Union that set national goals, budgets, and supervise the work of the various republics of the USSR, in consultation with Gosplan, the Soviet Ministry of Finance. Through the years there have been changes in the role of these Moscow ministries. Under Stalin there was tight centralized control with all marching orders coming from Moscow. Khrushchev relaxed the controls, allowing greater regional variation with republic governments permitted important decisions. Then Brezhnev tightened the reins again. Today there is a strong element of central government, meaning Communist Party, control over the plan and all budgets.

After the health plan and budget are initially written at the Ministry of Health, they are submitted for approval to the Health and Social Welfare Committee of the Central Communist Party. The party, acting through its legislative body, the Supreme Soviet (roughly similar, except for free elections, to our Senate), sends the health plan budget to a special preparatory committee made up of fifteen members of the Supreme Soviet and fifteen specialists from the Ministry of Health. For two months, beginning in early November, the preparatory committee meets and discusses how best to distribute the money allocated for medical care. Much of the budget is already designated for ongoing projects and for support of the thousands of hospitals and polyclinics. The rest is carefully structured around quotas and standards. There is little flexibility. The plan specifies everything: How many new thousand-bed hospitals should be built. How many patients a polyclinic *vrach* must see in her five-and-a-half hour working day. How many sutures it should take to close a laceration.

"The plan, the plan," a hospital administrator in Ufa lamented. "With the plan everything is possible and because of the plan nothing is possible."

The plan, and the many reports it requires, not only takes up a great deal of the administrators' and physicians' time (a survey of physician workload in a Moscow polyclinic concluded that the typical doctor spends as much time filling out forms as she does seeing patients), it also reduces flexibility. The need, whether for more beds or for an expanded clinic capacity, must get over an incredible series of bureaucratic hurdles before the changes can be made. Even when the changes are approved, there is likely to be no money for implementation until the next Five Year Plan begins.

The deterioration in infant mortality and life expectancy has somewhat upset this bureaucatic ritual. There have been attempts to divert more resources to the Central Asian republics where birth and infant mortality rates run high, but it has been a piecemeal approach since the origins of the problem remain undiagnosed.

One of the hallmarks of Soviet health planners is their preoccupation with numbers and complex formulas. I recall listening to a long presentation by a high-ranking ministry official on the best way to estimate the total number of hospital beds needed in a particular region. Like most Soviet bureaucrats, indeed like most Soviet doctors that I had met, he was a warm, intelligent, extremely attractive person. It was with great pride that he explained how his analysis took into account the many factors that influenced hospital use. The formula was logical and well presented. Coupled with a system to ensure that the beds were properly utilized and adequately supported by other hospital services, his work would have provided a firm base.

The problem is that the Soviets do not yet have the ability to go beyond the numbers, or "normative values" as they are called, to uncover the defects in their system. Shortly after Leonid Brezhnev replaced Nikita Khrushchev as premier in 1964, the Ministry of Health discovered large reservoirs of untreated disease. There was more tuberculosis, diphtheria, and polio than expected, along with persistent oubreaks of cholera. The morbidity and mortality from heart disease and cancer seemed overwhelming.

The response from Brezhnev and his right-hand man for domestic policy, Alexsei Kosygin, was a large increase in the number of physicians and middle medical workers. It was assumed that, regardless of the origins of the problem, more doctors would solve it. And to a certain extent it helped. Unfortunately, today, sixteen years later, the same "more is better" philosophy still exists.

For example, the current Five Year Plan for health calls for a 10 percent increase in the number of hospital beds, to bring the national total to about 3.2 million beds. Yet there is extensive evidence of poor utilization of existing beds. According to Soviet standards, the typical hospital bed in a large Soviet city should not be empty more than thirty days a year; beds in rural areas, no more than fifty-five days. These are standards which the Soviet government expects the country to meet. When they are not met, just as happens in the United States, the empty beds increase cost, adding about two-thirds of what the same bed would cost if it were occupied. Most of the Soviet problems with underused beds are in rural areas.

Soviet citizens, especially those in Soviet Georgia and Armenia, do not want to be hospitalized in rural hospitals even though they may be close to their homes. They think the physicians and services provided in rural hospitals are inferior to those available in the larger cities. Because of this problem, some of these small rural hospitals are empty 180 days or half the year while hospitals in cities like Yerevan and Tbilisi remain overcrowded. Christopher Davis, of the University of Birmingham, has found that from 1958 to 1973 the number of days Soviet hospital beds were not utilized in a year rose from sixty-three to sixty-seven in the countryside.

Moreover, the Soviet people today are among the most hospitalized in the world. According to recent surveys, 60 million persons, or one out of every four Soviet citizens, are hospitalized every year. Dr. Victor Golovteev, head of health-care planning and finance of the Ministry of Health, acknowledged on a recent visit to the United States that many of the hospitalizations are unnecessary.

"One problem," he explained, "is that many patients are not properly examined before being sent to the hospital. The polyclinic doctor decides the illness is not interesting or that he doesn't understand the problem. He sends the patient to the hospital, knowing that his colleague will find out what's wrong. This," Golovteev concluded, "falsely increases the demand for hospital beds."

Nevertheless, having set a goal of 3.2 million hospital beds, the bureaucracy behind the Five Year Plan is too large to stop suddenly and revise goals. Other problems such as a decreased life expectancy, although recognized by Soviet medical leaders, also seems to require more flexibility than the system seems capable of providing. Initial attempts at population research such as health planning studies are incomplete and do not provide clear guidance.

Dr. Urii Lisitsin, an aide close to Soviet Minister of Health Boris Petrovsky, told me of Petrovsky's personal concern over the rise in infant mortality rates. "Petrovsky asked me," he said, "what the reason was behind the increase. I had to tell him that we just didn't know."

Since 1964 the top medical leader of the USSR has been Boris Vasilevich Petrovsky, the Minister of Health. A gruff but kind fatherly figure, the seventy-two-year-old Petrovsky is the personification of the traditional Soviet Communist leader. Formerly physician to the elite Communist Party Fourth Department of medicine, Petrovsky reached his leadership position by a combination of scientific expertise and careful political maneuvering. Petrovsky is a close friend of Alexsei Kosygin, who until his resignation and death in 1980 was Prime Minister and the man directly in charge of the Soviet economy.

As Minister of Health, Petrovsky is used to running a bare-bones medical system, doing the best he can with limited resources. For sixteen years he has fought to improve the quality of Soviet medical research. He has continued the emphasis on preventive care by public education and by the symbolic gesture of prohibiting smoking in all Ministry of Health offices. He has spoken out repeatedly about the problems caused by low funding and inefficient use of personnel. Under Petrovsky's leadership the Soviet budget for health has increased from 6.7 billion rubles in 1965 to 18 billion rubles today. But the numbers alone are deceptive.

A 1981 publication of The Joint Economic Committee of the U.S. Congress, "Consumption in the USSR: An International Comparison" prepared by Gertrude Schroeder and Imogene Edwards estimates that, after removing rubles spent on physical culture, vacation sanatoriums along with one time expenses like building hospitals from the official Soviet health budget, actual expenditures for medical care in 1976 were 10 billion rubles, two thirds of the published total. This means that per person use of medical services in the USSR is roughly a third of that found in the United States.

Even more impressive than this comparison, which at best is a rough estimate, is the report's summary of how per capita medical spending in the USSR has failed to grow. During the last twenty years, from 1960 through 1980, when real, i.e., inflation corrected expenditures for medical care grew in the United States by 233 per cent the Soviets increased their spending by just 50 per cent. Today the USSR spends 2 per cent of its Gross National Product on health; we spend 9 per cent.

Soviet planners are so used to working within strict monetary limits that they refuse to consider budgetary increases in their projections. "There is no point in talking about more money," one of them told me. "We have a budget and that is all the money we will get. There are no cost overruns in Soviet medicine."

In addition to the effect of low financing on medical supplies, new technology, and research, another fundamental difference between medical care in the United States and the Soviet Union is the extent to which medical care takes over individual, religious, and family responsibilities.

In the United States, medical care now substitutes for many of the duties formally carried out by the family. Nursing homes, for example, are the fastest-growing item of medical care in the United States. In 1960, they accounted for only 2 percent of all medical expenditures; today, they total close to 10 percent. Yet nursing homes provide little in the way of formal medical services. They take care of old and handicapped persons, make sure they are fed, clothed, and not alone when they die. The family used to do those things at home.

The family in the Soviet Union is still expected to care for its old and troubled members. When there is no family, there is no help. Most people still die at home. Consumer demands for change are generally ignored.

"The doctors should have better equipment," was a frequent complaint I heard when talking with Soviet patients. "There should be more medicine. Operations shouldn't be so painful. There should be more people working in the hospitals," the complaints go. And as an old woman from Yerevan told me, "It is hard to be sick. A little comfort would be nice."

But these random comments are all that is known of consumer complaints. The Soviets do not consider patient satisfaction in evaluating medical services.

More importantly, the suffering and destruction during World War II and the isolation felt by the Russian people are too strong for the leaders to risk diverting any resources from defense to increase the "comfort" of Soviet patients. Comfort is something the Soviet leadership feels the country cannot yet afford.

For the same reason it is unlikely that any Soviet leadership, old or new, will substantially increase the budget for medical care. Nor will they drop the official line they have followed for years, that spending on medical care is sufficient to meet all basic needs. To the Soviet Union, this type of statement is necessary to protect its image at home and abroad.

It is necessary despite the fact that since the mid-sixties, Soviet studies have consistently demonstrated failures of basic preventive medical services. Today, by the Soviets' own accounting, tuberculosis still accounts for 3 percent of all hospital admissions and rheumatic fever, 1 percent. Vitamin deficiencies occur in infants and for many pregnant women, diet is inadequate. Important indicators of health are moving in the wrong direction.

Granted, many of these problems may not respond to traditional medical treatment. There are very real limits today to the power of medical care to improve the quality and length of human life. In the United States we have probably asked medical care to do too much: to assume religious and family responsibilities, to take away our fears of illness and death. In the process we have spent our resources extravagantly, even wastefully.

The Soviet Union has avoided that pitfall. For all of this century the Soviet government has followed the consistent policy that they do not need nor can they afford all the medicine that money can buy.

As a ministry official told me in a 1979 interview, "In the 1980s the United States will face a crisis in medical care because everybody wants to make money from the sick. In the Soviet Union we will have no such problem. Medical care will remain *besplatno.*"

Or as Dr. Lisitsin put it, "In the Soviet Union we are ashamed to talk about money when it comes to medicine."

16

Extraordinary Limits

The call came late on a busy Tuesday afternoon. I was not going to answer but the secretary said it was the Soviet Embassy, so I picked up the receiver in the middle of a crowded and noisy intensive care unit.

"Excuse me for interrupting," I heard Dr. Borisov say, "but I have a favor to ask. There are some Russian doctors in town, they are here for only a short time and, well, before they leave they would like to see an American hospital. I was wondering, would it be possible to bring them by tomorrow morning?"

Dr. Borisov is the medical attaché at the Soviet Embassy in Washington. I had met him shortly after his posting to Washington. A member of a small elite group of Soviet diplomats who rotate assignments in Paris, New York, and Washington with brief trips to Moscow, he is polished, confident, and experienced. Although I knew he would never permit a friendship to develop between us, I had told him to call if ever I could be of help. This phone call was his first request and, although short notice, I agreed to the meeting.

The next morning they arrived precisely at ten: three physicians, accompanied by Borisov and a lower ranking embassy official. The physicians stood huddled self-consciously in the hospital lobby, appearing awkward in two dark, wrinkled suits and one heavy black dress. Next to Borisov with his carefully tailored clothes, silk tie, and practiced manners, they seemed like poor relations. As I approached, Borisov added to their discomfort by quickly apologizing, saying he could not stay. He had another meeting at the State Department. After hasty introductions he disappeared into a waiting limousine.

Following their host's sudden departure the Soviet physicians, one the director of a large hospital, another the head of a coronary care unit, the third a professor of medicine, looked down at the floor or glanced nervously over their shoulder. To reduce anxiety I suggested we get started on the tour by visiting the intensive care unit. As we reached the ICU entrance the embassy official became uncomfortable at the prospect of seeing sick patients. He asked to be allowed to remain outside.

I explained to the physicians how our intensive care unit accepted and treated critically ill patients. I knew that many of the treatments and techniques we used in the ICU were rare in the Soviet Union. Some were not available at all. My purpose, however, was not to impress my visitors but to help them understand the differences between the Soviet and American approach to medical practice.

We began at the bedside of a fifty-one-year-old man who was recovering from coronary artery bypass surgery, an operation common throughout the U.S. but only recently performed in the USSR. I discussed indications for the procedure, how American physicians felt it relieved disabling chest pain, and reviewed the evidence that for some patients it might even prolong life.

"Of course," one of the Soviet physicians, the hospital director, responded, "we've read about this surgery. Such operations are beginning to be done in our country. Soon I am sure we will be doing more of them. But, of course," he laughed nervously, "not as many as you."

"Why?" I asked. "You have as much heart disease as we do."

"Yes," he said, "but we are not as convinced as you are of the surgery's value. And, as you know, it is very expensive. I have read that it costs more than $10,000 per person. I think it would be better to try to prevent heart disease."

The next patient had heart failure. To measure the progress of our treatment we were using a new catheter that, when combined with a small computer, provided instantaneous readings of how vigorously her heart was pumping. The Soviet doctors showed restrained fascination with the new technique. The woman physician, who treated many heart failure patients, said that while she wasn't able to measure cardiac output with such a catheter she could still estimate performance of her patients' hearts by injecting a drug into a vein and then waiting for it to reach the patient's mouth where it produced a strong metallic taste.

"Of course," she smiled, "your method is more accurate, but I am not sure it makes much difference in the end."

Our third case was an eighty-one-year-old man whose gallbladder, obstructed by a large stone, had become infected. Admitted to the ICU following emergency surgery the night before, he was in fragile condition. His lungs, heart and kidneys were damaged by the poisons released from his gallbladder. That morning it was all we could do to keep him alive.

I reviewed for the Soviet doctors how we were balancing our patient's need for a ventilator to assist his breathing versus his poor heart function and failing kidneys. After a long discussion, concentrating on the medical challenges presented in his care, one of the Soviet doctors motioned us away from the bedside. We formed a tight circle in the center of the ICU. In a hushed voice he asked me whether I thought the old man was going to live.

"I don't know," I admitted. "He has a lot of problems but he is still alert and since surgery was successful I think we have a chance. At least," I concluded, "it's too early to give up."

"But such extraordinary care," the Soviet doctor replied, "so much effort, so many decisions. Who decides that all this should be done? Who decides when to stop?"

I explained that the decision to admit the patient to the ICU had been mine and that along with the patient's surgeon I would also determine how far to go in treatment.

At that my Soviet visitor grabbed my arm, firmly pulling me closer to his face.

"Are there age limits for the intensive care unit?" he asked.

"No," I replied.

"Would you treat someone with cancer?"

"Yes, if we thought the acute problem he was having was reversible and if his tumor was not far advanced."

"Do you ever withold treatment from certain patients who you think will not live?"

"Of course," I said. "There are cases when we feel we are doing more harm than good. If so, we stop."

"Isn't it difficult to stop treatment once you've started?"

"Yes," I admitted, "It is very difficult, sometimes impossible."

"So how do you know, and why do you begin? This patient is eighty-one years old. He's had a good, long life; why add to his misery now?"

"But I am trying to save his life."

The Soviet doctor shook his head slowly.

"That is the difference," he said, speaking softly at first. "That is the difference. In America you think medicine can do everything. In Russia we understand its limits."

Living with limits is something the Russian, and more recently, the Soviet population has frequently had to do. Since the turn of the century a cycle of war, revolution, war, famine, epidemics, economic mismanagement, war again, and for the last twenty-five years, constant preparation for war has demanded frequent sacrifice by the people of the Soviet Union.

There is a saying in the USSR that no family was left untouched by the destruction of the Second World War. Everyone, even those not directly involved in the fighting, was injured. Today the scars of those injuries are constantly being reopened by a Soviet government intent on building a strong defense and on being able to withstand any attack.

"You must always be on the alert," schoolchildren are warned, "you must always be prepared to fight the enemy, to sacrifice for your homeland."

Sacrifice takes many forms. Only one out of every hundred Soviet citizens owns a car and most have never traveled more than a few hundred miles from their birthplace. The stores where they shop and the apartments where they live never satisfy their demands. The newspapers they read seldom provide much news and many of their greatest writers and artists have left to work in other countries where freedom of expression is unlimited.

This official policy of limits affects not only discretionary items like consumer goods, travel, and transportation but also more controversial areas such as medical care. Today one of the major differences between the United States and the Soviet Union is their investment in modern medicine.

Placing limits on the amount of medical care is part of every medical system. Public hospitals in the United States, usually located in large cities, have traditionally had smaller budgets, poorer services, and fewer doctors than private hospitals. Recently, however, this unofficial method of rationing medical care has come to be regarded here as a public embarrassment. In the 1960s the U.S. government developed two large medical insurance programs, Medicare and

Medicaid, which were aimed at getting old and poor Americans treated in private hospitals by private doctors.

From the standpoint of access these two programs have been enormously successful. Since Medicaid's passage the number of visits to a physician by low-income persons has increased. Medicare removed many of the financial barriers for medical care of persons over sixty-five.

Together these two programs have also placed the American government in the position of being the largest single financial supporter of medical care in the United States and most of the world (43 percent of the annual health budget of the United States now comes from government sources). But neither Medicare nor Medicaid has greatly changed the character of American medicine.

American medicine remains a private relationship between American patients and their doctors. Regardless of who pays the bill, an American doctor still controls all decisions regarding care. He alone is accountable for the results of his treatment.

The power and responsibility given to the American doctor is one characteristic which invariably amazes Soviet medical visitors to the United States. The ability of any American doctor to hospitalize his patient, recommend an operation, or prescribe almost any new treatment stands in stark contrast to the Soviet physician's inability to independently make such decisions.

This lack of responsibility reflects back to the early years of the Soviet medical system when no single interest group, certainly not physicians, dominated its development. Convinced that they had to reduce the social and political power of physicians, the new Soviet regime insisted that physicians join the Union of Medical Workers. This union, which included all medical workers, supported the government and effectively eliminated the political power of physicians.

Moreover, as far back as 1932, when the National Commission on the Cost of Medical Care met in the United States and designated the doctor as the centerpoint of American medicine, Soviet physicians were being drafted by their government as necessary but low priority employees. Women, and a few men, whose services were not necessary in factories or farms became medical students. They worked within a national medical care system supported by a government overwhelmed with the sudden responsibility of providing food, defense, transportation—everything for a struggling economy. During the 1930s and 1940s there were shortages of medicines, hospital beds, bandages and stethoscopes. From the beginning the Russian doctor had to work with less than he or she needed.

At the same time the collective attitude that was promoted as the basis of the new Soviet state, and that was encouraged in agriculture and industry as one way of coping with regional and national shortages, found its way into medical care. Independent decisions by physicians were discouraged and, as a result, individual responsibility slowly declined. As the years went by the dominance of national priorities over the needs of individuals not only changed the character of the doctor-patient relationship in Soviet Russia, it also limited the vision and challenges to which Soviet medicine and Soviet physicians aspired.

I remember making rounds with a Russian doctor in Siberia. Together we visited some of the patients in a small one-hundred-bed hospital near the Soviet Union's border with Mongolia. Located far from Moscow, the hospital is typical of the two-thirds of Soviet hospitals with small staffs, no laboratory, and fewer than a hundred beds.

In one of these beds was an eighteen-year-old girl recovering from injuries she had received in an automobile accident. Both of her legs were broken and as a result of the extensive muscle damage and blood loss, her kidneys had quit functioning. Toxins, normally cleared by the kidney, were building up in her bloodstream. Each day she was sinking deeper into coma. I asked my friend whether he planned to use an artificial kidney machine or another simpler form of dialysis where a special fluid is placed into the patient's abdomen to treat her kidney failure.

No, he replied simply, there would be no dialysis. No artificial kidney machine was available in the hospital and no physician on the hospital's staff knew how to perform abdominal dialysis. The girl would have to recover with conservative treatment.

"It must be frustrating," I said, "not to be able to do everything possible for your patient."

"But I am doing everything possible," my friend countered, "in this case we are carefully controlling all the fluid and minerals she receives. So, until her kidneys recover, she will not need dialysis."

"But it would be better and safer, if you had an artificial kidney machine," I said.

"Yes, of course, but you must understand that the Soviet Union is not as rich as the United States. We cannot have every treatment available at every hospital. We must use our wealth for other things, we must sacrifice, we must wait. . . . but things are not so bad."

Does the lack of modern and alternative treatments make a difference? In recent years there has been a trend in this country to question the wisdom of spending more and more of our limited national wealth on medical services. A number of studies have emphasized how most of the increase in costs has gone into hospital care and how new technologic innovations treat disease rather than maintain health.

Other critical studies have suggested that, as a result of our concentration on aggressive all-out treatment of serious diseases, we are spending much of our medical care dollar for a very small number of patients, those with chronic and often incurable diseases. Finally, critics of American medicine point out that we frequently accept and aggressively promote new operations and techniques before we know for whom and when they should be used. For all these reasons, the critics say, American medicine is becoming increasingly inefficient and unnecessarily expensive.

Viewed from this perspective the Soviet approach appears more logical. The Soviets apply strict limits to expenditures. They set out to decide what is good for the general health rather than for special interest groups. They emphasize prevention rather than treatment.

One way to answer the question of which approach is best is to compare results. The problem with such a comparison is that the challenges and the numbers are really not comparable. When the Soviet government took control of the medical system the United States had, in terms of health indices, a two-hundred-year head start. In 1917 there were no cholera or typhus epidemics in the United States. Large numbers of Americans were not starving. American medicine, although still not equal to the quality of practice in Western Europe, was developing a strong scientific base. It was also enjoying the financial support of a dynamic and growing economy.

Since then Americans have shown almost no restraint in their desire to spend more and more money on medical care and medical research. The Soviets, although trying to catch up, maintained rigid control over their expenditures, setting strict budgets for medical care and then sticking to them.

During the last thirty years (since approximately 1950, when the USSR began recovering from the devastation of World War II) this approach appeared not only to make sense but also to produce results. From 1950 through 1970 infant mortality fell and life expectancy increased in both countries. Beginning in 1971 this progress, whether real or created because of previous sloppy reporting, stopped in the USSR and today there are wide disparities between the United States and USSR. Today Soviet health indices resemble those of a developing rather than a developed country. Clearly something is wrong.

The recent deterioration in life expectancy for Soviet men could be the result of alcoholism alone but, more likely, it stems from a combination of factors. The Soviet Union does not manufacture as wide a variety of high blood pressure drugs as the United States. Soviet surgeons do not operate on many patients suffering from coronary artery disease. The average Soviet diet remains high in saturated fats and, despite a 1980 directive aimed at "limitation and, in the future, a ban on smoking in work places," the number of cigarettes consumed increases each year.

As a result death rates from heart disease, a major killer of young men, have not decreased in the USSR as they have in the United States.

But even without the numbers it is obvious that the various bureaus, ministries, institutions and individuals are not fulfilling the formal promise of Soviet medicine. Many physicians, treated as employees, have little enthusiasm for their jobs or patients. Factories charged with producing X-ray film ostensibly meet quotas but 75 percent of their product is unusable. Faced with inadequate drug supplies, pharmacists barter what they do receive for hard-to-get automobile parts. Researchers, frustrated with political considerations outweighing their scientific accomplishments, rewrite the same article over and over again. Soviet leaders are not getting the performance they need at the price they are willing to pay.

In an unusual article published in *Literaturnaya gazeta* on December 14, 1977, the results of a public opinion poll consisting of two thousand letters written by patients in Kiev, capital of the Ukranian republic, were analyzed. Two common themes emerged.

One was that Soviet practitioners were frustrated with the lack of alternatives and, as a result, insensitive to patient's feelings. A doctor was reported to have said, "You have a stomach ulcer and diabetes. You will not survive an operation. I simply don't know what to do with you."

This lack of concern extends, according to the article, to the patient's relatives. Families waiting for hours in hospital lobbies for some word are treated as an unwelcome intrusion by physicians and hospital staff. As the author of the survey article explains, "We love the patients, but as for their relatives—we have little sympathy."

The Soviet patient, while complaining about the lack of compassion, however, also understands the reason behind it. All Soviet medical care is a government service, comprehensive but impersonal. To obtain a better balance many patients told me they tried, through gifts or money, to create some attachment between themselves and their physicians. These secret payments provide more than a subsidy to the low salary the Soviet government allocates physicians; it hopefully establishes a bond, a tentative guarantee that, despite the system, they will get personal attention.

With the exception of this "grey market" system the Soviet citizen has little ability to influence the course of his medical care. Most Soviet citizens I spoke with would like better hospitals, sophisticated technology and more up-to-date treatments. But national decision making regarding the number of rubles spent on medical care is well beyond control of the Soviet physician, much less the average Soviet citizen.

In the United States the doctor, in exchange for a large fee, high social standing, and respect, is expected to provide a maximal effort on behalf of his patients. He is challenged to remain up-to-date. He can be sued if he makes a mistake.

The Soviet physician does not enjoy the positive rewards and does not fear the negative. Ultimate responsibility is not his; it rests with the system.

Prevention of rheumatic heart disease, for example, is possible with throat cultures and appropriate antibiotic treatment. The proper application of this type of system, the ability to do simple things well, is credited with significantly reducing rheumatic heart disease in the United States. In the Soviet Union, the availability of adequate laboratory facilities is one noticeable weak link in the chain. As a result, undetected streptococcal infections and the resulting rheumatic heart problems remain a recognized but as yet unsolved health risk for thousands of Soviet children.

This does not mean that all of the Soviet Union's difficulties could be eliminated with the purchase of more laboratory technology or with the expenditure of more money. As we are learning in this country, money has a progressively limited ability to buy better health. At the same time, however, it does appear that some of the deficiencies evident in Soviet medicine today could be improved with a better balance between the leadership's theoretical support for a comprehensive medical care system and its financial commitment to one.

Devoting more money to medicine would at this time present a challenge to Soviet leaders. The economy of the USSR is in precarious shape, productivity is down and, for the last few years, there has been little real growth in the Soviet Gross National Product from which any increase in health expenditures would have to come. Even a substantial increase in the Soviet health budget would not correct the inherent inefficiencies and educational deficits that years of low funding have produced. But, short of restructuring the entire system, an increase in funding is the most direct way to improve the type and quality of medical services in the USSR.

This is a different situation than the one we face in the U.S. American physicians and American medicine are enthusiastically, some say too enthusiastically, supported by the government. Responsibility for reducing this support rests on a small group of individuals and public leaders who are convinced that further money spent on medical care will weaken other sectors of the economy.

In the Soviet Union there are no public debates over medical care funding; no interest groups lobbying for more support. University physicians are politically ineffective because the very skills they need to press demands for more support, such as precise epidemiologic data, are the same skills they currently lack. The thousands of practicing physicians are, like their fellow citizens, unaware of what they are missing.

This is one reason past observors have referred to the Soviet medical care system as either an enormous success or a colossal failure. It truly is both. As a national program aimed at conserving scarce resources while providing basic services, it is a qualified success. From the perspective of a patient in need of special attention or individual emphasis it is frequently a failure.

There is evidence that a few Soviet leaders recognize this problem. Academicians like Moscow economist-physician Popov argue that more doctors and more office visits are not the answer to deteriorating health statistics in the USSR. High-ranking officials such as Deputy Minister of Health Chazov campaign openly for an increased research budget and more international exchanges of scientists.

Many younger and better trained Soviet physicians who have spent time in the United States or Western European countries also tell me of their desire to bring their new information and expertise home for Soviet patients. I recall leading a young Soviet surgeon on a tour of an American operating room. "Look at those instruments," he said softly, "with a set of such instruments I could be the greatest surgeon in Kishinev."

But there is little evidence that increased expenditures will soon be a part of Soviet medicine. The real, i.e., adjusted-for-inflation, budget for Soviet medical care shows little growth. To date the purchase of new medical technologies by the Soviet government has been erratic and has not improved the overall quality of care. The 1980 takeover of Afghanistan, and the resulting Olympic boycott, and the continued suppression of prominent dissidents, reduced enthusiasm for the exchange of U.S. and USSR medical scientists.

Meanwhile the Soviets continue to follow their old "Sputnik" approach. They support showcase programs of medical care in a few hospitals or research institutes where visitors are taken. The majority of their clinics and hospitals remain crowded with patients, filled with physicians, but empty of the equipment and other technical support needed to provide modern medical care.

Appendices

Selected Bibliography

Glossary

and

Index

Taking Care of Yourself in the USSR—
An Informal Guide for Travelers

The Soviet Union is a fascinating country. With its ancient Russian heritage still visible through its recently acquired Soviet veneer, the USSR remains one of the few places in the world that is truly different. The tourist will find little there that reminds him of home.

The same is true of their medical system. An American visitor who does not speak Russian will be bewildered in a Soviet polyclinic and overwhelmed by the unusual demands of their hospital system. Such differences, however, are not unique to the Soviet medical system. Whenever a person travels to another country, be it France, Mexico, South Africa, India, or the USSR, he will find important differences in the way medicine is practiced. Knowing about and preparing for these differences is an essential part of foreign travel. The information in this chapter will help you do this. As such, it is not meant to frighten the traveler or persuade him to cancel his trip.

Remember, thousands of Americans and other tourists enjoy the beauty and fascination of old Russia each year and return richer for the experience. The chances of getting ill are small and with the proper precautions, can be reduced even further. But precautions are necessary. Going into the Soviet system totally unprepared can lead to problems.

The story is told in Moscow of the American businessman who came to the USSR to sell oil-drilling machinery to the Soviets. He attempted to conduct his business the way he had formally done in the United States. After four weeks of unreturned phone calls, unproductive meetings, and constant shuffling from one ministry office to another, he was found sitting naked on the floor of his hotel room, babbling incoherently. When asked what was wrong he kept repeating, "Come back tomorrow, come back tomorrow."

In this case the American Embassy was called and the unfortunate man was quickly escorted back to the United States for treatment. After six months he had partially recovered and within a year he was back at work.

Fortunately, not many people react so violently to the Soviet way of doing business and few become psychotic. Other types of illness can occur. Knowing how to plan for and possibly prevent them is as important as knowing what to do once they occur. The Soviet Union presents some unique medical challenges.

Prescription Drugs

There is no way for you to have a prescription filled in the USSR. The Soviets have few drug combinations and do not produce many of the compounds we commonly use. What is more, an American prescription would be unintelligible to a Soviet pharmacist. Come prepared.

The first thing to do is obtain extra supplies of all your prescription drugs. If you are planning a two-week tour, pack enough high blood pressure pills to last four weeks. Carry the extra supply with you in a separate suitcase so you will not lose everything should one traveling bag be delayed.

It is also a good idea to carry a letter or brief statement from your physician, describing your major health problems along with the exact dosage of all medication.

Remember that many chronic conditions such as hypertension can be aggravated by the excitement and frustrations of international travel. The differences in time, customs, and food magnify the problem in the USSR. (Moscow is eight hours ahead of New York when that city is on Daylight Savings Time.)

There are no vaccination requirements to enter the USSR.

Over-the-Counter Drugs

Because of the large differences between drug names and preparations in the United States and the USSR, a few standard nonprescription drugs should be carried by *every* person traveling to the Soviet Union. These should include a bottle of aspirin or aspirin substitute, an antihistamine (can be used as a mild sedative if sleeping is difficult), a decongestant or cold capsule, a bottle of Pepto-Bismol®, and fifty tablets of Lomotil.

Travelers with a history of motion sickness can try to avoid the problem by taking anti-motion sickness pills or antihistamines before departure. This is especially important if your plans call for travel on Aeroflot, the Soviet Union's international airline. Aeroflot flights are always crowded, the planes uncomfortably warm, and most internal takeoffs are steep in order to conserve fuel. Aeroflot did not become the world's largest airline by putting its customers' comfort first.

Dental Care

Most Soviet dental care is crude and done without anesthetics. If a dental emergency such as a lost filling should develop while you are traveling in the USSR, treatment should be delayed until your return.

If the pain or discomfort will not let you continue, seek a temporary filling that can be easily replaced upon your return. The Soviet practice is to extract teeth if any problems develop, and restorative dentistry is limited to a few stomatologists (mouth specialists) in the larger cities. Besides, a permanent treatment could interfere with the treatment available once you are home. Finally, remember that it is inadvisable to fly within twelve hours of an extraction, root canal, or filling. The change in atmospheric pressure can cause pain from expansion of trapped gas.

Diarrhea

One of the more common and definitely one of the most uncomfortable problems a traveler faces is diarrhea. It intrudes into tours to the Hermitage Museum and can ruin a night at the Bolshoi theater.

The onset of traveler's diarrhea or the "trots," as it is ingloriously but accurately known, is sudden. The illness begins with cramps and nausea followed quickly by frequent and watery diarrhea. In most cases, the diarrhea is explosive but the illness is self-limited. Although the first few hours make you feel as if you are going to die, the symptoms improve within a day or two and most persons are weak but getting back to normal by the third day.

Many cases of diarrhea are noninfectious, resulting from eating strange foods, nervous tension, or simply becoming overtired. Such cases are best treated by rest and a bland diet, one avoiding fats and alcohols. But the major cause of traveler's diarrhea is infection and its source is the water.

All major Soviet cities, like their American counterparts, chlorinate their water supplies to provide protection against viral and bacterial waterborne disease. The Soviets also monitor the coliform counts of their water supplies to ensure that the number of bacteria (which are present in every water system) are at a safe level.

Even so, Soviet water, especially that available in the Central Asian republics,[1] can often be contaminated. Water in the major cities such as Moscow and Leningrad, while generally free of most bacteria, contains other problem-causing organisms (see next section).

The best solution is not to drink the water. This is an absolute rule that should be followed by every short-term traveler to the USSR.

Not drinking the water also means not using ice (which is rarely available in the USSR anyway) and avoiding salads and unpeeled fruit. Tap water used for brushing teeth and drinking should be boiled for 10 minutes and allowed to cool to room temperature in a clean container (Soviet current is 220 volts, 50 cycles, so appliances require converters).

A more practical method for water purification is to use iodine tablets (Potable-aqua® or Globaline®), which are available in most U.S. drugstores.

In Soviet hotels or restaurants, drink beverages such as tea or coffee made with boiled water. Bottled carbonated beverages, including Soviet mineral water, are safe, as are wine and beer.

If, despite these efforts, diarrhea still occurs, remember you must replace fluid loss. A glass of tea alternated with one of carbonated mineral water containing a quarter-teaspoon of baking soda (bicarbonate of soda) provides excellent fluid replacement.

Avoid solid foods and especially milk and other dairy products until the diarrhea stops.

Diarrhea is the body's way of eliminating the foreign, offending bacteria or virus, so drugs that stop the diarrhea before its job is completed only prolong the illness. This is why drugs like Lomotil that inhibit or stop intestinal activity are inappropriate as first-line treatment for traveler's diarrhea. Pepto-Bismol® is a better initial choice since it will not stop the diarrhea but will increase the amount of fluid absorbed by the intestine. Take one ounce of Pepto-Bismol® or, if not available, Kaopectate®, every half hour for four hours. If this treatment does not reduce the frequency of bowel

---

[1] The Kazak, Kirgiz, Turkmen, Uzbek, and Tadzhik republics.

movements, one tablet of Lomotil after each bowel movement can be used for two or three days, by which time the problem should be over.[2]

Remember that traveler's diarrhea, while initially devastating, is short-lived. The vast majority of cases last only a few days and do not require medical attention. Watch for warning signs that indicate more substantial problems—blood or mucus in the stool, fever with shaking chills, or persistent diarrhea (more than ten stools a day) leading to dehydration. If these develop, or if the diarrhea persists beyond a few days, you should get medical attention. (More on that later.)

Giardia

Besides unfamiliar bacteria and viruses, another important reason to avoid Soviet water is a disease called giardiasis.

Giardia lamblia, as they are known scientifically, are active creatures belonging to the class of intestinal protozoa. They are larger than bacteria, oval-shaped, and capable of attaching to the surface of the human intestine. Once attached, they can cause uncomfortable symptoms of fullness, bloating, cramping, and diarrhea.

According to Martin Wolfe, M.D., a specialist in tropical medicine and an international authority on giardiasis, the coliform counts the Americans and Soviets use to monitor their water supplies can be normal but giardia can still be present. Adequate chlorination and filtration are necessary to kill them. Thus, it is impossible to know where or when the risk of infection with giardia is present. Studies indicate that visitors to Moscow and Leningrad and other Soviet cities have been infected.

We do know that there is large individual variation in how people react to infection with giardia. Some become violently ill and lose substantial amounts of weight. In others the infection is silent, being

[2] Recent studies have suggested that the use of an antibiotic, doxycycline, may prevent traveler's diarrhea. It must be taken before leaving and once daily while traveling. Since doxycycline is associated with side effects (nausea, skin rashes, and even diarrhea itself), travelers should check with their physicians prior to its use. Another study, this one on tourists traveling to Mexico, found that prophylactic use of Pepto-Bismol® (four tablespoons four times a day) as soon as the person entered the country significantly reduced the chances of developing diarrhea. Again, if unsure, check with your doctor.

detected only when stool samples are examined for other reasons.

Stool testing is the way giardiasis is diagnosed. Since the incubation period (the time between ingesting the organism and beginning symptoms) is two weeks and often longer, most travelers will not become ill until they return home. Because of this long incubation time, all persons who have visited the USSR in the past year and have gastrointestinal problems, should have stool examinations to look for giardia. Treatment of symptomatic infection is by drugs which should only be administered under the supervision of a physician.

Food

Like drinking, eating can often be a problem while traveling in the Soviet Union. The typical meal in a Soviet restaurant contains more fat and grease than most Americans are accustomed to eating. Most soups, including the famous Russian borsch, are especially heavy with grease. If you order ham, you are likely to get a small piece of meat surrounded by a large circle of fat. *Bifsteki*, the Soviet's version of sirloin, comes topped with a fried egg. Potatoes usually are heavily coated with grease. The excellent dark bread is also heavy. Restaurants serve few vegetables and the typical salad is a few thin slivers of cucumber. Other sources of roughage or bulk are impossible to find on most menus.

These heavy, high-carbohydrate, fat-laden meals are exactly what you should not eat when traveling. To persons with a history of gallbladder or other digestive problems, they can spell disaster. Even persons with normal digestion will, after a week, be constipated and feel uncomfortably full and sluggish.

The alternatives to this restaurant diet are few. Most USSR tours are all-inclusive. As a general tourist you cannot choose the hotel where you will stay or the restaurants in which you will eat. Often menus are even chosen for you. But if you do have a choice and you are a tourist in Leningrad, the Hotel Astoria is the best hotel for service and food in the entire USSR. (Hitler planned to make it his headquarters if Leningrad had been captured during World War II). While in Moscow, an evening at the Aragvi restaurant, which specializes in Middle Eastern food, is a welcome break. (The doorman at the always crowded Aragvi will tell you there is no room.

Quietly hand him a few rubles and you will soon have a table.) There are other official Intourist restaurants where, in exchange for payment in dollars, good food and prompt service are available.

Whether you are visiting the USSR on business or pleasure, vodka drunk straight will be frequently offered, for example in the drinking of toasts. Although there is no known remedy for too much vodka, one way to prevent it from reaching your bloodstream as rapidly as it does your stomach is to eat heavily buttered bread or drink milk prior to the toast.

Brown-Bagging, Soviet Style

An alternative to the long wait and generally unexciting food found at most Soviet restaurants is to buy your own. Besides providing variety, shopping for your meals will give you some insight into the struggles of Soviet daily life.

Most Soviet stores are specialized—bread is sold at one, cheese and dairy products at another, fruit and vegetables at a third. Meat and chicken are also marketed separately. Since the short-term traveler has no facilities to prepare meat, the easiest meal is built around bread, cheese, and fresh vegetables. The latter are in short supply, very expensive ($1 cucumbers are not unusual), and the best selection is at the large markets on the outskirts of each city. Nevertheless, a taxi ride out to a vegetable market is one of the more interesting ways to spend the small amount of free time an Intourist tour permits.

Privately cultivated vegetable gardens make up only a small fraction of the USSR's cultivated land, but they produce more than a third of all vegetables and fruits sold. In fact, in his 1977 Constitution, Leonid Brezhnev recognized the importance of these peasant plots by guaranteeing their continued existence. Moreover, compared to the drabness of most Soviet stores, peasant markets are colorful, lively places to shop.

Early each morning, buses from the countryside begin arriving. In every seat is a kerchiefed *starushka* (older peasant woman). On her lap or between her legs she has a sack containing a few dozen apples, six or seven carefully nurtured cucumbers, three or four kilograms of potatoes, and a few bunches of gnarled carrots.

Often the sack is as large as the *starushka*. It is always better dressed. The *starushka* comes to market with a brown *babushka* (scarf) drawn tightly over her short-cropped hair. The layers of sweaters she wears are carefully chosen so the holes will not overlap. Her apron is stiff with chicken blood and frying grease from the many times it has been used to wipe her constantly busy hands.

The *starushka*'s weather-wrinkled face is frequently punctuated by open sores and small, permanently squinting eyes. But working with a diligence seldom found in the government-run stores, she carefully arranges her small pile of apples or precious cucumbers on the makeshift wooden counters. When a potential buyer shows the slightest hint of interest, the *starushka* holds the apple aloft, extolling its virtues. She has difficulty looking up herself for her back is bent from years spent cultivating and picking her crops.

The markets close down early; most of the choice produce is sold before noon. By three in the afternoon the peasant women are sitting in small groups, chewing on loaves of bread, waiting for the buses to take them back to the farm. A good day means five or ten one-ruble notes safely tucked into their sweaters or folded carefully in the bottom of their boots.

Once you have visited the local market and perhaps bought some cucumbers or a few tomatoes (wash them in boiled water before eating), you can return to the city to complete your shopping. Bread, like most other foods, is sold in a specialty store and dispensed by weight. The Soviets use the metric system and a convenient Russian phrase is *pol-kilo,* which means half a kilogram or a little over a pound.

Your last stop should be at a store selling dairy products. As a general rule, it is a good idea to avoid milk and dairy products in any country where sanitation and hygiene are poor. But the Soviet Union does an adequate job of pasteurization and many longtime Soviet travelers contend cheese and dairy products are the most reliable foods.[3]

Many varieties of cheese are available. Especially good is the cottage cheese, *tvorog.* While living in the USSR, one of my favorite combinations was *tvorog* mixed with sour cream (*smetana*) and a pinch of sugar. These items are occasionally available on restaurant

---

[3] An important exception is the Central Asian republics, where caution regarding all dairy products is advised.

menus and make an excellent breakfast. After you have recovered from a bout of diarrhea or if your stomach feels weary, buy a small bottle of Soviet yogurt, called *kifir*. *Kifir* does not come in fruit flavors, but the natural bacteria in it will often quiet a troubled gastrointestinal system.

A less troublesome but equally effective way to eat while touring is to skip dinner in the restaurant on the nights you are scheduled to go to the opera, ballet, or theater. All Soviet performances have long intermissions when you can go to the theater's *bufeti* (buffets). The *bufeti* sell an assortment of sandwiches, usually just cheese or meat in a roll. Washed down with a Soviet-style soft drink or, more in the Russian traditon, champagne, they provide a quick and easy meal.

While touring museums or art galleries, a quick lunch consists of meat-filled pies (*pirozhki*) sold at most street corners by white-capped women. Although *pirozhki* are deep-fried and greasy, they are the closest thing to a Big Mac you will find in the USSR.

For the more adventurous, a visit to a *pelmeni* café provides eating Russian-style. *Pelmeni* are meat-filled dumplings served either in a broth or with sour cream. Most *pelmeni* cafés are cafeteria-style: you simply pick up a tray and follow the person in front of you. A bowl with milk or *sok* (fruit juice) is less than one ruble.

Calling a Doctor—When and How

Compared to the United States, contacting a doctor is remarkably easy in the Soviet Union. All telephones in every major city come equipped with a special number (03) that can be dialed without depositing a coin. This number puts the caller in contact with the city's central ambulance dispatcher, and every Soviet ambulance comes with a physician. In an emergency, this is the fastest way to get help.

In nonemergency situations, the hotel or your tourist guide can direct you to one of the many outpatient facilities or polyclinics located in every Soviet city. Further, there are first-aid stations in many Moscow subway stations that, while not staffed by physicians, can provide emergency care. Every large museum, library, or other public place has a small clinic and, frequently, a physician available.

The problem is not where to find medical care, but when. The non-Russian-speaking visitor to the USSR should approach Soviet medicine with caution, not so much because medical care is poor but because it is so different.

In the first place, the Soviets will hospitalize patients with minor problems. This is especially true for anyone with stomach or abdominal pain.

Secondly, the Soviets operate almost as readily as they hospitalize. More than one unwary tourist with traveler's diarrhea who has asked to see a Soviet doctor has had his appendix removed before his diarrhea had time to stop. Even if you avoid the operating room, the chances are you will be in the hospital longer than you'd like.

Consider the experience of Jane, a twenty-six-year-old tourist vacationing in Tiblisi, in the Georgian Republic of the USSR. One early September evening, as Jane tells it, she and her husband ate dinner at a local Soviet restaurant. The meal consisted of eggplant and green beans cooked in garlic, bread and butter, white wine, and *shashlyk* (grilled lamb). Her husband had exactly the same dinner except that he ordered beefsteak instead of lamb.

An hour and a half later, Jane felt her stomach becoming uncomfortably full. Cramps and nausea began. Ninety minutes later she vomited and began having loose, watery diarrhea.

Both continued throughout the night, leaving her weak, sore, and exhausted by morning. Because she felt so terrible, she asked the *dezhurnaia* (hotel floor manager) to call a doctor. A little over an hour later, two female *vrachi* decided to put her in the hospital. Within the hour an ambulance arrived and took her to the local hospital where she was sent to the infectious disease ward. A blood sample and stool specimen were taken.

When her lunch arrived, the *babushka* who presented the boiled noodles, black bread, and butter urged Jane to eat. She did and found that, unlike that morning, her stomach would now accept food.

In the late afternoon her treatment arrived, 500 grams of a white elixir containing a mixture of calcium, belladonna, and ginger. By then her nausea, vomiting, and diarrhea were gone. Nevertheless, her Soviet doctors strongly recommended she stay in the hospital for six days "to completely recover."

Using her ability with Russian, Jane persuaded the Soviet doctors she was well enough to travel after just two days and that she had to rejoin her tour. As she left, the *vrachi* told her never to eat lamb again.

Jane's experience and that of dozens of other tourists emphasize why it is so important to try to tolerate the short-term discomfort associated with food poisoning and traveler's diarrhea. Someone without Jane's language ability would have had a far more difficult time leaving the hospital after only two days.[4]

Bumps and Bruises

According to Henry Feffer, M.D., professor of orthopedic surgery at the George Washington University and an experienced Soviet medical observer, the same approach toward hospitalization is found in orthopedics. Soviet surgeons will often hospitalize and operate on fractures that would be treated with a sling or a simple cast in this country.

In Dr. Feffer's experience, the Soviets are especially quick to use external fixation on many fractures. External fixation requires placing metal pins through both ends of a broken bone. The pins are then attached to a wire frame, immobilizing the arm or leg and requiring the patient to remain hospitalized in traction. In this way a simple fracture can lead to a prolonged hospital stay.

"Most orthopedic problems," says Dr. Feffer, "can be temporarily treated by a well-fitted plaster cast. Almost nothing has to be operated on immediately and I recommend that all travelers return home for surgery."

Because the Soviets put more emphasis on immediate treatment, minor muscular complaints and small injuries should not be treated while in the USSR. Make adjustments in your travel schedule and delay definitive care until you can return home. If you are too uncomfortable to continue sightseeing but feel well enough to travel, demand an early flight home. It is better to cut your vacation short than to enter a Soviet hospital for a minor problem.

The real problem, of course, is deciding what is minor. Decisions regarding medical treatment, the need for hospitalization, and surgery should not have to be made alone.

---

[4] Soviet policy says that foreigners should pay for hospital care at sixteen rubles ($25) a day. In my experiernce, the hospital seldom bothers to present a bill.

But since so few tourists speak Russian and almost no Soviet doctors—especially those riding the ambulances—know English, little communication takes place between American patient and Soviet *vrach*. One way to help is to arrange for a interpreter to be present when the doctor arrives or when you go to the polyclinic. Taking a patient's history is an important part of a medical evaluation, and you and the *vrach* should exchange more than nods and rough gestures.

This is especially important if the ambulance doctor or polyclinic physician recommends hospital admission. Ask the *vrach* what he thinks the diagnosis is. What kind of treatment will you get in the hospital? Could you purchase medication and stay at the hotel? Will there be need for an operation?

Once you have the answers, your next step should be to contact the American Embassy in Moscow.

The Embassy Doctor

In 1977 the State Department Medical Division began sending its own physician to staff the small outpatient clinic at the American Embassy in Moscow. Before that, the Moscow post had been filled by an Air Force flight surgeon approved by the Defense Intelligence Agency. As with other military personnel assigned to Moscow, the embassy physician was expected to perform intelligence gathering along with these medical duties.

Most of his intelligence work related to observing Soviet and foreign diplomats, looking for signs of alcoholism or other illnesses. Once an Air Force physician thought he spotted a malignant mole on Leonid Brezhnev's cheek while the Soviet premier was attending a diplomatic reception. Fortunately, this informal diagnosis turned out to be wrong.

The embassy physician was also expected to keep an eye on his American patients. Any of the embassy employees suffering from emotional disturbances, alcoholism, or marital problems were to be reported so they could be sent out of the country before the Soviets used such information against them.

Frank V. Keary is the current embassy physician. He is expected to remain in Moscow until mid-1982. He sees 125 patients a week in addition to his hospital rounds and administrative duties. Because he is busy and because medical supplies at the embassy are limited, the infirmary cannot be used as a clinic by tourists seeking prescription refills or treatment of minor colds or injuries.[5]

Where the embassy and Dr. Keary can be of help is when you or a member of your party is seriously ill and is considering entering a Soviet hospital. Although the State Department is *not* formally responsible for tourists and businessmen, past problems American citizens have had with Soviet hospitals have led the embassy to try and prevent such occurrences.

If you are in Moscow and become seriously ill, call the embassy immediately. Explain that you are an American about to enter a Soviet hospital and ask if the embassy physician could see you beforehand. If, after an examination, the doctor agrees that you should be hospitalized, arrangements can be made for you to take the short flight to Helsinki, Finland, where a 3,000-bed general hospital with Western-style medical practice is available. In many cases, the embassy doctor may be able to treat you from your hotel or suggest you cut your trip short and return home for more specialized care.

If you are in someplace other than Moscow and become ill, consider the possibility of returning to Moscow before entering a local hospital. Your Soviet *vrach* may disagree and say it is dangerous for you to travel, in which case your best course of action is to follow his advice while contacting the embassy and informing them of the hospitalization.

In the Hospital

Unless you become ill in Moscow, where most foreigners and all diplomats are admitted to Botkin Hospital, chances are you will be hospitalized alongside Soviet citizens in the closest hospital that has an available bed.

Once you are in the hospital, it is important to remember that your treatment is directly controlled by Soviet physicians. The em-

[5] The Department of State is very firm that tourist medical care is *not* their responsibility. Every tourist travels at his own, not government risk. The recommendations I make, therefore, are my own, not formal State Department policy.

bassy doctor can visit and consult on your care, but cannot order any changes. He cannot order your discharge, nor can he provide you with medication.

Given the past record of embassy physicians, the Soviets view many of his movements with suspicion and, despite the best of intentions, there may be little he can do to protect your interests.

You must do most of the protecting. Have an interpreter available at all times. Stay in close contact with the physicians in charge of your care. Demand as much medical information as possible and request details concerning future treatment plans. Keep the embassy notified of your progress or lack of it. Insist that once you have recovered you be permitted to return to Moscow.

Since our initial success in 1973 in evacuating James Torrence from Siberia, as described in Chapter 1, the Soviets occasionally permit critically ill Americans to be transported out of the country via military evacuation. As emphasized by our experience in Irkutsk, this is a difficult, complicated, and dangerous undertaking.

A better approach is to avoid, by good planning and careful questioning, ever becoming a Soviet hospital patient.

Important Moscow Telephone Numbers

American Embassy: 252-00-11
    Ulitsa Chaikovskovo 19/23
    Mon.–Fri. 9 A.M.–1 P.M., 2 P.M.–6 P.M.
American Embassy doctor: 252-00-11 Ext. 247
Tourists Clinic: 229-73-23 or 229-03-82
    Ulitsa Gertsena 12
Botkin Hospital: 255-00-15
    2nd Botkinsky Proyezd 5

24-hour pharmacists
    25th October Ulitsa 1: 295-18-46, (night) 221-49-42
    Tishinsky Pl. 6: 254-46-10
    First aid, ambulance: 03
Tracing people in Moscow hospitals: 294-31-52

Infant Mortality 1961-1980: Comparison of the USSR and U.S.

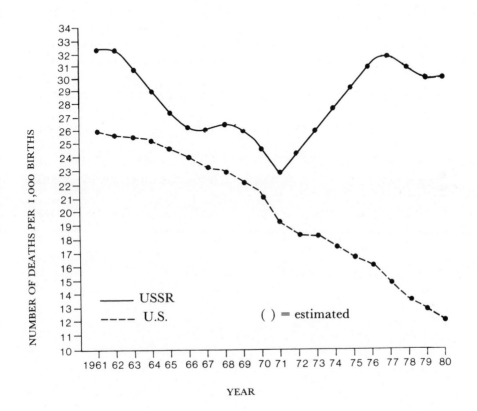

Adapted from Christopher Davis and Murray Feshbach, "Rising Infant Mortality in the USSR in the 1970's." U.S. Department of Commerce, Series p. 65, 74, 1980.

Age-Adjusted Death Rates 1961–1979: Comparison of the USSR and U.S.

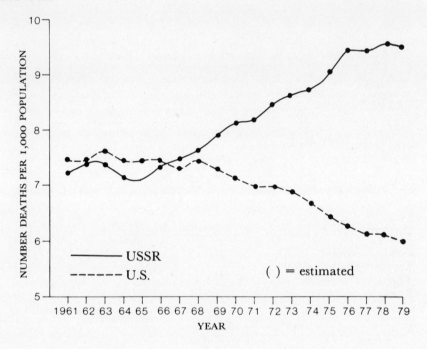

Adapted from Christopher Davis and Murray Feshbach, "Rising Infant Mortality in the USSR in the 1970's." U.S. Department of Commerce, Series p. 65, 74, 1980.

Geographic and Medical Comparison of the USSR and U.S.

	USSR	U.S.
Surface Area	8.5 million sq. miles	3.6 million sq. miles
Population (1980)	265.5 million	221.6 million
Rural Inhabitants	37%	25%
Total Hospital Beds per 10,000 Population	115	47
Total Physicians per 10,000 Population	38	19.3
Total Medical Care Expenditures—1979	18 billion rubles[1]	$212 billion
Percent Medical Expenditures Provided Through Government Funds	92[2]	43

[1] 1 ruble = $1.55. This total does not includes rubles spent for physical culture and a few other non-medical items. Medical care accounts for approximately two-thirds.
[2] Prescription expenses account for approximately 4 percent; personal expenditures for other items estimated at an additional 4 percent

Estimated Medical Personnel in the USSR and U.S. 1980

	USSR		U.S.	
Active Physicians	1,000,000		433,600	
General Physicians[1]	321,000	(32.1%)	140,486	(32.4%)
Pediatricians	115,000	(11.5%)	28,184	(6.5%)
Surgeons[2]	102,000	(10.2%)	104,064	(24%)
Ob-Gyn	59,000	(5.9%)	26,016	(6%)
Sanitary Physicians[3]	59,000	(5.9%)	5,638	(1.3%)
Psychiatrists	22,000	(2.2%)	29,484	(6.8%)
Other specialties[4]	322,000	(32.2%)	99,728	(23%)
Nurses[5]	1,185,500		1,599,000	
Feldshers	525,100		27,000 (Nurse Practitioners; Physician's Assistants)	
Laboratory Technicians	105,300		534,000	

[1] In USSR includes all physicians involved in primary care.
In U.S. includes general, family practitioners and general internists.
[2] Includes all subspecialties in both countries.
[3] In U.S. includes occupational and public health medicine.
[4] In USSR includes all other specialties not involved in primary care.
In U.S. includes unlisted and unspecified specialties.
[5] In U.S. includes registered practical nurses.

SELECTED BIBLIOGRAPHY

This selected bibliography, combined with the conservative use of footnotes in the text, aims at providing the specialist with information regarding sources while preserving enjoyment for the general reader. Those wanting more information about my research may write in care of the George Washington University Medical Center, 2300 K Street, N.W., Washington D.C. 20037.

General

Bulgakov, M. A. *Zapiski iunogo vracha.* Letchworth-Herts, England: Prideux Press, 1975.

Clarke, Roger A. *Soviet Economic Facts 1917–1970.* New York: John Wiley & Sons, 1972.

Field, Mark G. *Soviet Socialized Medicine; an Introduction.* New York: The Free Press, 1967.

Fry, John. *Medicine in Three Societies.* New York: American Elsevier Publishing Co., 1969.

Glass, Roger I. "A Perspective on Environmental Health in the U.S.S.R." *Archives of Environmental Health* 30 (August 1975): 391–395.

Glass, Roger I. "The SANEPID Service in the U.S.S.R." *Public Health Reports* 91 (March–April 1976): 154–158.

Goldman, Marshall I. *Environmental Pollution in the Soviet Union, The Spoils of Progress.* Cambridge, Mass.: The MIT Press, 1972.

Grinin, O. V., *Metodicheskie posobie po sotsialnoi gigiene i organizatsii zdravookhraneniia.* Moscow: Minzdravo RSFSR, 1974.

Hyde, Gordon. *The Soviet Health Service.* London: Lawrence and Wishart, 1974.

Jones, Albert. "An Evaluation of the Health Care System of the Union of Soviet Socialist Republics." Mimeographed. Washington, D.C.: The George Washington University, 1976.

Kaser, Michael. *Health Care in the Soviet Union and Eastern Europe.* London: Groom Helm, Ltd., 1976.

Komarov, Boris. *The Destruction of Nature in the Soviet Union.* New York: M. E. Sharpe, 1980.

Lisitsin, Y. *Health Protection in the U.S.S.R.* Moscow: Progress Publishers, 1972.

Lisitsin, Yu, and Bargin, K. *The U.S.S.R. Public Health and Social Security.* Moscow: Progress Publishers, 1978.

Metodicheskie ukazaniia po podgotovke ordinatorov i aspirantov po sotsialnoi gigiene i organizatsii zdravookhraneniia. Moscow: Minzdravo RSFSR, 1975.

Mickiewicz, Ellen. *Handbook of Soviet Social Science Data.* New York: The Free Press, 1973.

Navarro, Vincente. *Medicine Under Capitalism.* New York: Prodist, 1977.

Navarro, Vincente. *Social Security and Medicine in the U.S.S.R.: A Marxist Critique.* Lexington, Kentucky: Lexington Books, 1977.

Podolsky, Edward. *Red Miracle: The Story of Soviet Medicine.* New York: The Beechhurst Press, 1947.

Programa po organizatsii lechebo-pvofilakticheskoi pomoshchi materiam i detiam v SSSR. Moscow: Minzdrav. RSFSR, 1972.

Quinn, Joseph R. *Anatomy of East-West Cooperation: U.S.-U.S.S.R. Public Health Exchange Program 1958-1965.* Washington, D.C.: Government Printing Office, 1969.

Rabichev, L. Ya. *Ritmy zhizni v SSSR.* Kishinev: Karta Moldovenyaske, 1974.

Ryan, Michael. *The Organization of Soviet Medical Care.* Oxford: Basil Blackwell, Ltd., and London: Martin Robertson, Ltd., 1978.

Shitskova, A. P. "Results and Main Directions of Hygienic Studies in the Russian Federation." *Zdravookhraneniye Rossiskoi federatsii* (7 July 1977): 3–9.

Storey, Patrick B. *Medical Care in the U.S.S.R.: Report of the U.S. Delegation on Health Services and Planning.* Washington, D.C.: Government Printing Office, 1972.

U.S. Department of Health, Education, and Welfare, *A Bibliography on Medicine and Public Health in the U.S.S.R.* Washington, D.C.: Government Printing Office, 1975.

The Soviet Doctor

Ashurkov, E. *Slovo o doktore Chekhove.* Moscow: Medgiz, 1960.

Barsukov, M. I. *Velikaia Oktiabrskaia revolutsiia i organizatsiia sovetskogo zdravookhranenia.* Moscow: Medgiz, n.d.

Buford, W. H. *Chekhov and His Russia.* New York: Doubleday/Anchor, 1971.

Cabot, Hugh. "Russian Medicine Organized for War." *American Review of Soviet Medicine* 1 (December 1943): 158–165.

Curtiss, John Shelton. "Russian Sisters of Mercy in the Crimea, 1854–1855." *Slavic Review* 25 (March 1966): 84–100.

Deutscher, Isaac. *Lenin's Childhood.* London: Oxford University Press, 1970.

Entsiklopedicheskii Slovar. 1896 ed., Brokgauz, Efron, S. V. "Krasny; Krest," "Meditsina," "Sestra Miloserdie," "Zemstvo."

Fedyukin S. A. *Velikii Oktiabr i intelligentsiia.* Moscow: Nauka, 1972.

Field, Mark G. "Approaches to Correct the Underrepresentation of Women in the Health Professions: A U.S. Response to the U.S.S.R." *Proceedings of the International Conference on Women in Health, June 16–18, 1975.* Washington, D.C.: DHEW, 1976.

Gantt, W. Horsely. *Russian Medicine.* New York: Paul B. Hoeber, 1937.

Geizer, I. M. *Chekhov i meditsina.* Moscow: Mindzdravo RSFSR, n.d.

Gracher, F. F. *Zapiski voennogo vracha.* Leningrad, 1970.

Heim, Michael Henry, and Karlinsky, Simon. *Letters of Anton Chekhov.* New York: Harper & Row, 1973.

Hizhniakov, V. V. *Anton Pavlovich Chekhov kak vrach.* Moscow: Medgiz, 1947.

Johanson, Christine. "Autocratic Politics, Public Opinion and Women's Medical Education During the Reign of Alexander II, 1855–1881." *Slavic Review* 38 (September 1979): 426–443.

Kapustin, M. Ya. *Osnovnye voprosy zemskoi meditsiny.* Rikker, 1889.

Karpov, L. M. *Zemskaia sanitarnaia organizatsiia v Rossii.* Leningrad: Meditsina, 1964.

McGrew, Roderick E. *Russia and the Cholera.* Milwaukee: University of Wisconsin Press, 1965.

Marzeev, A. N. *Zapiski sanitarnogo vracha.* Kiev, 1965.

Meyer, J. M. *Knowledge and Revolution.* Netherlands: Van Corium/Assen, n.d.

Muller, James E.; Abdellah, Faye G.; Billings, F. T.; Hess, Arthur E.; Petit, Donald; and Egeberg, Roger O. "The Soviet Health System—Aspects of Relevance for Medicine in the United States." *New England Journal of Medicine* 286 (March 30, 1972): 693–702.

Muller, James, "The Formation of the Soviet Health Services." M. A. Thesis, Georgetown University, 1978.

Osipov, Popov, Kursan. *Russkaja zemskaia meditsina*. Moscow, 1899.

Payne, Robert. *Life and Death of Lenin*. New York: Simon and Schuster, 1964.

Polivonov, M. P. *Russkoe zemstvo, ego istoriia i ideinoe znachenie*. 1970.

Polner, Tikhon J.; Obolensey, Vladimir; and Turin, Sergius P. *Russian Local Government During the War and the Union of Zemstvos*. New Haven: Yale University Press, 1930.

Pondoev, Gavriel Sergevich. *Notes of a Soviet Doctor*. London: Chapman & Hall, 1959.

Romashov, F. N. "Higher Medical Education in the USSR." *Journal of the American Medical Association* 230 (October 28, 1974): 617.

Rufanov, I. G., and Rostotskii, I. B. "Medical Care in the Red Army and Navy." *American Review of Soviet Medicine* 2 (December 1943): 362–369.

Ryan, T. M. "Primary Medical Care in the Soviet Union." *International Journal of Health Services* 2 (February 1972): 243–253.

Schultz, Heinrich. "Changes in Soviet Medical Ethics as an Example of Efforts to Find Stable Moral Values." *In Religion and the Search for New Ideals in the USSR*. pp. 49–61. Edited by William C. Fletcher and Anthony J. Strover. New York: Frederick A. Praeger, n.d.

Segal, Boris M. "Therapist and Patient in Contemporary Soviet Society." New York: Radio Library Research, 1977.

Semashko, N. A. *Health Protection in the USSR*. London, 1934.

Shreider, G. I. *Nashe gorodskoe obshchestvennoe upravlenie*. St. Petersburg: Izd. "Vostok," 1902.

Sidel, Victor W. "Feldshers and Feldsherism." *The New England Journal of Medicine* 17 (April 25, 1968): 934–992.

Sigerist, H. E. *Medicine and Health in the Soviet Union*. New York: Citadel Press, 1947.

Skalona, V. Iu. *Po zemskim voprosam*. St. Petersburg, 1905.

Skalona, V. Iu. *Zemskie voprosy*. Moscow, 1882.

Skorokhodov, L. *Kratkii ocherk istorii russkoi meditsiny*. Leningrad, 1926.

Smirnov, Aleksandr. *Pervaia russkaia zhenshchina-vrach*. Moscow, 1960.

Smirnov, E. I. "The Organization of Medical Care for The

Wounded." *American Review of Soviet Medicine.* (August 1944):
9–14.

Stites, Richard. *The Women's Liberation Movement in Russia: Feminism, Nihilism, and Bolshevism, 1860–1930.* Princeton: Princeton University Press, 1978.

Storey, P. B. "Continuing Medical Education in the Soviet Union." *New England Journal of Medicine* 285 (August 9, 1971): 437–447.

Trofimov, V. V. *Zdravookhranenie Rossiskoi Federatsii za 50 let.* Moscow: Meditsina, 1967.

"USSR Switches to Group Practice." *Journal of the American Medical Association* 236 (July 19, 1976): 312

Veresayev, V. *The Confessions of a Physician.* Translated by Simeon Linden. London: Grant Richards, 1904.

Veselovskii, Boris. *Istoriia zemstva za sorok let.* St. Petersburg: O. N. Popova, 1909.

Zguta, Russel. "Witchcraft and Medicine in Pre-Petrine Russia." *The Russian Review* 37 (October 1978): 443–448.

Soviet Hospitals

Arkhangelsky, G. V., ed. *Manual for Nurses.* Moscow: Mir Publishers, 1978.

Bogatyrev, I. D. "Establishing Standards for Outpatient and Inpatient Care." *International Journal of Health Services* 2 (February 1972): 45–49.

Hobbs, G. A. "Personal View." *British Medical Journal* (November 26, 1977): 1413.

Sidrys, Linas A. "Opthalmology in Lithuania." *Journal of the American Medical Association* 239 (May 1978): 2181.

"Soviets Intensify Hospital Construction." *Journal of the American Medical Association* 277 (March 4, 1974): 1071.

"Xerography Popular in USSR." *Journal of the American Medical Association* 225 (September 17, 1973): 1541.

Medical Research

Abelson, Philip H. "United States-Soviet Scientific Relationship." *Science* 201 (September 1978): 1.

Breo, Dennis L. "Former Tailback Prompts Treatment Controversy

Over Spinal Cord Injuries." *American Medical News,* 2 March 1979, p. 13.

"Can Cancers Be 'Dissolved'?" *New York Times,* 12 October 1946, Sec. 1, p. 18.

"Cancer Solvent Tested in Russia." *New York Times,* 11 October 1946, Sec. 1, p. 6.

Cuny, Hilaire. *Ivan Pavlov, The Man and His Theories.* New York: Paul S. Ericksson, 1965.

Fitzpatrick, William H. *Nutrition Research in the U.S.S.R. 1961–1970.* Washington, D.C.: Government Printing Office, 1972.

Fitzpatrick, William H. *Soviet Research in Pharmacology and Toxicology.* Washington D.C.: Government Printing Office, 1974.

Gorodilova, V. V., and Hollinshed, A. "Melanoma Antigens That Produce Cell-Mediated Immune Responses in Melanoma Patients: Joint U.S.–U.S.S.R. Study." *Science* 190 (October 24, 1975): 391.

Greenberg, D. S. "Scientific Exchange: The Reluctant Russians." *The Washington Post,* 6 June 1978, Sec. 1, p. 13.

Holden, Constance. "Russians and Americans Gather to Talk Psychobiology." *Science* 200 (May 1978): 631–634.

I. P. Pavlov v vospominaniakh sovremmenikov. Leningrad: Nauka, 1967.

"K R for Cancer." *New York Times,* 13 October 1946, Sec. 4, p. 11.

"K R News." *New York Times,* 23 March 1947, Sec. 1, p. 9.

Kiselinchev, A. *Marksistko–Leninskaia teoriia otrazheniia i uchenie I. P. Pavlova o vyshei nervnoi deiatelnosti.* Moscow: Inostrannoi Literatury, 1956.

Levin, David, ed. *Cancer Epidemiology in the U.S.A. and the USSR.* Washington, D.C.: Government Printing Office, 1980.

Mansurov, Nikolai Sergeevich. *I. P. Pavlov i borba za materializmom v estestvoznanii.* Moscow: Sovetskaia Moskva, 1955.

Marx, Jean L. "Regeneration in the Central Nervous System." *Science* 209 (July 18, 1980): 378–380.

Medvedev, Zhores A. *Soviet Science.* New York: W. W. Norton and Company, 1978.

Mostofi, F. Kash; William, Marjorie J.; and Hartmann, William H. "Pathology in the Soviet Union." *Journal of the American Medical Association* 243 (January 18, 1980): 248–251.

Muller, James E. "Diagnosis of Myocardial Infarction: Historical

Notes From the Soviet Union and the United States." *The American Journal of Cardiology* 40 (August 1977): 269–271.

Muller, James E. "Experiment in Moscow." *Notre Dame Magazine* 6 (October 1977): 11–20.

Napalkov, N. P.; Tserkovnyi, G. F.; Mevabishvili, V. M.; Preobrazhenskaia, M. N.; Shabashova, N. Ya; and Guliyeva, L. M. "U.S.S.R. Mortality Due to Malignant Neoplasms." *Voprosy Onkologii* 1 (January 1977): 3–11.

Nolting, Louvan E.; and Feshbach, Murray. "R & D Employment in the U.S.S.R." *Science* 207 (February 1, 1980): 493–503.

Oganessyan, Spartak; Zaminian, Tatiana; Bay, Nelly; and Petrosian, Vladimer. "Structural and Fundamental Changes of the Contractile Proteins in Experimentally-induced Cardiac Hypertrophy in Animals, and Heart Failure in Man." *Journal of Molecular and Cellular Cardiology* 5 (1973): 1–24.

"Paraplegics Seek Russian Connection." *Medical World News* 18 (September 1978): p. 28.

Petrushevskii, S. A. *Filosofskie osnovy ucheniye I. P. Pavlova.* Moscow: Akademii Nauk SSSR, 1949.

"Quadriplegic Still Paralyzed after Russian Enzymes." *Medical World News* 8 (January 1979): pp. 21–25.

Relman, Arnold S. "Moscow in January." *New England Journal of Medicine* 302 (February 28, 1980): 532–534.

Roskin, G. "Toxin Therapy of Experimental Cancer." *Cancer Research* 42 (April 1946): 363–365.

Segall, Harold N. "Dr. N. C. Korotkoff: Discoverer of the Auscultatory Method for Measuring Arterial Pressire." *Annals of Internal Medicine* 65 (July 1965): 147–149.

Sheinin, Y. *Science Policy: Problems and Trends.* Moscow: Progress Publishers, 1978.

"Soviets Tie Research to Medical Schools." *Journal of the American Medical Association* 227 (February 11, 1974): 678.

U.S. Department of Health, Education and Welfare. *Documents from the Sixth Session of the U.S.–U.S.S.R. Joint Committee for Health Cooperation, October 24–28, 1977.* Mimeographed. Washington, D.C., 1977.

U.S. Department of Health, Education and Welfare. *Machine Diagnosis and Information Retrieval in Medicine in the U.S.S.R.* Washington, D.C.: Government Printing Office: 1973.

"U.S.-Soviet Science Cooperate on Drugs." *New York Times,* 9 October 1946, Sec. 1, p. 9.

"Vaccine Held Cure on Animal Cancer." *New York Times,* 24 October 1946, Sec. 1, p. 18.

"WHO's 12-Nation Hypertension Meeting." *Medical World News* (April 3, 1978): 21–24.

Chapters 5-13

Allen, Martin G. "Psychiatry in the United States and the U.S.S.R.: A Comparison." *American Journal of Psychiatry* 130 (December 1973): 1333–1337.

Austes, Simon L. "Impressions of Psychiatry in One Russian City." *American Journal of Psychiatry* 124 (October 1967): 538–542.

Atkinson, Dorothy; Dallin, Alexander; and Lapidus, Gail Warshofsky, eds., *Women in Russia.* Stanford: Stanford University Press, 1977.

Benet, Sula. *How to Live to Be 100.* New York: Dial Press, 1976.

"Biulleten ispolnitelnogo komiteta Moskovskogo gorodskogo soveta deputatov trudiashchikhsia." Moscow, February 1976.

"Bogomolets Serum." *New York Times,* 8 June 1946, Sec. 1, p. 20.

"Bolezn nomer tri." *Literaturnaia gazeta* (Moscow) 31 March 1976, p. 3.

"Bolezn nomer tri." *Literaturnaia gazeta* (Moscow), 19 May 1976, p. 10.

Bukovsky, Vladimer. *To Build A Castle: My Life As A Dissenter.* Translated by Michael Scammell. New York: Viking Press, 1977.

"Butylochka Vynuchalochka." *Krasnaia zvezda* (Moscow), 26 January 1979, p. 4.

Conelly, Violet. *Medical Problems in the BAM Zone.* Munich: Radio Library Research, 1976.

Corson, Elizabeth O'Leary, ed. *Psychiatry and Psychology in the U.S.S.R.* New York: Plenum Press, 1976.

David, Henry L. *Family Planning and Abortion in the Soviet Union and the Countries of Central and Eastern Europe.* New York: The Population Council, 1970.

Davis, Christopher, and Feshbach, Murray. "Rising Infant Mortality in the U.S.S.R." Washington D.C.: Department of Commerce, 1980, p. 19, No. 74, 1980.

Dilman, Y. M. *Why Death Comes*. Translated by Eugene Victor Prostov. Leningrad: Meditsina Publishing House, 1972.

"Do dobra ne dovedet." *Trud* (Moscow) 5 January 1979, p. 2.

Field, Mark G. "The Re-Legalization of Abortion in Soviet Russia." *New England Journal of Medicine* 255 (August 1956): 421–427.

Field, Mark G., ed. *Social Consequences of Modernization in Communist Societies*. Baltimore: The Johns Hopkins University Press, 1976.

Forgatson, Edward H., and Forgatson, Judtih H. "Innovations and Experiments in Uses of Health Manpower—A Study of Selected Programs and Problems in the United Kingdom and the Soviet Union." Santa Monica, Calif.: The Rand Corporation, 1969.

The Great Soviet Encyclopedia. Translation of the Third Edition S.V., "Bogomolets, Aleksandr Aleksandrovich."

Gorman, Mike. "Soviet Psychiatry and the Russian Citizen." *International Journal of Psychiatry* 8 (August 1969): 841–857.

Hindle, J. F.; Plower, L. W.; and Taylor, R. G. "Accident and Emergency Services in Russia." *British Medical Journal* 1 (February 1975): 445–447.

Kazanetz, Etely Philippovich. "Differentiating Exogenous Psychiatric Illness from Schizophrenia." *Archives of General Psychiatry* 36 (July 1979): 740–745.

Komarov, Boris. *Unichtozhenie Prirody*. Frankfurt-Main: Possev-Verlag, 1978.

"Kogo obkradyvaet pianitsa." *Sotsialisticheskaia Industriia* (Moscow), 12 January 1979, p. 4.

Kourenoff, Paul M., and St. George, George. *Russian Folk Medicine*. New York: Pyramid Books, 1971.

Kurganoff, I. A. *Women in the USSR*. Ontario: S.B.O.B.R. Publishing House, 1971.

Kurm, Helga. "Sexual Education of Adolescents." Translated by Nicholas Petroff. *Nauka i tekhnika* No. 2 (February 1978): 36–38.

Lamaze, Fernand. *Painless Childbirth*. Translated by L. R. Celestin. London: Burke Publishing Co., 1958.

Leaf, Alexander. *Youth in Old Ages*. New York: McGraw-Hill Book Company, 1975.

Madison, Bernice. "The 'Problemy' That Won't Go Away." *The Wilson Quarterly* 2 (Autumn 1978): 94–103.

Martin, James. "The Fetal Alcohol Syndrome: Recent Findings." *Alcohol Health and Research World* (April 1977): 8–12.

Mazess, Richard B. "Health and Longetivity in Vilacabomba, Ecuador." *Journal of the American Medical Association* 240 (October 13, 1978): 1781.

Messel, M. A. *Urban Emergency Medical Service of the City of Leningrad.* Washington, D.C.: DHEW, 1975.

Meyer, Herbert E. "The Coming Soviet Ethnic Crises." *Fortune,* August 1978, pp. 156–166.

"Network in U.S. Trying to Restore Health of Moscow Infant." *The Washington Post,* 13 May 1978, Sec. 1, p. A3.

"New Serum Helps Heal War Wounds." *New York Times,* 7 January 1944, Sec. 1, p. 8.

"Oberegaia zdorove podrostka." *Pravda* (Moscow), 15 January 1979, p. 3.

"Opasnoe zastole." *Sovetskaia Rossiia* (Moscow), 10 January 1979, p. 4.

Postanovlenie TSK VLKSM o borbe s pianstvom sredi molodezhi. Munich: Radio Svoboda, 1974.

Reich, Walter. "Diagnosing Soviet Dissidents." *Harpers,* July 1978, pp. 31–37.

Rockstein, Morris, ed. *Theoretical Aspects of Aging.* New York: Academic Press, 1974.

Scribner, R.; Raithaus, L.; and Ivanov, Dr. P. "Emergency Medical Service in the Soviet Union." *The Journal of Trauma* 14 (July 1976): 447–451.

Segal, Boris M. "The First Level of Soviet Psychiatric Services." New York: Radio Library Research, 1977.

Segal, Boris M. "The Incidence of Suicide in the Soviet Union." New York: Radio Library Research, 1977.

Segal, Boris M. "Traditions and Values of Psychiatry in the U.S.S.R." New York: Radio Library Research, 1977.

Shapiro, Jane P. "Consumerism in the Countryside: Policy Trends in the Brezhnev Era." Presented at the International Conference on Attitudinal and Behavioral Changes in Rural Life, Lincoln, Nebraska, April 14, 1978.

Shapiro, L. B., and Ostrovskii, I. A., eds. *Organization of Emergency*

Medical Care. Foreword by Patrick B. Storey. Baltimore: The Johns Hopkins University Press, 1975.

Shurygin, G. I. "Characteristics of the Mental Development of Children of Chronic Alcoholic Mothers." *Pediatriia* 11 (November 1974): 71–73.

"Soviet Biologist Sees 150-Year-Life If His New Serum Is Used Properly." *New York Times,* 7 June 1946, Sec. 1, p. 1.

Storey, Patrick B. *The Soviet Feldsher as a Physician's Assistant.* Washington, D.C.: DHEW, 1972.

Streissgath, Ann Pytkowicz; Landesman-Dwyer, Sharon; and Martin, Joan C. "Teratogenic Effects of Alcohol in Humans and Laboratory Animals." *Science* 209 (July 18, 1980): 353–362.

"Surgery Advance in Cancer Claimed." *New York Times,* 26 October 1946, Sec. 1, p. 30.

Terris, Milton. "Ambulatory Care in the USSR." Paper presented at the American Public Health Association, Washington, D.C., 1977.

Torrey, Dr. E. Fuller. "Emergency Psychiatric Ambulance Services in the USSR." *American Journal of Psychiatry* 128 (August 1971): 153–157.

Treml, Vladimer. "Alcohol in the U.S.S.R.: A Fiscal Dilemma." *Soviet Studies* 26 (April 1975): 161–177.

Treml, Vladimer G. "Production and Consumption of Alcoholic Beverages in the USSR: A Statistical Study." *Journal of Studies on Alcohol* 36 (March 1975): 285–320.

"Tsena Butylki." *Literaturnaia gazeta* (Moscow), 31 March 1976, p. 3.

"Umeite vlastovat soboiu." *Sovetskaia Rossiia* (Moscow), 17 November 1978, p. 4.

"Use of Technology in Emergency Health Care in the USSR." *Proceedings of a USSR/Control Data Corporation Seminar, June 21–22, 1979.* Chicago, Illinois.

"Utochnim pozitsii." *Sovetskaia Rossiia* (Moscow), 20 December 1978, p. 3.

U.S. Department of Health, Education, and Welfare. *Critical Review of the Fetal Alcohol Syndrome.* Presented at NIAAA Press Conference, Washington, D.C. June 1, 1977.

Willis, David K. "Soviet Scourge: Hard Drinking." *The Christian Science Monitor,* 10 January 1978, p. 2.

Whitney, Craig R. "Brezhnev: Summit For An Ailing Leader." *The New York Times Magazine*, 10 June 1979, p. 29.

Solzhenitsyn

Bjorkgren, Hans. *Aleksandr Solzhenitsyn: A Biography*. New York: The Third Press, 1972.

Lebedz, Leopald, ed. *Solzhenitsyn: A Documentary Record*. Bloomington, Indiana: Indiana University Press, 1973.

Lopukhina-Rodzyanko, T. *Dukhovnye osnovy tvorchestva Solzhenitsyna*. Frankfurt am Main: Possev-Verlag, 1974.

Maier, John G.; Mitteneyer, Bernard T.; and Solon, Michael H. "Treatment and Prognosis in Seminomas of the Testis." *The Journal of Urology* (January 1968): 72–78.

Maier, John G., and Sulok, Michael H. "Radiation Therapy in Malignant Testis Tumors." *Cancer* 32 (November 1973): 1212–1216.

Nielsen, Niels Christian. *Solzhenitsyn's Religion:* Nashville: Nelson, 1975.

Reshetovskaya, Natalya. *Sanya: My Life with Aleksandr Solzhenitsyn*. New York: The Bobbs-Merrill Company, 1975.

Rothberg, Abraham. *Alexandr Solzhenitsyn: The Major Novels*. Ithaca: Cornell University Press, 1971.

Solzhenitsyn, Aleksandr. "An Interview." *The Kenyon Review* 1 (Summer 1979): 8–17.

Solzhenitsyn, Aleksandr. *Bodalsia telenok s Dubom*. Paris: YMCA Press, 1975.

Solzhenitsyn, Aleksandr. *Cancer Ward*. New York: Farrar, Straus, and Giroux, 1969.

Solzhenitsyn, Aleksandr. *Sobranie sochinenii*. Vol. 5. Frankfurt am Main: Possev-Verlag, 1971.

Free of Charge—Medicine and Money in the USSR

Babanovskii, I. V. *Voprosy finansirovaniia zdravookhraneniia v SSSR*. Moscow: Meditsina, 1976.

Bergson, Abram, ed. *Productivity and the Social System—The USSR and the West*. Cambridge: Harvard University Press, 1978.

Byrenkov, S. P. "The Economics of Public Health at the Present Stage." *Sovetskaia meditsina* 6 (June 1976): 3–10.

Central Intelligence Agency. National Foreign Assessment Center. "A Dollar Cost Comparison of Soviet and U.S. Defense Activities, 1967–77." Washington, D.C., January 3, 1978.

Central Intelligence Agency. National Foreign Assessment Center. "The Soviet Economy in 1976–77 and Outlook for 1978." Washington, D.C., August 1978.

Field, Mark G. "American and Soviet Medical Manpower: Growth and Evolution, 1910–1970." *International Journal of Health Services* 5 (March 1975): 455–473.

Golovteev, V. V.; Kalia, P. I.; and Pustovoi, I. V. *Osnovy ekonomiki sovetskogo zdravookhraneniia.* Moscow: Meditsina, 1974.

Kurm, Helga. "Seksualnoe prosveshchenia podrostkov." *Nauka i tekhnika* (February 1978): 36–38.

Lidov, I. P.; Stochik, A. M.; and Tserkovny, G. F. *Soviet Public Health and the Organization of Primary Health Care for the Population of the U.S.S.R.* Moscow: Mir Publishers, 1978.

Lisitsin, Yu. *Rol profilaktiki v okhrane zdorovia naseleniia.* Moscow: Obshchestvo "Znanie" RSFSR, n.d.

Lockle, Paul. "Analyzing Soviet Defense Spending: The Debate in Perspective." *Survival* 20 (September–October 1978): 209–219.

Ministerstvo finansov SSSR Biudzhetnoe upravlenie. *Gosudarstvennyi biudzhet SSSR i biudzhety soiuzkh respublik: 1971–1975 gg.* Moscow: Financy: 1976.

"Operatsionnaia na remonte." *Pravda* (Moscow), 24 June 1976, p. 2.

Petrovsky, Boris V. *Uspekhi sovetskogo, zdravoohraneniia za gody deviatoi piatiletki.* Moscow: Meditsina, 1976.

Popov, Georgii. *Ekonomika i planirovanie zdravookhranenie.* Moscow: MGU, 1976.

Popov, Georgii A. *Questions of Theory and Methodology of Health Services Planning.* Moscow: Meditsina Publishing House, 1967.

Sivard, Ruth Leger. *World Military and Social Expenditures 1980.* Leesburg, Virginia: WMSE Publications, 1980.

U.S. Congress. Joint Economic Committee. *Soviet Economy in a New Perspective, A Compendium of Papers.* Washington, D.C.: Government Printing Office, 1976.

U.S. Department of Commerce, Bureau of the Census, Foreign Demographic Analysis Division. *Wages in the U.S.S.R. 1950–1960:*

Health Services by George Hoffberg. Washington, D.C.: April 1968.

Wren, Christopher S. "Russia in Entropy." *Harpers,* June 1978, pp. 31–38.

Taking Care of Yourself

U.S. Department of Commerce. *Foreign Service Health Status Study. Evaluation of Health Status of Foreign Service and Other Employees From Selected Eastern European Posts.* Washington, D.C.: National Technical Information Service, 1978.

The Library of Congress method for transliteration of modern Russian with the diacritical marks omitted has been employed throughout the text. Any deviations from the Library of Congress System II occur only in the transliteration of certain familiar terms as well as a number of personal and place names. This is done for the convenience of those readers not familiar with Russian pronunciation. The bibliography is rendered exclusively according to System II.

GLOSSARY

akusherki, midwives
appenditsit, appendicitis
apteka, apothecary; pharmacy

babushka, grandmother; used colloquially in reference to an older matronly woman
besplatno, free of charge
Bogoroditsa, the Theotokos; Mother of God; Madonna
bolnitsy, houses of pain or suffering; hospitals
bolnichnyi, sick list
bufeti, Soviet snack bars which sell open-faced sandwiches, juices and *pirozhki*

cheredovanie, rotation of physicians between hospitals and polyclinics on an every-other-day system

dacha, summer house or vacation retreat
detski sad, nursery school
dezhurnaia, combination of floor maid and junior manager in a hotel or apartment building
dispanserizatsiia, a follow-up clinic for people with special medical needs
dolgozhitel, centenarian; one who has lived an exceptionally long life
dom kultury, house of culture
dvukhdnevnaia sistema, rotation of physicians between hospitals and polyclinics on a half-day basis

epidemiia, an epidemic

feldsher, physician's assistant

gastronom, grocery store
golubchik, an affectionate expression; endearment; roughly 'my dear'

gospodin, mister; in use before 1917; now replaced by "tovarishch" or "comrade"

iazva, ulcer
idti pod nozh, go under the knife
intelligentsia, the educated, intellectual or artistic elite
issyk kul, mandrake root

kabinet, office; receiving room for official business
kandidat, doctor of medical science
kasha, a gruel made of wheat or buckwheat
kerosinka, kerosene; slang term for low-grade vodka
khirurg, surgeon
kifir, a thinner version of yogurt popular in the USSR
klizma, a colonic irrigation
kumiss, fermented pregnant mare's milk first introduced into Russia by the invading Tatars in 1240.

molodoi chelovek, young man

nachalstvo, the ruling members of the communist party; the Soviet elite of privileged party officials
nadomniki, retarded individuals who are not placed into institutions
na levo, a method of unofficial and sometimes illegal "under the table payment" for goods or services rendered
narkoz, anesthetic
narodnichestvo, a populist movement that sprang up in Russia in the 1870's. The so-called *"narodniki"* felt compelled to turn to the peasant masses and to lead them to a better future

393

neotlozhnaya, minor emergency services number

novy god, the New Year

ordinatura, residency training at the end of medical school

otpusk, vacation

pelmeni, meat-filled dumplings served either in a chicken broth or with sour cream. *Pelmeni* are especially popular in Siberia

peritonit, rupture of the appendix; peritonitis

pirozhki, small meat- or vegetable-filled pies

platnye polikliniki, polyclinics that charge a fee for treatment

podrazdelenie, army troop unit

pokazukha, an object, act or mannerism used for the express purpose of boasting or showing-off

prepodovatel, high school instructor

profsouz, trade union

putevka, resort tickets to a sanitorium given to workers by their trade union

rak, cancer

samogon, a type of Russian moonshine

sanitarnye vrachi, public health physicians

setka, a shopping net made of plastic or fabric brought by the customer to carry groceries; also *"avoska"*

Skoraya Meditsinskaya Pomoshch, quick medical assistance system or 'Skoraya' for short

smetana, sour cream

sok, fruit juice

sosed, neighbor

sostradanie, co-suffering; empathy

sovkhoz, state farm collective, larger in size and more centrally controlled than the *kolkhoz*

spravka, an official written excuse from work

srednaya shkola, high school

srednii vrach, average doctor

starushka, an old woman

sto gram 100 grams

stoikost, firmness, steadfastness; perseverence

terapevt, general internist

travy, herbs; herbal preparations

tvorog, a type of loose cheese popular in the USSR; similar in appearance and taste to farmer's cheese

uchastok, a rural district; section of land

verst, unit of measurement used in pre-Soviet Russia. 1 verst = 3,500 ft. or approximately .66 mile.

vnutrikozhnye ukoly, intradermal injections

vrach, the lowest ranking physician in the USSR

vytrezviteli, sobering-up stations run by the local militia (police).

zagavarivat, prescribed magical formula of phrases used to talk or whisper away a disease; the phrases or spells were kept in strict secrecy by the znakharka or wise-woman

zemstvo system, characterized by the law of 1864, enacted by Tsar Alexander II; it represented a strong modernization and democratization of local government as well as an effort to meet the pressing needs of rural Russia

zhenskii konsultatsii, women's consultation center

zhivot, belly or stomach

zholochnye kamni, gallstones

znakharka, a village wise-woman

INDEX

395